Demystifying Epilepsy:
A Multidimensional Perspective

Dr. Clotilda Mujeyi Chinyanya (DBA)

Copyright © 2025 by Dr. Clotilda Mujeyi Chinyanya
All rights reserved. No part of this publication may be reproduced, distributed, or transmitted in any form or by any means - electronic, mechanical, photocopying, recording, or otherwise without the prior written permission of the publisher, except in the case of brief quotations embodied in critical reviews and certain other noncommercial uses permitted by copyright law.

Title: Demystifying Epilepsy: A Multidimensional Perspective
Author: Dr. Clotilda Mujeyi Chinyanya
ISBN (Paperback): 9798999613707
ISBN (eBook): 9798999613714

This book is a work of nonfiction. While every effort has been made to ensure the accuracy of the content, the publisher and author make no representations or warranties about the completeness or suitability of this material for any purpose.

Library of Congress Control Number: 2025916304
Library of Congress Cataloging-in-Publication Data
Name: Chinyanya, Clotilda Mujeyi, author
Title: Demystifying Epilepsy / Clotilda Mujeyi Chinyanya.
Includes bibliographical references and index.
RC372 .C45 2025
DDC Number— 616.853
First Edition

Interior design by Kuzivakwashe Chinyanya
Cover design by Victor Mupangami
Edited by Selena Class and Kuzivakwashe Chinyanya
Cover Concept by Kundai-Munashe, Kudakwashe, and Kuzivakwashe Chinyanya
Publisher: Self-published

For permissions, inquiries, or bulk orders, contact:
demystifyepilepsy@gmail.com
Printed in the United States of America

Medical and Legal Disclaimer

Demystifying Epilepsy was created with the utmost care to provide accurate, thoughtful, and accessible information for individuals, families, and communities affected by epilepsy. While every effort has been made to ensure the reliability of the content, the author and publisher make no representations or warranties regarding its completeness, accuracy, or applicability to individual circumstances. This includes any implied warranties of merchantability or fitness for a particular purpose.

The information in this book is not intended as a substitute for professional medical advice, diagnosis, or treatment. Readers are strongly encouraged to consult a qualified healthcare provider before making any decisions about epilepsy care or related health matters.

Any strategies, perspectives, or resources shared reflect knowledge available at the time of writing and may not be suitable for every situation. Additionally, website links or external references provided may change or become outdated over time.

The author and publisher disclaim liability for any loss, injury, or damages, including but not limited to special, incidental, or consequential damages, that may arise from the use or misuse of the information contained within this book.

Preface

As a family living with someone with epilepsy, we have witnessed the physical, emotional and social toll of epilepsy. We have also witnessed the strength and resilience of a woman who lives a full life regardless of a diagnosis. This book, *Demystifying Epilepsy: A Multidimensional Perspective*, is a shining reflection of this resilience.

Experiencing the complete journey from a single audacious idea over a decade ago, to the impactful resource you are reading today, has been exhilarating and inspiring. A lot of late nights, research and cups of tea have been poured into the process of writing this book. Edit after edit, the author never wavered from her determination to remind the world that behind every diagnosis is a person with dreams, dignity, and a voice that deserves to be heard.

We are proud of this work, and even prouder of the exceptional woman behind it. If this book results in one person being treated with more compassion and understanding, or helps one family feel less alone, then it has done its job.

With love,
Vitalis, Kudakwashe, Kundai-Munashe, and Kuzivakwashe

Acknowledgments

Writing *Demystifying Epilepsy* has been one of the most meaningful journeys of my life. The book began as a personal mission to understand and explain this condition. However, it has grown into a resource that I hope will empower, educate, and uplift many. This book would not have been possible without the support, encouragement, and contributions of so many people I have encountered and interacted with in the past 26 years that I have lived with the condition of epilepsy.

To the individuals and families living with epilepsy who inspired this book - thank you. Your stories, resilience, and courage are the heart of this work. You reminded me that behind every diagnosis is a person with dreams, fears, and the right to live with dignity. To the readers, advocates, caregivers, and healthcare workers who dedicate themselves to understanding and supporting those affected by epilepsy, this book is for you. May it serve as a tool to demystify outdated beliefs, spark conversation, reduce the epilepsy treatment gap, eliminate all forms of stigma, and foster compassion.

To the epilepsy foundations, Epilepsy Action, epilepsy advocacy groups, support organizations, the International Bureau for Epilepsy, and the International League Against Epilepsy, whose public resources and research helped shape the content of this book, your commitment to awareness, education, and care is inspiring. You are making a difference every day, and I am proud to contribute in my own way. To all researchers and scholars, whose materials I used to support the material shared in this book, I thank you and appreciate all the work you are doing to provide facts on epilepsy.

I am deeply grateful to the medical professionals, researchers, and educators who shared their insights, offered guidance, and patiently answered my questions. Your expertise helped ensure this book remains grounded in evidence while accessible to a broader audience. Special thanks to Ruth Chapereka, Dr. Rugare Mugumbate, Dr. Gerald Madziyire, who reviewed sections of the manuscript and provided critical feedback that helped strengthen the clarity and accuracy of the final work. This book is self-published, and I am especially grateful to the individuals who supported the behind-the-scenes process, especially my editors, Selena and Kuzi; cover design, Victor Mupangami; proofreading, Peggy Zvavamwe; including all those who assisted with formatting, typesetting, and navigating the complexities of independent publishing. Your talents and generosity were essential.

A heartfelt thank you to my family and friends, who stood by me during countless late nights, long edits, and moments of self-doubt. Your patience, encouragement, and unwavering belief in this project gave me the strength to see it through.

Finally, to everyone who chooses to see the person beyond the condition: thank you. Let us continue to build a world where epilepsy is met not with fear or stigma, but with knowledge, empathy, and respect.

Dedication

To my mother, **Scolastica Ruzvidzo**, whose steadfast love, strength, and prayers have carried me beyond what words can measure.

To my husband, **Vitalis**, for your unwavering, loyal, and enduring love even through the storms of every seizure. Thank you for being my constant, my calm, and my courage.

To our children, **Kuda, Kundai, and Kuzi**, your belief in me, your gentle nudges, and your endless encouragement gave me the strength to finish this book. You are my reason, my joy, and my hope.

This book was written in love, for the ones who walk beside me in light and in dark, and for all those seeking to see epilepsy more clearly.

Author's Foreword

Epilepsy is one of the most common neurological conditions, affecting 65 million people worldwide, yet it remains misunderstood, often surrounded by fear, stigma, and misinformation. I wrote *Demystifying Epilepsy* to challenge misconceptions surrounding diagnosis, causes, treatment, triggers, stigma, or life stages like childhood and womanhood. Though not a medical textbook, this research-based resource offers practical insights for people with epilepsy, their families, healthcare providers, and communities, while reminding us all that behind every seizure is a real person with emotions, dignity, and a full life.

At its heart, this book aims to empower. It provides knowledge that can help individuals with epilepsy navigate their condition with confidence, advocate for better care, and find solidarity in shared experiences. This work draws on extensive research, professional experience, and the lived realities of those affected by epilepsy. While it does not replace clinical guidance, it fills a critical gap in everyday understanding, especially at the primary healthcare level where timely recognition, support, and referral are crucial.

Readers are welcome to approach the book in the way that suits them best. You can read it cover to cover or dive into specific chapters most relevant to your interests, whether you're looking to understand the basics of epilepsy, treatment options, the impact of stigma, or strategies for living well. It is my hope that *Demystifying Epilepsy* will contribute meaningfully to a more informed, compassionate, and empowered approach to epilepsy around the world. I would be keen to receive your feedback and suggestions for further research through any channel of your choice:

email: demystifyepilepsy@gmail.com
Facebook: https://www.facebook.com/share/1PgiVjHSVa/?mibextid=wwXIfr
Instagram: https://www.instagram.com/demystifyingepilepsy/
LinkedIn: https://www.linkedin.com/company/demystifying-epilepsy-llc/
Website: https://www.demystifyingepilepsy.com

Dr. Clotilda Mujeyi Chinyanya (DBA) - Phoenix, Arizona, 2025

TABLE OF CONTENTS

CHAPTER 1 – HOW IT ALL STARTED FOR ME 1
CHAPTER 2 – WHAT IS EPILEPSY? 7
CHAPTER 3 – DIAGNOSIS OF EPILEPSY 31
CHAPTER 4 – EPILEPSY IMITATORS 42
CHAPTER 5 – SEIZURE TRIGGERS 56
CHAPTER 6 – EPILEPSY TREATMENT OPTIONS 66
    Pharmacotherapy: anti-epilepsy drugs 66
    Epilepsy surgery 98
    Ketogenic diet in epilepsy treatment 105
CHAPTER 7 – COMPLEMENTARY AND ALTERNATIVE MEDICINE 117
CHAPTER 8 – SUDDEN UNEXPECTED DEATH IN EPILEPSY (SUDEP) 140
CHAPTER 9 – STATUS EPILEPTICUS 153
CHAPTER 10 – EPILEPSY MYTHS AND MISCONCEPTIONS 160
CHAPTER 11 – EPILEPSY AND RELIGION 181
CHAPTER 12 – EPILEPSY IN CHILDREN 204
CHAPTER 13 – EPILEPSY IN WOMEN AND GIRLS 229
CHAPTER 14 – STIGMA IN EPILEPSY 246
CHAPTER 15 – ACCOMMODATIONS FOR PWE 262
PERSONAL ACKNOWLEDGEMENTS 282
ABOUT THE AUTHOR 284

List of Figures

Figure 1: ILAE 2017 classification of seizure types expanded version 11
Figure 2: Framework for classification of the epilepsies 19
Figure 3: Pharmacokinetics illustrated 74
Figure 4: An illustration of drug level maintenance in the blood 78
Figure 5: Ayurveda systems of the body 119

List of Tables

Table 1: Old to new terminology 17
Table 2: Epilepsy syndromes associated with encephalopathy or PND 23
Table 3: Seizure warnings, symptoms, after-seizure 63
Table 4: Drug choice 69
Table 5: Seizure medication list 69
Table 6: Effects of older AEDs on newer AEDs 81
Table 7: Interactions between enzyme-inducing AEDs and other drugs 86
Table 8: Types of epilepsy in Ayurveda 120
Table 9: Childhood epilepsy syndromes 206
Table 10: Clinical characteristics of childhood epilepsy syndromes 209
Table 11: Possible teratogenic effects of AEDs 237
Table 12: AEDs excreted in breast milk and their effects on breastfed babies 240

List of Commonly Used Abbreviations:

AEDs:	Anti-epileptic drugs
CAM:	Complementary and alternative medicine
CBD:	Cannabidiol
CT:	Computed tomography
DRE:	Drug-resistant epilepsy
EEG:	Electroencephalogram
ESF:	Epilepsy Support Foundation
ILAE:	International League Against Epilepsy
LMICs:	Low- and middle-income countries
MRI:	Magnetic resonance imaging
PWE:	People/Person with epilepsy
SE:	Status epilepticus
SUDEP:	Sudden unexpected death in epilepsy

All Bible references are from the following version:

Stanley, C. 2009. *The Charles F. Stanley Life Principles Bible: New American Standard Bible.* Nashville: The Lockman Foundation

CHAPTER 1 – HOW IT ALL STARTED FOR ME

On Monday January 11, 1999, I woke up and started getting ready for work. I had worked at Harare Central Hospital for 8 years. As far as I was concerned, today was like any other day. My family's odd behavior, however, made me feel like something was not right. After breakfast, my husband Vitalis, and I proceeded to the garage. When we opened the garage door, I saw an unfamiliar car parked inside our garage.

I asked Vitalis, "Where is our car, and whose car is this?"

I was certain that we owned a Mazda Familia, but a Toyota Corolla was parked in our garage. My sister, Massie, who had strangely been following me closely, started crying.

Vitalis asked, "What car are you talking about?"

"Our Mazda," I replied.

"Remember, we sold the Mazda to uncle Kwenda 3 months ago after we bought the Corolla."

I did not respond. Nothing made sense to me. I did not remember the Corolla at all.

Immediately, Vitalis asked me to get in the car and drove me to the Avenues Clinic casualty department. Through history taking, it became clear that I could not remember things that had happened in the past 6 months, but I could remember things that had happened a year ago or more. I was disoriented and frightened. What was going on? The doctor attending to me wanted to rule out a brain tumor first. He ordered a computed tomography (CT) scan, and I was rushed to the radiology department. The results were out within an hour: I had no brain tumor. I was referred to a specialist physician for further management. They ordered an electroencephalogram (EEG), and I was asked to return after 3 days to get the EEG results. The EEG technician told me to reach out to him if I needed any clarifications after seeing my physician.

The physician was a well-respected doctor who was the head of medicine at one of the central hospitals in the country. I felt I was in good hands. If anyone could find out what was causing my memory loss, it was him. When I got into the examination room, he did not discuss or explain the EEG results. He prescribed phenobarbitone 90mg, to be taken at night. My job as a pharmacy technician made me familiar with phenobarbitone and its uses.

"Why are you giving me phenobarbitone? Do I have epilepsy?" I asked.

"The EEG did not reveal much, but I want to try phenobarbitone to see if the symptoms will be resolved," replied my highly regarded physician.

I started taking phenobarbitone 90 mg that night, on January 14, 1999.

What happened on January 11 remained a mystery to me. I did not remember having a seizure prior to the memory loss. I did not remember any weird feelings before waking up. Now, I was on phenobarbitone despite the inconclusive EEG. I wondered why I was exposing myself to the terrible side effects of this drug. Why would a physician want to just try a drug on me before he was sure of the diagnosis? I started losing faith in my physician. I reached out to the EEG technician who had previously offered to discuss the EEG results and told him that the physician had found the EEG to be inconclusive. He asked me what treatment I was on. I told him I was put on phenobarbitone and had been taking it for 2 weeks. The EEG technician said he could no longer discuss the results because I had already begun treatment. He said that I should have come back immediately and not waited for 2 weeks. I went home frustrated and just decided to stop taking the phenobarbitone. I was not going to expose myself to the side effects of this drug for an unknown condition. If my physician had given me a diagnosis, I would gladly take the drug knowing it would treat or help me manage my condition. My physician had not given me a diagnosis. He explicitly stated he was just trying this drug to see if my condition improved after taking it. I was not going to do that!

Abruptly stopping phenobarbitone was a big mistake. Two days later I started having auras and seizures, especially at night. I was puzzled. Were the seizures the result of the sudden withdrawal of medication or was this a sure sign that I had epilepsy? January 11, 1999 remains a significant date to me because life as I had known it up to that day would never be the same.

I was beginning a new life journey into the unknown. The seizures usually occurred at night and started with an aura. I would alert Vitalis that the seizure was coming and then pass out. I was terrified. My heart raced when I felt the impending seizure. The seizures usually lasted a minute or two according to observers, but the after-effects were ongoing. I did not resume taking medication. I was in denial. My inner voice told me I did not have epilepsy. "Where would the epilepsy be coming from? I have no family history of epilepsy, so it cannot be epilepsy," I told myself.

Being a person of faith, I sought spiritual answers to this mysterious illness I was suffering from. It was mysterious because in my opinion, even the physician could not come up with a diagnosis after history-taking and several tests. The next obvious thing to me was that the seizures could be spiritual. I went to church. My pastors and fellow congregants prayed for me, yet the condition persisted. My whole family supported me in prayer. Even our children, Kuda and Kundai, who were only 7 and 3 years old at that time, would fast and pray. I remember someone asking Kundai why she was not eating. She replied that she was praying for mom to get well. What followed was a period of 13 months of seizures, denial, struggle, dejection, fear, confusion, pregnancy, a baby (Kuzi), and finally comprehension.

It then took me another 5 years to come to accept my epilepsy diagnosis. By that time, I was a successful businesswoman running a pharmaceutical wholesale and healthcare product manufacturing company. I was awarded businesswoman of the year in 2003 by the Zimbabwe National Chamber of Commerce for Harare. Despite my success in business, I felt broken inside because of epilepsy. After years of feeling inadequate, I began connecting with others living with epilepsy at the Epilepsy Support Foundation (ESF) in Harare, Zimbabwe.

Belonging to this support group and seeing ways I could add value helped me come out of my shell. I did not know that I could help anyone as I felt I was the one in need of help. The director at the Foundation then, Jacob Mugumbate, went out of his way to help me find my place at the Foundation. He asked me to help them on issues of adherence to treatment, focusing on women and children. I gladly accepted, as the role was suited to my skills as a pharmacy technician. I then resolved to help other people deal with the condition of epilepsy and began to talk openly about my condition. When I accepted this task, I did not know that by helping others I was also helping myself in my healing journey.

I started meaningfully helping women and young girls. In that process, I learned about the issues that some of those women were going through. Some women in the support group did not have epilepsy, but had children with epilepsy. The main issues we encountered were around stigma, marriage, divorce, over-protective parents, women's health issues, and economic empowerment. I sought resources to help all of us navigate through the challenges we all faced. We met every Friday, and I would organize speakers on different topics that affected this group of women and girls. I established relationships with obstetricians, gynecologists, pediatricians, neurologists, nutritionists, psychologists, and sociologists, to name a few. These professionals would come to meet our support group at the ESF and present on specific topics and answer questions.

Our group became empowered. We would laugh at each other's stories and even made fun of each other about our different experiences with epilepsy. It was our own safe space. We were so happy and free in this group. One lady whose seizures were triggered by excitement had a seizure as we were coming to the end of one fun session. We had had a great presenter. The session was filled with laughter, and everyone was excited. After the seizure, we all gathered to offer her support.

She said, "I told you that when I get excited, I have a seizure."

We told her that in a previous session, we had encouraged people to avoid seizure triggers. "How can I avoid being happy?" she asked.

We still laughed at her response because we wanted to keep the mood light, but deep down in my heart, I felt conflicted. How could and why should someone avoid being happy to prevent triggering their seizures? It would have been better if the seizures were triggered by sadness. How could someone seek help to fend off excitement and happiness? This was her reality.

I also became a regular speaker, through the ESF, at the Children's Rehabilitation Unit (CRU) at Harare Central Hospital. I would go to the CRU at least once per month. I also spoke twice at the Tose Respite Home in Harare. At the CRU and Tose, I met with parents of children with different epilepsy syndromes and co-morbidities. I was always assigned to speak on drug adherence, and I articulated that topic with excellence, especially considering I had suffered for 13 months with uncontrolled seizures due to non-adherence. I found a purpose through meeting with these parents. Some found hope that if someone with epilepsy like Clotilda could still do what she did, then their children could have purpose and a bright future. I was a successful businesswoman living with epilepsy. It was my choice to disclose my condition, because if I had not told them, they would have never known. I always disclosed my condition as I felt it made more sense when speaking with parents whose children had the condition but had never seen anyone with epilepsy living independently. As I worked with these different groups, in as much as I was helping them, I was also receiving internal healing and gaining acceptance of my condition. Even after moving to the United States, I became an epilepsy awareness ambassador with the Epilepsy Foundation and actively participate in local programs, both at state and federal level. I keep in touch with the Zimbabwe ESF and represent my country as a committee member of the Zimbabwe chapter of the International League Against Epilepsy.

No one deserves to go through what I went through due to ignorance. I dedicated my life to researching more about my condition, with a special focus on women and children. I wanted to be able to help parents of children with epilepsy, as well as women with epilepsy. Most of the information in this book applies to all population groups, but there are two chapters dedicated to children and women. The information in this book will help demystify the condition of epilepsy. It will help dispel all the myths and misconceptions and help people better manage the condition. The information in this book may help in reducing the epilepsy treatment gap, which is defined as the ratio of people with recurring seizures not receiving suitable treatment.[1] The epilepsy treatment gap can be as high as 100% (meaning no one is on treatment) in some parts of certain countries.[1] Such a gap is not ideal for a condition that can be managed with medication.

References:

1. Kwon, C., Wagner, R. G., Carpio, A., Jette, N., Newton, C. R., & Thurman, D. J. (2022). The worldwide epilepsy treatment gap: A systematic review and recommendations for revised definitions –A report from the ILAE Epidemiology Commission. *Epilepsia, 63*, 551- 564. https:doi.org/10.1111/epi.17112

CHAPTER 2 – WHAT IS EPILEPSY?

Not everything that shakes is a seizure - Not every seizure is epilepsy – Not every seizure needs to be treated.
Selim R. Benbadis

Lucretius, a Roman philosopher and poet who died in the year 55 B.C., described epilepsy as follows:
Epilepsy violently disrupts both body and mind, causing sudden seizures that leave a person convulsing, disoriented, and mentally scattered. Though recovery follows as the body stabilizes, the mind, like the body, requires care and healing to fully regain its strength.[1]

Introduction

Epilepsy is one of the oldest medical conditions, and one of the most common neurological disorders, affecting over 65 million people globally.[2,3,4] The disorder has long been documented in many different regions of the world, suggesting that people have known about it for a long time. The Greek philosopher Hippocrates discussed epilepsy in his book, *On the Sacred Disease,*[2] in 400 B.C. The term epilepsy originates from the Greek verb *epilambanein*, which means "to be snatched," or "to be surprised."[5] A Persian doctor, Avecinna, is credited for naming the condition "epilepsy,"[6,7] meaning being seized or controlled by an external power.[8] Epilepsy is recorded in the earliest medical writings from Babylon, India, and Persia. For example, it appeared in Ayurvedic texts dated 1200 B.C., where it is listed as one of the first eight diseases to be identified.[9] Epilepsy appeared in Babylonian writings 3,000 years ago.[10] According to The Hammurabi Code of 1780 B.C., no person with epilepsy could marry or testify in court.[5] In the same Code, the purchase of a slave was nullified if the slave suffered an epileptic attack within the first 3 months of purchase.[5]

Epilepsy has historically been misunderstood and feared, often attributed to supernatural causes, leading to the isolation and discrimination of those affected. Even into the mid-20th century, people with epilepsy (PWE) faced significant challenges, including denial of rights and forced sterilizations.[11] Even though we understand a lot more about epilepsy, misconceptions persist globally.

Epilepsy is one of the most prevalent neurological disorders, affecting people of all ages, races, and socio-economic statuses, and both sexes. Many people know a family member, relative, friend, acquaintance, colleague, or schoolmate with this condition. The greatest epilepsy burden is found in low and middle income countries (LMIC).[12,13] Studies have found that 80% of PWE live in LMICs.[13,14] In an ideal world, with proper diagnosis and treatment, 70% of all PWE could live seizure-free on anti-epilepsy drugs (AEDs).[13,14] The number may never be achieved with the epilepsy treatment gap at 100% in some areas as previously mentioned. Several factors contribute to the wide epilepsy treatment gap, as will be discussed later.

At this stage, let me introduce proper language. A person is not an epileptic, but a person with epilepsy. What is epileptic is the seizure, where a seizure is described as either epileptic or non-epileptic. However, a person is not epileptic. This will become clearer as I go through the chapters of this book, starting with this chapter. This chapter explores what epilepsy is and how it is understood in different communities. To give a well-rounded view, I'll look at both scientific explanations and cultural beliefs about epilepsy.

Scientific view of epilepsy

Epilepsy has always been referred to as a "disorder," but the International League Against Epilepsy (ILAE) in 2014 changed its definition to "brain disease" so as not to trivialize its seriousness.[15] The effects of epilepsy are neurological, cognitive, psychological, and social.[13] PWE have repeated seizures that frequently occur unexpectedly.[13] In 2014, the ILAE came up with a practical clinical definition of epilepsy as follows:

Epilepsy is a disease of the brain defined by any of the following conditions:

(1) At least two unprovoked (or reflex) seizures occurring more than 24 hours apart;

(2) One unprovoked (or reflex) seizure and a probability of further seizures similar to the general recurrence risk (at least 60%) after two unprovoked seizures, occurring over the next 10 years;

(3) diagnosis of an epilepsy syndrome.
Epilepsy is considered to be resolved for individuals who either had an age dependent epilepsy syndrome but are now past the applicable age or who have remained seizure-free for the last 10 years and off anti-seizure medicines for at least the last 5 years.[15]

Epilepsy, also known as a seizure disorder, is diagnosed when a person has had at least two unprovoked seizures. Provoked seizures are single seizures that may occur as the result of trauma, low blood sugar, low blood sodium, high fever, alcohol, or drug abuse. Fever-related (or febrile) seizures may occur during infancy and are usually outgrown by the age of 6. Two seizures can be defined as epilepsy, but one seizure can lead to an epilepsy diagnosis if it is supported by an EEG and a person can be started on treatment.[16] Epilepsy is therefore a syndrome of recurrent seizures. Clinicians understand epilepsy as a "network disease,"[17,18] meaning seizures can start from any part of the brain or connections between the different parts of the brain, like the limbic network, thalamocortical networks, and neocortical network.

Understanding epilepsy starts with a good grasp of seizures because the definition of epilepsy is a description of seizures. A seizure is a short-term event triggered by excessive, synchronized neuronal activity in the brain, producing a sudden burst of electrical impulses that temporarily affect a person's awareness, sensations, or behavior.[17,18,19] A seizure is not a disease, but a sign or a symptom of one. Some seizures are subtle while others are theatrical and incapacitating. Some seizures can be linked to brain injury, central nervous system infections, stroke, family tendencies, traumatic brain injuries, or immunology;[13] however, at least 50% of seizures cannot be linked to any known cause.[12] Epilepsy does not present in the same way for everybody, because it is a syndrome of seizures, and an individual may experience different seizure types, such that the epilepsy manifests differently each time. The type of seizure determines the manifestation of the epilepsy. Recognizing the different ways epilepsy seizures present is critical for onlookers to be able to assist.

Epilepsy seizures can be put into three broad categories: focal (formerly known as partial), generalized, and unknown.[8,18] Focal seizures originate from a specific location in the brain and may or may not affect the consciousness of the person. Generalized seizures involve both hemispheres of the brain. When it is not possible to put seizures in either of these two categories, they are classified as unknown. Seizures usually last no more than a few seconds, though some can last up to 2 minutes. What is of substance here is that though the seizure may only last a few seconds, the effects usually last longer and can take the form of stupor and confusion as consciousness is regained. In *status epilepticus* (SE) the seizure extends beyond 5 minutes and is a medical emergency that can have long-term consequences if it lasts more than 30 minutes.[20] When someone has a seizure that lasts more than 5 minutes, immediate action is required as the possibility of SE is high. Any delays could lead to irreversible neurological damage or even death.

Types of seizures

Not all seizures are epileptic seizures.[12,21] Seizures can occur due to causes unrelated to epilepsy, including non-epileptic seizures (NES, formerly psychogenic non-epileptic seizures), syncope, paroxysmal movement disorders, sleep disorders, transient ischemic attacks, or complicated migraine to name a few.[6,21,22] Epilepsy imitators are real and to do justice to the topic, I will cover them separately in Chapter 4. I will just mention that it is important to establish that a seizure is an epileptic seizure before starting treatment. Giving someone a wrong diagnosis and therefore wrong treatment can have unintended results.[6] Not only will seizures persist, but there is also a risk of exposing the patient to unnecessary side effects and stigma. Also, the imitator remains untreated.

From the time of Hippocrates, people have given importance to the description of seizures.[18] Historically, seizure classifications were either described in terms of the region of the brain from which they originated or the age of the patient.[18] These classifications have changed with time as new knowledge is gained on the condition. Neuroscience advancements have profoundly transformed the understanding of epilepsy, transitioning the focus from specific brain regions to a wider, network-oriented view. In 2016, the taskforce on seizure classification set-up by the ILAE came up with an operational classification of seizures.[18] The classification is designed to evolve as new knowledge is gained.

New seizure classification is critical in the diagnosis and treatment of epilepsy because it enhances the understanding of the condition, opening new avenues for diagnosing, monitoring, and treating epilepsy. The ILAE further classified seizure types into meaningful groups. The first publication of seizure classification was in 1960, and over the years, different classifications have been used, until the operational classification of seizures was introduced in 2016.[23] The ongoing classification revisions aim to make it clearer for clinicians on ways to treat and manage epilepsy. The new classification comes with three major groups: focal, generalized, and unknown onset. The sub-categories are motor, non-motor, retained or impaired awareness for focal seizures.[18] Figure 1 shows these classifications from the ILAE.

Figure 1: ILAE 2017 classification of seizure types expanded version

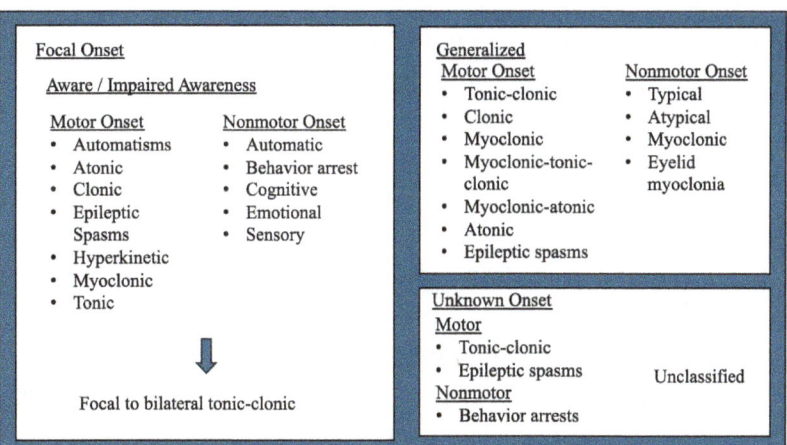

Adapted from Fisher RS *et al.* (2017). Operational classification of seizure types by the International League Against Epilepsy: Position Paper of the ILAE Commission for Classification and Terminology. *Epilepsia*, 58(4): 522–530. https://doi.org/10.1111/epi.13670 [18]

The new ILAE classification sought to revise terminology that was either misleading or unacceptable.[24] The old classifications left out many types of seizures that are now included. The new classification recognizes the two major groups, that is, focal and generalized. The third group, called "unknown onset," is only used until the seizures can be classified into one of the two groups, i.e., it acts as a temporary grouping. According to the ILAE,[24] the terminology has changed quite significantly, and they came up with a table to guide people on the new terminology, based on the old terminology. The frequently used terms are illustrated in Table 1.

Focal-onset seizures

Here is a summary of focal seizures according to the ILAE 2017 operational classification.[24] Focal seizures, previously known as partial seizures, originate in and affect a specific part of the brain. The manifestation of these seizures ranges from very subtle to striking motor movements, even leading to compromised consciousness. Focal seizures are classified into two main subtypes: motor onset and non-motor onset. The two subtypes are further classified based on level of awareness.[25]

- Symptoms of focal motor onset seizures:
    - *Tonic: Muscle stiffness. Abnormal sustained contractions and posturing of the limbs characterize tonic movements.*
    - *Clonic: Continuous jerking or twitching of different muscles.*
    - *Atonic: Loss of muscle tone in limbs.*
    - *Myoclonic: Asymmetrical jerks of limbs.*
    - *Hyperkinetic: Uncontrolled movements.*
    - *Epileptic spasms: Rhythmic body movements of waist and arm extensions.*
    - *Automatisms: Repetitive motor activities like lip-smacking, tapping, or swallowing.*[25]
- Symptoms of focal non-motor onset seizures:
    - *Autonomic: Changes in blood pressure, heart rate, sweating, skin color, or gastrointestinal upset.*
    - *Behavioral arrest: Cessation of movement.*
    - *Cognitive: Odd feelings, like jamais vu, déjà vu, hallucinations, and visualization of illusions.*
    - *Emotional: Feelings of joy, fear, dread, or anxiety. The person may laugh (gelastic seizures), or cry (dacrystic seizures).*
    - *Sensory: Abnormal visual, hearing, smell, or pain sensations.*[25]
        - Ighodaro et al.
- Focal-onset aware seizures (formerly simple partial seizures)[24]

    o Awareness is retained during the seizure.
    o Seizures can progress to become focal-onset aware seizures with impaired awareness if consciousness is altered during the seizure.
- Focal-onset impaired awareness seizures (formerly complex partial seizures)[24]
    o Seizures result in loss of, or compromised consciousness.
    o May start as focal-onset aware before progressing to impaired awareness.

In addition to these two main subtypes, the ILAE 2017 classification also recognizes "focal-onset to bilateral tonic-clonic seizures" (previously known as secondary generalized seizure). The focal-onset to bilateral tonic-clonic seizures begin as focal seizures that progress into generalized convulsive seizures.[26] Most people with focal seizures usually have all three types: the focal non-motor, the focal motor, and the focal-onset to bilateral tonic-clonic seizures.[26] A person with focal seizures may not present the same way every time they have a seizure.

Generalized-onset seizures
The following is a summary of the generalized-onset seizures according to the ILAE 2017 operational classification.[24] Generalized seizures originate in and affect both hemispheres of the brain at the same time from the onset of the seizure. They are further categorized into several subtypes based on their clinical features and EEG findings. Generalized seizures are categorized by motor and non-motor only. Awareness is not a general descriptor of these seizures as most of them impair awareness.[24] Generalized onset seizures are shown in Figure 1, categorized under motor and non-motor. The following describes how these seizures manifest:[22,24,27,28]

Symptoms of generalized motor onset seizures:
- Generalized tonic-clonic seizures (formerly grand mal seizures)
    o The most frightening seizure type among observers.
    o Characterized by generalized muscle stiffening (tonic phase), prolonged rhythmic jerking of limbs (clonic phase), and a deep sleep at the end.

- o Tongue biting, urinary incontinence, and postictal confusion are common features.
- o Most people only know this type as epilepsy and do not consider any other seizure types as epileptic seizures.
- o Alternatives, like clonic-tonic-clonic and myoclonic-tonic-clonic can also manifest.
- Generalized clonic seizures
  - o Usually start and end with prolonged rhythmic jerking of limbs, head, neck, face, and trunk, leading to loss of consciousness.
  - o Common in infants.
- Generalized tonic seizures
  - o Sudden muscle stiffness.
  - o Consciousness may be impaired during the seizure.
  - o A distinct sound may be made.
  - o Common in people with intellectual impairment.
- Generalized atonic seizures (akinetic seizures or drop attacks)
  - o Sudden loss of muscle tone often leading to a person dropping to the ground.
  - o If muscle tone is lost in the legs, the patient may collapse onto their buttocks, or forward onto their knees and face.
- Generalized myoclonic seizures
  - o Present as intermittent jerks on both sides of the body.
  - o Involve a single or series of muscle jerks or twitches.
  - o In severe cases, the patient can involuntarily drop or throw objects.
  - o Most people say they feel like being subjected to a momentary electrical shock.
  - o Each jerk typically lasts milliseconds.
- Generalized myoclonic-atonic seizures (formerly myoclonic-astatic)
  - o Typically, this is a myoclonic seizure followed by an atonic seizure.
  - o Short jerking of limbs or trunk, with a subsequent loss of muscle tone.
  - o Affects the head and limbs, leading to an abrupt fall.
- Generalized epileptic spasms (formerly infantile spasms)
  - o Abrupt contraction of muscles, lasting 1–2 seconds.

- o Happen in succession, normally on waking up.

Symptoms of generalized non-motor onset seizures:
- Absence seizures (formerly petit mal seizures)
    - o Brief episodes of altered consciousness characterized by staring spells and a lack of responsiveness.
    - o No motor activity associated with absence seizures.
    - o Seizure duration can be a few seconds to 30 seconds; recovery is quick.
    - o Occur several times a day and are more prevalent in children.
    - o Patient may not know they have seizures but have issues accounting for some of their time.
    - o Seizures can be further divided into typical and atypical absences based on clinical features and EEG patterns.
- Generalized typical absence seizures
    - o Sudden beginning and cessation of altered awareness that varies in severity.
    - o Memory of occurrence during the seizure may be distorted.
- Generalized atypical absence seizures
    - o Less sudden starting and ending compared with typical absence seizures.
    - o May lose muscle tone of head, trunk, or limbs.
    - o Normally noticed in people with intellectual disabilities.
    - o Patient may continue with activities, but with errors and less speed.
- Generalized myoclonic absence seizures
    - o Jerking of shoulders and arms, resulting in raising of arms during the seizure.
    - o Last 10–60 seconds.
    - o Awareness may be impacted from full awareness to unconsciousness.
- Generalized absence with eyelid myoclonia seizures
    - o Short, repetitive, fast myoclonic jerks.
    - o Seizure duration is less than 6 seconds.
    - o Several seizures occur in a day.
    - o Awareness is usually retained.

Old and new terminology

Table 1 helps reconcile the new terminology to the old that most people have been used to for a long time. The new classification shows that even when a seizure is focal, it can also be tonic, atonic, clonic, myoclonic, or epileptic spasms.[18,24] In the generalized seizure category, new seizure types have been included: absence with eyelid myoclonia, myoclonic-atonic, and clonic-tonic-clonic. Awareness is a key descriptor for both focal- and unknown-onset seizures. Awareness in a focal seizure describes the person being conscious of what is happening even if they seem frozen or unresponsive. The language used to describe seizures has been revised, eliminating some terms that were a source of stigma and bringing more clarity to some existing terms, as shown in Table 1.

Table 1: Old to new terminology

Old Term for Seizure	New Term for Seizure [choice] (optional)
Absence	(Generalized) absence
Atonic	[Focal/generalized] atonic
Aura	Focal aware
Clonic	[Focal/generalized] clonic
Complex partial	Focal with impaired awareness
Convulsion	[Focal/generalized] motor [tonic-clonic, tonic, clonic], focal to bilateral tonic-clonic, tonic-clonic
Drop attack	[Focal/generalized] atonic, [focal/generalized] tonic,
Frontal lobe	Focal
Grand mal	Generalized tonic-clonic, focal to bilateral tonic-clonic, tonic-clonic unknown onset
Infantile spasms	[Focal/generalized/unknown] onset epileptic spasms
Myoclonic	[Focal/generalized] myoclonic
Occipital/parietal/partial lobe	Focal
Petit mal	Absence
Psychomotor	Focal impaired awareness
Rolandic	Focal aware motor, focal to bilateral tonic-clonic
Secondarily generalized tonic-clonic	Focal to bilateral tonic-clonic
Simple partial	Focal aware
Temporal lobe	Focal aware / impaired awareness
Tonic	[Focal/generalized] tonic
Tonic-clonic	[Generalized/unknown] onset tonic-clonic, focal to bilateral tonic-clonic

Adopted from Fisher RS, Cross JH, D'Souza C, et al. (2017). Instruction manual for the ILAE 2017 operational classification of seizure types. *Epilepsia*, 58, 531– 542. https://doi.org/10.1111/epi.13671[24]

Mentioning the old terminology is important because many people were diagnosed using those terms and may need help connecting them to the new ones. The updated classification also highlights the wide range of seizure types, each with its own distinct features.

Classification of epilepsy

Once an epilepsy diagnosis has been made, the epilepsy must be classified. Classification assumes an epilepsy seizure has been identified. The way seizures are classified not only guides treatment choices but also helps ensure that each person receives a plan tailored to their specific condition. Figure 2 is a visual presentation of classifying epilepsy based on the clinical settings. The classification involves the seizure type, epilepsy type, and epilepsy syndrome.[27,29]

Figure 2: Framework for classification of the epilepsies

Seizure Types
- Focal
- Generalized
- Unknown

Epilepsy Types
- Focal
- Generalized
- Combined Generalized / Focal
- Unknown

Epilepsy Syndrome
- Common syndromes include:
- Childhood absence epilepsy
- West syndrome
- Dravet syndrome

Etiology
- Structural
- Genetic
- Infectious
- Metabolic
- Immune
- Unknown

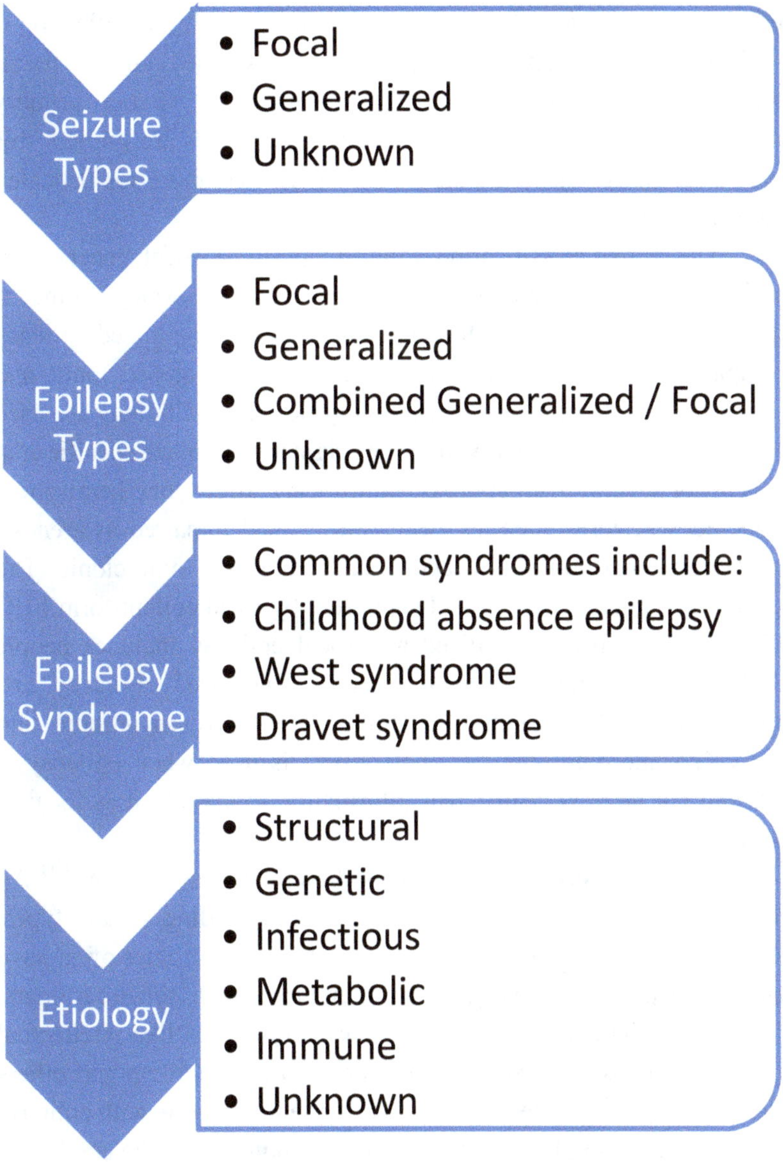

Adapted from Scheffer IE, *et al*. (2017). ILAE classification of the epilepsies: Position paper of the ILAE Commission for Classification and Terminology. *Epilepsia*, 58(4):512–521. https://doi.org/10.1111/epi.13709 [29]

Epilepsy classification starts with identification of an epileptic seizure, which eliminates NES.[29] Classification of epilepsy involves three levels. As illustrated in Figure 2, the first level of classification is the seizure type. The seizure types, as already discussed, fall into focal-onset, generalized-onset, and unknown-onset.[27,29] At the primary healthcare level, and in most LMICs where resources are limited, this may be all they are able to do due to lack of access to more sophisticated diagnostic equipment.

The second classification is the epilepsy type: focal, generalized, combined generalized and focal, and unknown.[27,29] Many forms of epilepsy will present with different seizure types. Generalized epilepsy encompasses seizure types like absence, myoclonic, atonic, tonic, and tonic-clonic.[29] Both clinical criteria and typical EEG findings are used for diagnosis. Focal epilepsy, whether it originates from one specific area (unifocal) or several distinct areas (multifocal), affects one hemisphere and includes seizures such as focal aware, focal impaired awareness, focal motor, focal non-motor, and focal to bilateral tonic-clonic. The diagnosis is clinically determined supported by focal epileptiform EEG findings.[29] Combined generalized and focal epilepsy includes people with both generalized and focal seizures, diagnosed clinically and supported by EEG. Common examples are Dravet syndrome and Lennox–Gastaut syndrome.[27,29] "Unknown" is used when epilepsy is diagnosed but there is insufficient information to classify it as focal or generalized.[27,29]

The third classification type is the epilepsy syndrome.[27,29] An epilepsy syndrome is a collection of features, including seizure types, EEG, and co-occurring imaging features.[29] These syndromes often have age-related aspects, such as age at onset and remission, seizure triggers, and diurnal variation, and may include co-morbidities like intellectual and psychiatric issues.[29] Some syndromes can be outgrown and others persist for a lifetime.[27] Identifying a syndrome in someone with epilepsy often influences both the prognosis (expected outcome of the condition) and treatment approach.[27] Some syndromes show seizure worsening with specific medications, which can be prevented through early diagnosis of the syndrome.[27] Examples of epilepsy syndromes include childhood absence epilepsy, West syndrome, and Dravet syndrome.[27,29]

Etiology (causes) of epilepsy - Scientific view

When a person is diagnosed with epilepsy, the clinician will need to isolate the cause of the epilepsy because this determines the treatment options. The ILAE categorized the causes into six main groups. The categories as illustrated in Figure 2 are: structural, genetic, infectious, metabolic, immune, and unknown. It is possible for someone's epilepsy to fall into several etiologic categories.[29]

Structural causes are due to brain abnormalities linked to epilepsy. These abnormalities can be acquired, such as from stroke, traumatic brain injury, hippocampal sceloris, tumors, or a porencephalic cyst, or genetic, like cortical or vascular malformations.[27,29,30] Accurate magnetic resonance imaging (MRI) studies are crucial for detecting these causes and can help clinicians decide if epilepsy surgery will be an option if pharmaceutical treatments fail.[29]

Genetic causes emanate from identified or presumed genetic mutations, with seizures being a fundamental symptom.[27,29,30] While the specific genes involved are not fully known, genetic etiology can be inferred from family history, clinical research, or identified molecular mutations.[27,29] New mutations not inherited from parents (*de novo*) can cause epilepsy, and while they may not appear in a family history of seizures, they could be passed to future generations.[27,29] Additionally, having cells with both mutated and normal genes (mosaicism) can influence epilepsy severity.[27,29]

Infectious etiology is the most common cause of epilepsy globally, but more prevalent in LMICs.[27,29] The infectious cause results in epilepsy that can be linked to a known infection where the primary symptoms are seizures.[27,29] Epilepsy may be caused by prenatal brain injury from the mother's infection, insufficient nutrition during pregnancy, or oxygen deprivation at birth.[24,30] The most common infections that can cause epilepsy include neurocysticercosis,[31] tuberculosis, human immunodeficiency virus (HIV), cerebral malaria, subacute sclerosing panencephalitis, cerebral toxoplasmosis, toxocariasis, schistosomiasis, Lyme disease, Zika virus, and cytomegalovirus.[24,27,29] Prevention of these infections could reduce the incidence and burden of epilepsy, especially in LMICs.[27]

Metabolic epilepsy arises from a known or suspected metabolic disorder in which seizures are a primary symptom. Examples include biotinidase and holocarboxylase synthase deficiency, cerebral folate deficiency, creatine disorders, folinic acid-responsive seizures, glucose transporter 1 deficiency, mitochondrial disorders, peroxisomal disorders, porphyria, uremia, aminoacidopathies, and pyridoxine-dependent seizures.[27,29] While many metabolic epilepsies are genetically based, some, such as cerebral folate deficiency, may be acquired. Identifying specific metabolic causes is crucial for developing targeted treatments and preventing intellectual impairment.[29]

Immune epilepsy can be linked to an immune disorder where the primary symptom is seizures.[29] Autoimmune describes a situation in which the body fails to differentiate foreign substances from its own cells and thus attacks its own healthy cells. Immune epilepsies occur in both children and adults. An immune etiology is a condition where there is proof of autoimmune-mediated inflammation in the central nervous system.[29] The autoimmune etiologies include anti-NMDA receptor encephalitis, voltage-gated potassium channel antibodies, GAD65 antibodies, GABA-B receptor antibodies, AMPA receptor antibodies, steroid-responsive encephalopathy associated with thyroid disease, and celiac disease.[27] Diagnosis includes antibody testing and is a critical step in developing targeted immunotherapy for treatment.[29]

Unknown etiology is when the cause of the epilepsy is not known. Identifying the causes sometimes requires advanced diagnostic tools and resources that may not be available in LMICs. The known causes account for 30% of all known epilepsy cases, the rest, which is 70%, is due to unknown causes.[30,31] This could be the reason why this condition has puzzled even those in the medical fraternity to the extent that it is not easily understood. The unexplained cases are then attributed to supernatural causes. This is common regardless of whether people are educated or religious, which will be discussed in later chapters.

Encephalopathy

According to the ILAE Diagnostic Manual,[27] encephalopathy is a brain disorder that can lead to disorientation, restlessness, mood alterations, or even coma in severe cases. It may be temporary or cause lasting damage, with various types caused by infections, toxins, or underlying conditions. Treatment is based on the specific cause. Developmental encephalopathy (DE) describes a condition characterized by impairments in cognition, neurology, or mental health due to an underlying cause. Epileptic encephalopathy (EE) arises when epileptic activity leads to the encephalopathy. If both developmental problems and epileptic activity are factors, the condition is called developmental and epileptic encephalopathy (DEE). For adults with DE, the appropriate term is progressive neurological deterioration (PND), as they have already completed developmental milestones. Table 2 shows the epilepsy syndromes that are always linked to DE, EE, DEE, and PND in almost all cases.

Table 2: Epilepsy syndromes associated with encephalopathy or PND

Neonate / Infant	Childhood	Any age
Early infantile developmental and epileptic encephalopathy	Epilepsy with myoclonic atonic seizures Lennox–Gastaut syndrome	Progressive myoclonus epilepsies Rasmussen syndrome
Epilepsy of infancy with migrating focal seizures	Developmental and/or epileptic encephalopathy with spike-wave activation in sleep	
Infantile epileptic spasms syndrome	Febrile infection-related epilepsy syndrome	
Dravet syndrome	Hemiconvulsion-hemiplegia-epilepsy syndrome	

Adapted from International League Against Epilepsy (2024). Diagnostic Manual. www.epilepsydiagnosis.org/index.html [27]

Etiology of epilepsy – (Worldview)

Epilepsy, a condition affecting both humans and animals, has been feared and misunderstood for centuries. Epilepsy has stirred several disagreements and garnered interest from various parties. It has drawn the attention of truth-seekers, religious leaders, doctors, and scientists alike. Historically, epileptic seizures were often viewed with superstition, leading to beliefs that those affected were either possessed by demons or controlled by divine forces.[32] These superstitious beliefs still dominate in many communities to this day.

Ayurveda is considered the oldest healthcare system in the world.[33] In Ayurvedic medicine, epilepsy was thought to be caused by both internal and external factors.[34] These factors include internal bleeding, fever, excessive sexual intercourse, sporting activities, unclean food, uncleanliness, psychological disturbances due to extreme fury, worry, desire, or apprehension.[34] Other causes of epilepsy in Ayurvedic medicine include eating unhealthy food; prolonged mourning and fury; inner fear and hatred; unethical observance and pastime; incapacitated intellect; and fluctuations in excitement of *doshas*[35] (the three categories of substances that are believed to be present in a person's body and mind, the balance of which influences health). Other diseases were also believed to cause epilepsy.[34]

In Saudi Arabia, while epilepsy can be medically explained, the predominant belief is that it is caused by God or Allah, either as a test or punishment.[36] This belief fosters acceptance, as many affected individuals see it as God's will. Others link epilepsy to cultural and psychosocial factors.[36] Therefore, treatment approaches should be comprehensive enough to address all these aspects.

The earliest recorded mention of epilepsy in China appears in the *Inner Canon of Huangdi*, where it was referred to as *Dian Xian*, a term that disparagingly described a person with seizures as being crazy.[37] In China, traditional beliefs predominantly regard epilepsy as a mental illness instead of a neurological disorder, and it is heavily stigmatized.[37,38] Some PWE in China believe anger, genetics, or brain injury to be the cause of their condition.[39] In both China and Vietnam, some people think epilepsy is caused by imbalances in the liver.[40] Generally, in these communities, almost everyone agrees that epilepsy is not contagious, but they have differing views on its hereditary nature. In the two countries, spiritual explanations are uncommon, and very few people seek help from traditionalists.[40]

In India, the epilepsy treatment gap is 50% and this could be attributed to a belief that epilepsy is a supernatural condition.[41] In their study, Pal et al.[41] found that only 14.5% of PWE in India consulted a medical practitioner when they had a seizure. The rest sought spiritual help through Shamanism. Shamanism is a religious system where practitioners enter a trance to connect with spirits thought to influence the living.[41] Certain families turned to spiritualists who use divine ash or *Vibhuti*, perform exorcisms or *Jhada-phuk*, recite hymns or *mantra*, and participate in rituals such as *tantra-mantra*, temple visits, orate religious scripts, prayers, and pilgrimages.[41] Shamanism encompasses traditional beliefs and practices that enables practitioners to allegedly diagnose, heal, and sometimes cause suffering by connecting with spirits through traversing the *axis mundi* and forming special relationships or gaining control over these spirits.[41]

In Latin America, both rural and urban communities generally believe epilepsy to have supernatural origins.[42] Rather than being recognized as a medical condition, it is frequently viewed as bewitchment or divine vengeance, and is a shameful condition to have.[42] In ancient American Inca culture, people believed a heart disease referred to as *Sonko-Nanay* in the Quechua language was responsible for causing epilepsy.[43] The Tzeltal native community of Mexico refers to epilepsy as *tub tub ik'al*.[44] In this community, epilepsy is believed to be acquired in adulthood and usually affects only one person per family. They fear *tub tub ik'al* as it has no cure. In this culture every person is assigned an animal spirit at birth that trains them in witchcraft.[44] They believe that this animal spirit may be conquered by other animal spirits, leading to epilepsy. In Brazil, the Kayamura tribe believes that epilepsy, known as *teawurup*, is caused by animal spirits.[44] When they kill an armadillo, they believe the spirit of the animal will seek vengeance by attacking a member of the family in the form of epilepsy.[44] In the Bolivian Andes, a tribal group called Uru refers to epilepsy as *tukuri*. They believe epilepsy can be caused by witchcraft, head injuries or sleep deprivation.[44]

According to Carod-Artal and V'azquez-Cabrera,[44] in sub-Saharan Africa, epilepsy is viewed as a supernatural condition. In Mauritania, they associate epilepsy with evil spirits, witchcraft, having caught it from an infected person, or a consequence of malnutrition (*iguindi*).[44] In Nigeria, a study conducted by Komolafe et al.[45] revealed that the people of Western Nigeria have identified three main causes of epilepsy as supernatural, contagion, and psychical. The supernatural causes include spiritual attack, a spell, covetousness, or bewitchment generally sent by people jealous of someone's achievement. The terms used for epilepsy in that region are *giri, warapa* and *ogun oru*.[45] These terms are said to be a source of stigma. In Southwest Nigeria, traditional healers consider epilepsy to be a deeply stigmatized and feared illness among the Yoruba people.[46] They explain its causes through a variety of factors such as natural, hereditary, and supernatural influences. Divination is essential to diagnose each case and treatments are progressively administered. Cases attributed to supernatural causes are deemed the most challenging to treat.[46] Traditional healers in Uyo, Nigeria, believe epilepsy is caused by witchcraft, spiritual attacks, and divine retribution for sins.[47] In Ghana, causes of epilepsy ranged from physical causes like hunger and starvation to spiritual and unknown.[48] In South Africa, witchcraft and evil spirits were also identified as the key causes of epilepsy and impacted the treatment protocol.[49] In Zimbabwe it is called *pfari or zvifa zvifa* (literally translated as dying several times) in Shona or *izithuthwane* in Ndebele. The main etiologies for epilepsy in Zimbabwe are evil spirits, demons, and witchcraft.[50] Other traditionalists classify it as a manifestation of an avenging spirit (*ngozi*) or goblins (*zvikwambo*). The usual first line of treatment based on these beliefs includes consulting pastors, prophets, spirit mediums, herbalists, prayers, and herbs.[50]

All these different worldviews discussed in this section are important because they help explain why people make certain treatment choices. With 70% of epilepsy cases having no known cause, it is only logical for people to seek explanations beyond science. The idea of disease is intricately connected to the cultural understanding of the body and the identifiable origins of illnesses.[51] Cultural knowledge about health and its maintenance is embedded in belief-based practices, experiences, and basic rules that help explain and manage unusual situations.[51]

Conclusion

In conclusion, epilepsy remains a complex neurological condition that has evolved in its understanding and treatment throughout history. Early records, such as those from Hippocrates, shifted the perception of epilepsy from a divine punishment to a medical disorder, laying the groundwork for future advancements.[2] Over centuries, misconceptions and cultural beliefs influenced how epilepsy was perceived and managed, varying across different societies and impacting patients' lives.[8,9] The modern definition provided by the ILAE highlights epilepsy as a brain disorder characterized by enduring predispositions to generating epileptic seizures.[15] Continued research into the mechanisms of seizures, types of epilepsy, and associated risk factors has greatly expanded our understanding of the condition.[17,18]

Despite progress in scientific knowledge and medical interventions, epilepsy remains a significant public health challenge worldwide, with disparities in awareness and access to care.[12,13] Efforts to reduce stigma and educate communities are essential to improve the quality of life for PWE and foster a supportive environment.[5,45] As we look to the future, ongoing research and interdisciplinary collaboration hold promise for better diagnostic tools, treatments, and a deeper understanding of this multifaceted condition. Shortly before this book went to print, the ILAE released an updated seizure classification, which can be accessed using this link: Updated Classification of Epileptic Seizures 2025

References:

1. *Lucretius, T.C.*, trans. Cyril Bailey. (1910). *On the Nature of Things, Oxford:* Clarendon Press, https://oll.libertyfund.org/titles/bailey-on-the-nature-of-things
2. Hippocrates. (400 B.C). *On the sacred disease.* Translated by Adams, F. https://onemorelibrary.com/index.php/en/books/technology/book/medicine-314/on-the-sacred-disease-2433
3. Kanner, A.M., & Bicchi, M.M. (2022). Antiseizure medications for adults with epilepsy: A review. *JAMA,* 327(13), 1269–1281. https://doi:10.1001/jama.2022.3880
4. LaRoche, S.M., & Helmers, S.L. The new antiepileptic drugs: Scientific review. *JAMA.* 2004;291(5):605–614. https://doi:10.1001/jama.291.5.605
5. International League Against Epilepsy. (2003). The history and stigma of epilepsy. *Epilepsia, 44*(6), 12-14. https://doi.org/pdf/10.1046/j.1528-1157.44.s.6.2.x
6. Lennox, W.G. (1960). Epilepsy and related disorders. Boston: Little Brown & Co.

7. Lim, K.S., Li, S.C., Casanova-Gutierrez, J., & Tan, C.T. (2012). Name of epilepsy, does it matter? *Neurology Asia, 17*(2), 87-91. https://www.neurology-asia.org/articles/neuroasia-2012-17(2)-087.pdf
8. Akhtar, S.W. and Aziz, H. (2004). Perception of epilepsy in Muslim history; with current scenario. *Neurology Asia. 9 (Supplement 1): 59 – 60.* https://www.academia.edu/download/82397420/20043_059.pdf
9. Brown, E. (2010). Ayurveda and the "Sacred Disease" : Treating epilepsy with ancient Ayurvedic wisdom. www.chopra.com/files/docs/teacherdownloads/.../Epilepsy,%20Erin%20brown.pdf
10. A dialogue with historical concepts of epilepsy from the Babylonians to Hughlings Jackson: Persistent beliefs. https://www.sciencedirect.com/science/article/pii/S152550501100148X
11. Kaculini, C.M., Tate-Looney, A.J. & Seifi, A. (2021). The history of epilepsy: From ancient mystery to modern misconception. *Cureus, 13*(3):e13953. https://doi.org/10.7759%2Fcureus.13953
12. Beghi, E. (2020). The Epidemiology of Epilepsy. *Neuroepidemiology*, 54:185–191. https://doi.org/10.1159/000503831
13. World Health Organization. (2019). Global Epilepsy Report: Epilepsy – A public health imperative. https://www.ilae.org/files/dmfile/19053_Epilepsy_A-public-health-imperative-For-Web.pdf
14. World Health Organization. (2023). Epilepsy. https://www.who.int/health-topics/epilepsy#tab=tab_1
15. Fisher, R. S., Acevedo, C., Arzimanoglou, A., Bogacz, A., Cross, J. H., Elger, C. E., ... & Wiebe, S. (2014). ILAE official report: a practical clinical definition of epilepsy. Epilepsia, 55(4), 475-482. https://doi.org/10.1111/epi.12550
16. Benbadis, S.R. and Riaz, A. (2012). "VIREPA Course on Clinical Pharmacology and Pharmacotherapy: Treatment in Newly Diagnosed Patients." Stockholm: *International League Against Epilepsy.*
17. Blumenfeld, H. (2014). What is a seizure network? Long-range network consequences of focal seizures. In: Scharfman, H., Buckmaster, P. (eds). Issues in Clinical Epileptology: A View from the Bench. *Advances in Experimental Medicine and Biology. 813*, 63-70. https://doi.org/10.1007/978-94-017-8914-1_5
18. Fisher, R. S., Cross, J. H., French, J. A., Higurashi, N., Hirsch, E., Jansen, F. E., ... & Zuberi, S. M. (2017). Operational classification of seizure types by the International League Against Epilepsy: Position Paper of the ILAE Commission for Classification and Terminology. Epilepsia, 58(4), 522-530. https://doi.org/10.1111/epi.13670
19. Fisher, R. S., Boas, W. V. E., Blume, W., Elger, C., Genton, P., Lee, P., & Engel Jr, J. (2005). Epileptic seizures and epilepsy: definitions proposed by the International League Against Epilepsy (ILAE) and the International Bureau for Epilepsy (IBE). Epilepsia, 46(4), 470-472. https://doi.org/10.1111/j.0013-9580.2005.66104.x
20. Trinka, E., Cock, H., Hesdorffer, D., Rossetti, A. O., Scheffer, I. E., Shinnar, S., ... & Lowenstein, D. H. (2015). A definition and classification of status epilepticus–Report of the ILAE Task Force on Classification of Status Epilepticus. *Epilepsia, 56*(10), 1515-1523. https://doi.org/10.1111/epi.13121
21. International League Against Epilepsy. (2022). Epilepsy imitators. https://www.epilepsydiagnosis.org/epilepsy-imitators.html
22. Kodankandath, T.V., Theodore, D. & Samanta, D. (2024). Generalized Tonic-Clonic Seizure. [In: StatPearls [Internet]. Treasure Island (FL): *StatPearls Publishing*, https://www.ncbi.nlm.nih.gov/books/NBK554496/

23. Berg, A. T., Berkovic, S. F., Brodie, M. J., Buchhalter, J., Cross, J. H., van Emde Boas, W., ... & Scheffer, I. E. (2010). Revised terminology and concepts for organization of seizures and epilepsies: report of the ILAE Commission on Classification and Terminology, 2005–2009. *Epilepsia*, *51*, 676–685. https://doi.org/10.1111/j.1528-1167.2010.02522.x
24. Fisher, R. S., Cross, J. H., D'souza, C., French, J. A., Haut, S. R., Higurashi, N., ... & Zuberi, S. M. (2017). Instruction manual for the ILAE 2017 operational classification of seizure types. Epilepsia, 58(4), 531-542. https://doi.org/10.1111/epi.13671
25. Ighodaro, E. T., Maini, K., Arya, K., & Sharma, S. (2023). Focal onset seizure. In *StatPearls [Internet]*. StatPearls Publishing. https://www.ncbi.nlm.nih.gov/sites/books/NBK500005/
26. Senelick, R. (2012). "Types of Seizures and Seizure Symptoms" in: http://www.webmd.com/epilepsy/guide/types-of-seizures-their-symptoms
27. International League Against Epilepsy. (2024). *Diagnostic Manual*. https://www.epilepsydiagnosis.org/index.html
28. Ball, D.E., Mielke, J., Adamolekun, B., Mundanda, T. and McLean, J. (2000). Community leader education to increase epilepsy attendance at clinics in Epworth, Zimbabwe. *Epilepsia*. 41(8):1044-5. https://doi.org/10.1111/j.1528-1157.2000.tb00292.x
29. Scheffer, I.E., Berkovic, S., Capovilla, G. et al. (2017). ILAE classification of the epilepsies: Position paper of the ILAE Commission for Classification and Terminology. *Epilepsia*, *58*:512–521. https://doi.org/10.1111/epi.13709
30. Hoffman, M. (2024). Causes of epilepsy. https://www.webmd.com/epilepsy/epilepsy-causes
31. Carpio, A., & Hauser, W. A. (2009). Epilepsy in the developing world. *Current Neurology and Neuroscience Reports*, *9*(4), 319-326. https://dspace.ucuenca.edu.ec/bitstream/123456789/22129/1/scopus%20146.pdf
32. Melody, M.T. (1959). Epilepsy and social attitudes: An historical review of the evolution of these attitudes, with emphasis on developments during the years 1935 to 1958, https://research.library.fordham.edu/dissertations/AAI30557756
33. Brown, E. (2010). Ayurveda and the "Sacred Disease": Treating epilepsy with ancient Ayurvedic wisdom. www.chopra.com/files/docs/teacherdownloads/.../Epilepsy,%20Erin%20brown.pdf
34. Manyam, B.V. (1992). Epilepsy in Ancient India, *Epilepsia*, 33(3):473-175. https://doi.org/10.1111/j.1528-1157.1992.tb01694.x
35. Krishnamurthy, M.S. (2014). Epilepsy – Ayurvedic understanding and its treatment. http://easyayurveda.com/2014/04/23/epilepsy-ayurvedic-understanding-treatment/
36. Alkhamees, H. A., Selai, C. E. and Shorvon, S. D. (2015). The beliefs among patients with epilepsy in Saudi Arabia about the causes and treatment of epilepsy and other aspects', *Epilepsy & Behavior*, *53*:135–139. https://doi.org/10.1016/j.yebeh.2015.10.008
37. Ding, D., Zhou, D., Sander, J. W., Wang, W., Li, S., & Hong, Z. (2021). Epilepsy in China: Major progress in the past two decades. *The Lancet Neurology*, *20*(4), 316-326. https://doi.org/10.1016/S1474-4422(21)00023-5
38. Lai, C., Huang, X., Lai, Y.C., Zhang, Z., Liu, G., and Yang, M. (1990). Survey of public awareness, understanding, and attitudes towards epilepsy in Henen Province, China. https://doi.org/10.1111/j.1528-1167.1990.tb06304.x
39. Li, S., Wu, J., Wang, W., Jacoby, A., de Boer, H., & Sander, J. W. (2010). Stigma and epilepsy: The Chinese perspective. *Epilepsy & Behavior*, *17*(2), 242-245. https://doi.org/10.1016/j.yebeh.2009.12.015
40. Jacoby, A., Wang, W., Vu, T. D., Wu, J., Snape, D., Aydemir, N., ... & Baker, G. (2008). Meanings of epilepsy in its sociocultural context and implications for stigma: Findings from ethnographic studies in local communities in China and Vietnam. *Epilepsy &*

Behavior, *12*(2), 286-297.
https://www.sciencedirect.com/science/article/pii/S1525505007003599
41. Pal, S. K., Sharma, K., Prabhakar, S., & Pathak, A. (2008). Psychosocial, demographic, and treatment-seeking strategic behavior, including faith healing practices, among patients with epilepsy in northwest India. *Epilepsy & Behavior*, *13*(2), 323-332. https://doi:10.1016/j.yebeh.2007.12.023
42. Burneo, J. G., Tellez-Zenteno, J., & Wiebe, S. (2005). Understanding the burden of epilepsy in Latin America: a systematic review of its prevalence and incidence. *Epilepsy Research*, *66*(1-3), 63-74. https://doi:10.1016/j.eplepsyres.2005.07.002
43. Burneo, J. G. (2003). Sonko-Nanay and epilepsy among the Incas. *Epilepsy & Behavior*, *4*(2), 181-184. https://doi.org/10.1016/S1525-5050(03)00035-0
44. Carod-Artal, F.J. and Vázquez-Cabrera, C.B. (2007). An anthropological study about epilepsy in native tribes from Central and South America. *Epilepsia, 48*(5):886–893. https://doi.org/10.1111/j.1528-1167.2007.01016.x
45. Komolafe, M. A., Sunmonu, T. A., Fabusiwa, F., Komolafe, E. O., Afolabi, O., Kett, M., & Groce, N. (2011). Women's perspectives on epilepsy and its sociocultural impact in southwestern Nigeria. *African Journal of Neurological Sciences*, *30*(2). https://www.ajol.info/index.php/ajns/article/view/77320
46. Ademilokun, T.F., & Agunbiade, O.M. (2021). Aetiological explanations of epilepsy and implications on treatments options among Yoruba traditional healers in Southwest Nigeria. *African Sociological Review, 25*(1), 86-111. https://www.ajol.info/index.php/asr/article/view/246707
47. Abasiubong, F.U.D., Ekott, J., Bassey, E. & Nyong, E. (2009). Knowledge, attitude and perception of epilepsy among traditional healers in Uyo, Nigeria. *Global Journal of Community Medicine* 2(1-2). DOI:10.4314/gjcm.v2i1-2.47928
48. Deegbe, D.A., Aziato, L., and Attiogbe, A. (2019). Beliefs of people living with epilepsy in the Accra Metropolis, Ghana, *Seizure*, *73*, 21-25. https://doi.org/10.1016/j.seizure.2019.10.016
49. Keikelame, M.J. (2016). Perspectives on epilepsy on the part of patients and careers in a South African urban township. Stellenbosch University. https://scholar.sun.ac.za/bitstreams/6a0acda3-f468-46ad-b97c-053d614b7bc6/download
50. Mutanana, N. (2018). Indigenous Practices for Sustainable Management of Epilepsy in Zimbabwe. https://doi.org/10.13140/RG.2.2.33243.52004
51. Iancu, L. (2019). The magical and sacred medical world: World view, religion and disease in Magyarfalu. Cambridge Scholars Publishing, Newcastle. P. 59-77.

CHAPTER 3 – DIAGNOSIS OF EPILEPSY

Epilepsy is primarily diagnosed clinically through patient history, but it is often overdiagnosed, frequently due to misinterpreting a normal EEG as abnormal, especially when history is unclear. Reversing a misdiagnosis is difficult, highlighting the need for better EEG training and caution against relying too heavily on tests over clinical judgment.[1]
Ushtar Amin and Selim R. Benbadis

Introduction

Accurate diagnosis of epilepsy is the most critical step in its treatment and management. Misdiagnosis can lead to inappropriate therapy and even worsen the patient's condition.[2,3] Differentiating epilepsy from epilepsy imitators remains a significant challenge due to overlapping symptoms and varied presentations.[4,5] Clinicians need to use all strategies to ensure patients receive the best care tailored to their specific type of epilepsy. It has been observed that 20–30% of people who do not respond to AEDs do not suffer from epilepsy at all.[1] They were started on treatment because of a misdiagnosis. Without a proper diagnosis, even the best medicines do not add any value to patients.[6]

Epilepsy is not easy to diagnose as there are many conditions that imitate or mimic an epileptic seizure. Epilepsy is sometimes over-diagnosed when people cannot distinguish between a seizure and epilepsy.[7] In some instances, the epilepsy is subtle, and many people will not be able to tell that it is really epilepsy. Several seizure types can be easily misconstrued as epileptic seizures, and chapter 4 goes deeper into epilepsy imitators. Benbadis[8] summarizes it as follows: "not everything that shakes is a seizure, not every seizure is epilepsy, not every seizure needs to be treated." The most important thing to remember is that several things can cause seizures, but they are not epilepsy.

Clinical assessment

Diagnosis of epilepsy lies exclusively on history.[1] The initial clinical evaluation is crucial for diagnosing epilepsy accurately. The comprehensive history-taking process should include information such as how the seizures started, how often they happen, how long they last, any triggers, and a description of events preceding or following the seizure.[8,9,10] Obtaining an eyewitness account from someone who has observed the seizures can also be valuable, as it provides an objective view of the seizure characteristics, which may be missing from the patient's perspective.[5,10] The doctors use the information to make a diagnosis or start investigations. If the history is not very good, the chances of a misdiagnosis are greater.

The family should be encouraged to utilize technology to help them explain what happens during a seizure episode. Video recordings, available on most smartphones, have become a critical tool, especially in LMICs where other diagnostic tools may be unavailable. Though it may sound insensitive to ask a parent to take a video of their child during an epileptic seizure, it is the easiest way for the clinician to not only conclude a seizure is epileptic, but to identify the type of epilepsy as well. If the clinician is not sure about a diagnosis, the video can be shared with a colleague for a second opinion. Video filming helps when eyewitnesses fail to properly account for the whole seizure. Eyewitnesses may not be able to properly explain to the doctor what really transpired because medical terminology does not often appear in our everyday language. One example of medical terminology causing a communication barrier happened when a patient was asked by a doctor if she experienced auras. She told the doctor that she did not know what an aura was. The doctor explained what an aura is, leading the patient to admit that she had indeed experienced an aura before every seizure. Not all patients will be forthcoming in saying they do not understand what the physician is asking. Many will just reply with a yes or a no, which can contribute to misdiagnosis. The clinician attending to the patient is requested to take time in taking the history of the patient. If there is no video, eyewitnesses must be asked as many questions as possible. If the eyewitness to the seizure is not present, the doctor must phone that person to get a proper history.

After thorough history-taking, and if the clinician is satisfied they are dealing with an epileptic seizure, they should start with the seizure classification, as outlined by ILAE.[11] Seizures are categorized based on their onset (focal, generalized, or unknown) and clinical presentation.[2,11] Proper classification helps clinicians identify epilepsy syndromes, which have specific prognoses and treatment protocols. For example, generalized seizures often indicate a broader brain involvement and may be associated with syndromes such as juvenile myoclonic epilepsy, whereas focal seizures may suggest localized brain abnormalities or structural causes.[2,4]

Physical and neurological examinations should also be part of the clinical assessment to identify any signs indicative of underlying neurological disorders.[4] Clinicians evaluate mental state, intellectual function, muscle control, and involuntary responses, which can provide clues that guide further testing and diagnostic imaging.[4,9] Additionally, clinicians must watch out for anything that could suggest epilepsy imitators.[5]

Role of electroencephalography

Besides proper history taking, there are other tests that can be used to confirm the diagnosis of epilepsy. All new patients clinically diagnosed of epilepsy should undergo an MRI of the brain to exclude other things like tumors. Most individuals with epilepsy have a normal MRI. Every patient diagnosed with epilepsy should have a standard EEG examination.[8] EEG remains a cornerstone in the diagnostic process for epilepsy. Routine EEGs are conducted to identify specific waves that indicate epilepsy.[11,12]

At this point, it is necessary to highlight that many PWE will have a normal EEG, especially those with focal epilepsy.[13] Additionally, the EEG's sensitivity may be limited, as not all patients with epilepsy will show abnormal findings during a routine test.[14] In a project sponsored by the International Bureau for Epilepsy (IBE), two of the five individuals who shared their experiences with epilepsy said their EEG results were negative, despite having epilepsy.[19] This is why an EEG should not be used as the sole tool for diagnosing epilepsy. Some clinicians will not begin treatment until they have EEG results, which can be a problem in LMICs where an EEG machine may not be available. Clinicians' over-dependence on EEGs increases the risk of an incorrect assessment or treatment delay. The other contributing factor to misdiagnosis using EEGs is the skills gap,[1] especially in most LMICs where there are no or few neurologists. I would advise a clinician who is not knowledgeable on interpreting EEGs to avoid using this test. Interpreting EEG results can be complex, and requires special expertise.[1,14] For instance, certain brain waves could be misinterpreted as epileptic waves.[1,12,14] To improve diagnostic accuracy, video EEG monitoring or ambulatory EEG may be used if available. This test captures seizures in real time, providing a more complete clinical picture.[5,9] Ambulatory EEG is costly and in some geographical locations worldwide, may not be covered by medical insurance. Additionally, this test is not available in most LMICs.

The importance and usefulness of an EEG goes beyond diagnosing epilepsy. EEGs help with epilepsy classification and monitoring the effectiveness of ongoing treatment.[11] Accurate interpretation of an EEG provides tremendous benefits to epilepsy management. If the EEG confirms an epilepsy diagnosis, it can also help identify the type of epilepsy and pinpoint the area of the brain where the seizures originate. Clinicians can also conduct EEGs at specific times, such as after sleep deprivation or during sleep, to increase the chances of capturing epileptic activity.[12] These alternative ways of testing are useful when standard EEGs fail to detect abnormalities while clinical suspicion remains high.[1,14]

Imaging and advanced diagnostic tools

Neuroimaging is often used in addition to EEG to identify brain abnormalities that could be the source of seizures. Several imaging tests like MRI, CT scan, functional MRI (fMRI), and positron emission tomography (PET) can be used. However, MRI is the preferred imaging choice because it is the best for detecting brain abnormalities, tumors, and other lesions.[4,10] CT scans are ideal in emergency situations, but they have less diagnostic sensitivity than MRI.[4] Other tests like fMRI and PET are useful for providing additional insight into brain function and seizure location.[15,16] New technologies like magnetoencephalography

(MEG) and next-generation sequencing (NGS) are enhancing diagnostic capabilities. MEG provides high-resolution mapping of electrical activity, which is beneficial for evaluation before surgery.[16] Genetic mutations causing certain epilepsy syndromes can be identified using NGS.[15,17]

Genetic testing in epilepsy diagnosis

Clinicians now use genetic testing, especially when traditional tests fail to provide useful information.[15,17] Genetic tests help in identifying epilepsy syndromes that have a genetic origin. Accurate identification of these syndromes influences treatment choices and expected outcomes.[17] Some syndromes like Dravet syndrome and genetic generalized epilepsy (GGE) can be diagnosed using genetic testing.[14] Results of these tests are not easy to interpret and the tests are also very expensive, contributing to the limited use of genetic tests in clinical practice.[17] Nonetheless, when resources are available, they help in tailoring treatment to individual patients, reducing the risk of ineffective or harmful interventions.[15]

The value of going through all these tests described in this chapter is to ensure a proper diagnosis is made and appropriate treatment is started.

Misdiagnosis risks

Misdiagnosis is a prevalent challenge in epilepsy, with significant implications for patient care. Several studies suggest 20–30% of patients initially diagnosed with epilepsy are later found to have non-epileptic conditions.[3,18] Several factors contribute to these high rates of misdiagnosis, like poor history-taking, or misinterpretation of EEG or findings of any other tests.[1,3]

Misdiagnosis can have serious consequences. Patients can be exposed to unnecessary and potentially harmful treatments, including AEDs with a variety of undesirable side effects such as cognitive impairment, fatigue, or mood changes.[3,9] Moreover, the psychological burden of being wrongly labeled as having epilepsy can affect a patient's quality of life and lead to stigma.[3,4] Differentiating epilepsy from conditions that mimic seizures is important, because different epilepsy imitators require different treatment options.[5,18]

Misdiagnosis can be reduced if clinicians use multiple diagnostic tools to validate patient history. These tools may not be available in all situations, may be expensive, and require special skill to use and interpret.[5] When these tools and capable interpreters are available, clinicians should use them to ensure there is no misdiagnosis. Collaboration among different clinical specialists like neurologists, neuropsychologists, and cardiologists can help reduce misdiagnosis.[3] Additionally, repeat assessments and continuous monitoring may be necessary for ambiguous cases.[1,18] The most important thing is to treat the right condition.

Diagnostic criteria for special populations

Diagnosing epilepsy in children and older adults presents unique challenges, because it requires age-specific considerations. Seizures can present differently in children compared to adults.[10] For instance, certain syndromes such as infantile spasms or childhood absence epilepsy have specific observable and EEG characteristics that need expert evaluation to be accurately identified.[10,11] It is critical to diagnose epilepsy early in children because any delays could result in potential cognitive or developmental delays associated with untreated epilepsy.[9,10] EEG will be an essential tool for capturing age-specific patterns like hypsarrhythmia (highly abnormal brain wave), seen in West syndrome.[10,11]

Conversely, diagnosing epilepsy in older adults can be complicated by other age-related conditions that obscure the presence of seizures.[4,18] Conditions such as transient ischemic attacks or dementia that normally affect older adults make it difficult to make an accurate diagnosis of epilepsy.[4] Besides history-taking, an accurate diagnosis is more likely when combined with an EEG and MRI.[18] For clinicians without these extra tools, they will need to do more with clinical information to determine a correct diagnosis.

Drug-resistant epilepsy (DRE), a condition where two or more AEDs fail to adequately control seizures, is another area that demands a specialized diagnostic approach.[16] In such cases, a thorough reassessment involving advanced imaging, long-term video EEG monitoring, and genetic testing is necessary to identify potential surgical treatment options.[16,17] DRE in children could be resolved through surgery if the diagnosis is made early and the type of seizures are appropriate for a surgical approach. Surgery may help prevent developmental delays if this is done early enough.[10,16]

Comprehensive diagnostic approaches

In an ideal world, a complete and thorough diagnostic approach includes clinical history, EEG findings, neuroimaging, and genetic testing to create a complete diagnostic profile.[9,13] If all these tools are available, the possibility of an accurate diagnosis is increased, therefore increasing chances of proper management of the condition.[13] According to the ILAE's diagnostic guidelines, a clinical evaluation, EEG, and MRI, or any other type of imaging, should be done to either support or rule out epilepsy.[2,13] The process of combining different diagnostic tools helps clinicians better understand the type of epilepsy and therefore determine the best way to manage it.[9,12] Clinicians may know about these tools and tests, but they may not be available, or when available, too costly for their patients.

Clinical practice should prioritize continuous re-evaluation of patients, as epilepsy can evolve over time, requiring adjustments in diagnosis and treatment plans.[9,12] Every person with epilepsy will need an individualized plan of treatment depending on their seizures and the changing nature of the epilepsy, especially in children and older adults.[4,13]

After diagnosis

Once a diagnosis of epilepsy is made, the type of epilepsy must be identified. Doctors should avoid starting a patient on AEDs unless they are certain the patient has epilepsy. When the patient suspects that the doctor is unsure about a diagnosis, they are less likely to take any prescription given.[19] The clinician must explain the diagnosis to the patient and their family. This interaction should include the epilepsy type, causes of the epilepsy if known, treatment options, and possible outcomes. They must explain whether the type of epilepsy is a life-long condition or if it can be outgrown. Compliance to treatment will need to be emphasized, but the possible side effects should also be highlighted, so that the patient can know what to expect. The patient must be told about acceptable and unacceptable side effects. This is crucial because someone may continue to take an AED even when the side effects are of a serious nature. If possible, especially in LMICs where emergency rooms may not be available or accessible, physicians should give patients their personal phone number so that they can call them in an emergency.

If the clinician does not explain, or seems uncertain about their management plan, the probability of the patient seeking alternative treatment methods is high. If you ask people why they went to a spiritualist or traditional healer, the most likely answer they will give you is that even the medical professionals were puzzled by their condition. The patient is left with the idea that only alternative treatment methods could help them. Some people have gone untreated because they had no confidence in their clinician, so if a diagnosis has been reached, it is very important to communicate with the patient and give them the opportunity to ask any questions and provide honest answers. In my experience, I went on for 13 months refusing to take AEDs because my doctor had trivialized this important step, providing a diagnosis. Even though I continued having seizures, that alone was not enough to convince me to take AEDs. I needed a diagnosis first.

On the topic of treatment, it is known that some AEDs are more specific to certain types of epilepsies than others and that some AEDs specific for focal epilepsies can worsen some generalized epilepsies. It is pointless to have a policy that says all newly diagnosed patients should be commenced on phenobarbitone (sometimes known as phenobarbital) when there are better drugs to treat that type of epilepsy, especially in LMICs where this often happens. If the patient does not respond to this treatment, there is greater risk of losing this patient to faith and traditional healers. People must take their time to identify the type of epilepsy and prescribe the best possible AED for that epilepsy in consideration of all other factors like pregnancy, age, sex, other medical conditions the patient may be suffering from, and other medicines the patient may be taking.

It is advisable to start on a broad-spectrum AED. Always start on the lowest dose possible and increase with need. A patient should not be put on two or more drugs (polytherapy) unless it is necessary to do so. It is generally agreed that the majority of PWE will respond well to one AED (monotherapy). Polytherapy should be avoided as it increases risks of interactions, side effects, toxicity, and poor compliance. Diagnosis is the key to treatment of epilepsy. Therefore, clinicians must take their time and use all available tools to come up with a diagnosis. It is very inconvenient to be changed from one AED to another while a doctor figures out the correct treatment through trial and error. Diagnosis is like laying the foundation to a building: if clinicians take their time on the foundation stage, the possibility of prescribing the proper treatment is very high.

Conclusion

Accurate diagnosis of epilepsy involves several processes, including history-taking, clinical assessment, EEG, imaging, and genetic testing. Fifty percent of PWE become seizure-free on the first therapy as long as the diagnosis is accurate. Choosing this initial AED is crucial because once someone is seizure-free, it is not advisable to change their AED as this may disrupt their lifestyle again. If they were driving, they can no longer do so until they have settled on the new AED. The alternative AED may not work, and the physician might be forced to move the patient back to the old AED that had previously been discontinued. Clinicians must strive to prescribe the best drug available the first time.

Addressing challenges such as misdiagnosis and the need for specialized diagnostic criteria in children and older adults is essential for effective management.[3,4] As diagnostic technologies continue to advance, they promise to enhance the accuracy of epilepsy diagnosis and support personalized treatment strategies.[15,16] Continued research and collaboration across medical disciplines will be crucial in improving diagnostic accuracy and patient care.

References:

1. Amin, U., & Benbadis, S. R. (2019). The role of EEG in the erroneous diagnosis of epilepsy. *Journal of Clinical Neurophysiology*, *36*(4), 294-297. https://doi.org/10.1097/WNP.0000000000000572
2. Fisher, R. S., Cross, J. H., French, J. A., Higurashi, N., Hirsch, E., Jansen, F. E., ... & Zuberi, S. M. (2017). Operational classification of seizure types by the International League Against Epilepsy: Position Paper of the ILAE Commission for Classification and Terminology. *Epilepsia, 58*(4), 522-530. https://doi.org/10.1111/epi.13670
3. Oto, M. M. (2017). The misdiagnosis of epilepsy: appraising risks and managing uncertainty. *Seizure*, *44*, 143-146. https://doi.org/10.1016/j.seizure.2016.11.029
4. Thijs, R. D., Surges, R., O'Brien, T. J., & Sander, J. W. (2019). Epilepsy in adults. *The Lancet*, *393*(10172), 689-701. https://doi.org/10.1016/S0140-6736(18)32596-0
5. Elger, C. E., & Hoppe, C. (2018). Diagnostic challenges in epilepsy: seizure under-reporting and seizure detection. *The Lancet Neurology*, *17*(3), 279-288. https://doi.org/10.1016/S1474-4422(18)30038-3
6. Coebergh, J. (2013). Accurate diagnosis and long-term management is problem in epilepsy, not cost of drugs. *BMJ: British Medical Journal (Online)*, *346*. https://doi.org/10.1136/bmj.f3920
7. Carpio, A., & Hauser, W. A. (2009). Epilepsy in the developing world. *Current neurology and neuroscience reports*, *9*(4), 319-326. https://doi.org/10.1007/s11910-009-0048-z
8. Lennox, W. G., & Lennox-Buchthal, M. A. (1960). Epilepsy and related disorders. Little, Brown.
9. Milligan, T. A. (2021). Epilepsy: A clinical overview. *The American Journal of Medicine*, *134*(7), 840-847. https://doi.org/10.1016/j.amjmed.2021.01.038
10. Minardi, C., Minacapelli, R., Valastro, P., Vasile, F., Pitino, S., Pavone, P., ... & Murabito, P. (2019). Epilepsy in children: from diagnosis to treatment with focus on emergency. *Journal of Clinical Medicine*, *8*(1), 39. https://doi.org/10.3390/jcm8010039
11. Koutroumanidis, M., Arzimanoglou, A., Caraballo, R., Goyal, S., Kaminska, A., Laoprasert, P., ... & Moshé, S. L. (2017). The role of EEG in the diagnosis and classification of the epilepsy syndromes: a tool for clinical practice by the ILAE Neurophysiology Task Force (Part 1). *Epileptic Disorders*, *19*(3), 233-298. https://doi.org/10.1684/epd.2017.0935
12. Tatum, W. O., Rubboli, G., Kaplan, P. W., Mirsatari, S. M., Radhakrishnan, K., Gloss, D., ... & Beniczky, S. (2018). Clinical utility of EEG in diagnosing and monitoring epilepsy in adults. *Clinical Neurophysiology*, *129*(5), 1056-1082. https://doi.org/10.1016/j.clinph.2018.01.019
13. International League Against Epilepsy. (2022). Diagnostic Manual. https://www.ilae.org/education/diagnostic-manual
14. Seneviratne, U., Cook, M. J., & D'Souza, W. J. (2017). Electroencephalography in the diagnosis of genetic generalized epilepsy syndromes. *Frontiers in Neurology*, *8*, 499. https://doi.org/10.3389/fneur.2017.00499
15. Dunn, P., Albury, C. L., Maksemous, N., Benton, M. C., Sutherland, H. G., Smith, R. A., ... & Griffiths, L. R. (2018). Next generation sequencing methods for diagnosis of epilepsy syndromes. *Frontiers in Genetics*, *9*, 20. https://doi.org/10.3389/fgene.2018.00020
16. Anyanwu, C., & Motamedi, G. K. (2018). Diagnosis and surgical treatment of drug-resistant epilepsy. *Brain Sciences*, *8*(4), 49. https://doi.org/10.3390/brainsci8040049

17. Weber, Y. G., Biskup, S., Helbig, K. L., Von Spiczak, S., & Lerche, H. (2017). The role of genetic testing in epilepsy diagnosis and management. *Expert Review of Molecular Diagnostics*, *17*(8), 739-750. https://doi.org/10.1080/14737159.2017.1335598
18. Sarecka-Hujar, B., & Kopyta, I. (2018). Poststroke epilepsy: Current perspectives on diagnosis and treatment. *Neuropsychiatric Disease and Treatment*, 95-103. https://doi.org/10.2147/NDT.S169579
19. International Bureau for Epilepsy. (2012). The dilemma of epilepsy – Personal short stories. https://www.ibe-epilepsy.org/wp-content/uploads/2012/07/IBE-Story-Book-Final.pdf

Chapter 4 – Epilepsy Imitators

False-positive epilepsy diagnoses are common. Clinicians should carefully rule out other conditions before starting treatment, as unnecessary use of AEDs can lead to side effects and affect driving and employment.
Ying Xu, et al.[1]

Introduction

Epilepsy imitators are conditions that mimic epileptic seizures but are not caused by abnormal electrical activity in the brain. These imitator disorders can present with symptoms like seizures, such as involuntary movements, altered awareness, or unusual behaviors, increasing chances of misdiagnosis.[2,3,4] Separating epileptic seizures from non-epileptic events is critical for effective treatment and patient outcomes. Misdiagnosis can cause inappropriate management strategies.[5] Conditions imitating epilepsy include a wide range of neurological, psychological, and systemic disorders, each with its distinct underlying causes and clinical manifestations. Many seizures resemble epilepsy, leading to misdiagnosis, incorrect treatment, ongoing seizures, or even death. Proper diagnostic techniques discussed in the previous chapter, using all necessary tools, help in separating epilepsy from imitators. History-taking remains the chief cornerstone to diagnosing epilepsy.[6] Understanding epilepsy imitators is critical for clinicians to prevent the consequences of misdiagnosis and provide targeted, effective treatment. Some people can experience both epileptic and non-epileptic seizures, so it is crucial to identify and treat both types.

Consequences of misdiagnosis

The consequences of epilepsy misdiagnosis include, but are not limited to:
- Unnecessary side effects from AEDs
- Emotional and psychological distress due to a wrong diagnosis
- Delayed treatment of the actual condition
- Worsening of actual condition
- Stigma

- Unwarranted life restriction like no driving, or job limitations
- Waste of resources

Epilepsy imitator categories

What else could it be? The ILAE[6] categorizes these conditions that mimic epilepsy into six distinct groups as follows:
- Syncope and anoxic seizures
- Behavioral, psychological, and psychiatric disorders
- Sleep-related conditions
- Paroxysmal movement disorders
- Migraine-associated disorders
- Miscellaneous events

I will now explain each group and how these seizures could be mistaken for epilepsy.

Syncope and anoxic seizures

Syncope, or fainting, is a brief loss of consciousness caused by a sudden decrease in blood and oxygen supply to the brain.[2,3,5,6] Syncope can be more puzzling when accompanied by brief convulsive movements. The key differences between epilepsy and syncope are the warning signs associated with syncope such as lightheadedness or sweating before the event and quick recovery afterward.[2,5] Anoxic seizures cause collapse and stiffening from brainstem dysfunction, unrelated to epilepsy.[6] Syncope is common. Forty percent of people with syncope experience neurologically influenced types such as vasovagal syncope, reflex anoxic seizures, or breath-holding spells.[6] This section covers different types of syncope and anoxic seizures.

- *Vasovagal syncope,* a common fainting type across all ages, is triggered by standing, stress, or dehydration. Symptoms include lightheadedness, nausea, and sweating. Brief stiffening or movements may occur but differ from seizures.[1,2,6,7] Confusion, tongue biting, or incontinence can follow. It often runs in families, and tilt table testing helps confirm diagnosis, while EEG is less useful.[6]
- *Reflex anoxic seizures or pallid syncope* begin in infancy and may develop into vasovagal syncope. These seizures are triggered by sudden stimuli like a bump, causing overstimulation of the vagus nerve

leading to low blood pressure, a drop in heart rate, loss of consciousness, tensing of muscles, and tonic-clonic movements. Recovery is swift, though some children may sleep afterward. Though it is a frightening experience, patient outcomes are usually good. Rarely, they may trigger a secondary tonic-clonic seizure, known as an anoxic-epileptic seizure.[6]

- *Breath-holding attacks* are common in preschoolers. They usually happen after crying, leading to breath-holding, followed by low oxygen in the blood, and a brief loss of consciousness or anoxic seizures. These events are generally harmless.[8,9] Recovery is quick, and the prognosis is good. These attacks are more common in children with iron deficiency anemia and video-EEG monitoring is needed to distinguish these from true epileptic seizures.[6,8]
- *Hyperventilation syncope* is caused by rapid breathing and presents with brief unconsciousness, with or without a seizure.[6] When blood carbon dioxide is low, hyperventilation occurs, causing shifts in blood pH. This results in the narrowing of blood vessels in the brain, impacting the nervous system.[3]
- *Compulsive Valsalva* is triggered by fast breathing and breath-holding.[6] This is normally self-induced in people with developmental impairments, like autism. Compulsive Valsalva is believed to create pleasurable feelings.
- *Neurological* causes of syncope include structural defects in the cerebellum (Chiari malformation), neurological disorders causing exaggerated startle responses (hyperekplexia), and sudden extreme pain disorder. Neuroimaging is advised for patients with headaches and sensory symptoms, as surgery may be curative.[6]
- *Imposed upper airways obstruction* is a rare but serious cause of infant syncope. It usually happens when specific individuals are present and linked to feigned illness. Events happen slowly compared with other syncope types.[6]
- *Orthostatic intolerance leads to posture-related syncope.* This condition is identified by intolerance to specific upright postures like standing or sitting. People with this type of syncope experience vertigo, faintness, poor vision, sweating, headache, and general discomfort.[6]

- *Long QT syndrome and cardiac syncope* can lead to death. This type of syncope can be induced by fear, exercise, or water exposure. Symptoms include syncope during sleep, family history, and sudden death. Patients must be referred to a cardiologist for management.[6]
- *Hypercyanotic spells* usually occur in infants born with heart defects. Symptoms include fast breathing, blue skin, weakness, and possible tonic-clonic episodes. They are triggered by fast breathing, rapid heart rate, or fluid loss. Recognizing and managing these spells is critical to prevent severe oxygen deprivation and death.[6]

Behavioral, psychological, and psychiatric disorders
- *Daydreaming/inattention* – Daydreaming in children can resemble absence seizures but differs in important aspects. Unlike absence seizures, daydreaming doesn't involve eyelid flickering and can be interrupted by external cues like hearing their name. The child may appear to stare blankly or freeze, and some may show repetitive movements, especially if they have developmental or attention issues.[6]
- *Self-gratification*, common in infants and preschool girls, may mimic seizures with signs like rhythmic hip movements, staring, and flushed cheeks. They typically occur during quiet moments and can be hard to diagnose, especially if the child seems distressed. Parents prefer the term "self-gratification."[6]
- *Eidetic imagery, or childhood preoccupation*, involves children deeply engaging in vivid imaginary stories, with staring, movements, or whispering that can last several minutes. These episodes may resemble seizures but are longer, more detailed, lack a postictal state, and can cause frustration if interrupted.[6]
- *Tantrums* and rage episodes in young children are not seizures. They involve intense, prolonged outbursts over minor triggers, with screaming, destructive behavior, and partial memory loss. Afterward, the child may feel ashamed or remorseful.[6]
- *Out of body experiences* occur in people of all age groups. The person feels like they are seeing themself from above. This can be accompanied by seizures, migraines, or the experience can happen independently.[6]

- *Panic or anxiety attacks* are brief, intense episodes of fear with symptoms like breathlessness, palpitations, and dizziness, often mistaken for seizures. Triggers may be unclear, but EEG can help differentiate them from focal seizures.[3,6,7]
- *Dissociative states* range from mild detachment to severe unresponsiveness. In the mild form, dissociation can help the body cope with stress after an anxiety episode. However, when a dissociative state becomes severe, especially after trauma, individuals may become disconnected from self, even leading to memory loss, with no obvious triggers.[6]
- *Non-epileptic seizures* (NES, formerly psychogenic non-epileptic seizures), also known as pseudo-seizures, are clinical episodes of movement, behaviors, and sensations that closely resemble epileptic seizures, but have no link to abnormal cortical electrical discharges.[2,3,10] Their causes vary and may involve psychological factors that cannot be identified. Key distinctions include a lack of epileptiform discharges on EEG and symptoms often linked to psychological triggers.[7,11]
    - Accurate diagnosis is essential to avoid inappropriate treatments and ensure suitable psychological care, often requiring video-EEG monitoring.[6] Pseudo-seizures account for 90% of epilepsy misdiagnosis and syncope accounts for 9%.[12] A detailed and thorough history-taking is the most critical component of this diagnosis.[3] The following characteristics help distinguish these seizures from epileptic seizures:
    - They happen frequently in a day.
    - They are non-responsive to AEDs.
    - They are triggered by unusual seizure triggers and can even happen in the doctor's waiting room. They can start during history-taking.
    - Onset and termination of seizure is very gradual.
    - Movements are not synchronous, side-to-side head movements, pelvic thrusting, stuttering, and weeping (W.G. Lennox).[12]
- *Hallucinations* in psychiatric disorders are complex and involve multiple senses. Sensory hallucinations from focal seizures, on the other hand, are simple, and limited to a specific region of the brain.

Seizures may include complex hallucinations, which can be differentiated by their episodic nature and accompanying seizure features.[6]
- *Fabricated or factitious illness* can mimic epilepsy, often leading to misdiagnosis due to reliance on witness accounts. Factors may include psychological issues or financial gain. Suspicions arise if the clinical history is inconsistent, seizures are only witnessed by one person, or EEGs remain normal despite frequent seizures.[6]

Sleep-related conditions
- *Sleep-related rhythmic movement disorders*, such as body rocking and head banging, are usually harmless, self-soothing movements seen in infants during sleep transitions. However, if they persist in older children or throughout the night, frontal lobe seizures should be considered. Video review is key for diagnosis.[6]
- *Hypnagogic jerks* (sleep starts, or hypnic jerks) are involuntary muscle twitches that occur as a person falls asleep. They're more common in individuals with motor or developmental disorders and may disrupt sleep if frequent. These jerks can sometimes be confused with myoclonic seizures or epileptic spasms.[6,13]
- *Arousal parasomnias*, including night terrors, sleepwalking, and confusional arousals, occur during deep non-REM sleep, usually in the first third of the night. They can range from minor movements to dramatic episodes involving fear and agitation, where individuals may walk, shout, and fail to recognize family members, which are often mistaken for seizures. These events are linked to stress, lack recollection, and often have a genetic link. Diagnosis typically involves video review.[6]
- *REM sleep disorders* involve loss of normal muscle paralysis during dreaming, leading to physical actions like kicking or shouting. These episodes usually occur in the final third of sleep. Careful history-taking and neurological evaluation, particularly in older adults or those with brainstem issues, are important to rule out frontal lobe seizures.[6]
- *Benign neonatal sleep myoclonus* is a harmless condition in infants, often mistaken for seizures. It only happens during sleep and involves brief, variable limb jerks. The infant's behavior and development

remain normal, and the movements stop when baby is woken up unlike myoclonic seizures, which signal serious neurological issues.[6,13,14]
- *Periodic leg movements in sleep* are more common in older people but can affect all ages, often linked to restless legs syndrome. These repetitive movements can disturb sleep and may resemble myoclonic seizures. Family history and deficiencies in iron, magnesium, or folate should be evaluated, and treatment may include medication.[6]
- *Narcolepsy-cataplexy* is a lifelong neurological disorder characterized by blurred boundaries between sleep states and wakefulness, often starting in adolescence. It involves excessive daytime sleepiness, sudden and brief muscle weakness triggered by strong emotions, and hallucinations that occur between sleep states. Diagnosis requires detailed sleep history, video evidence, and tests like polysomnography, while genetic factors and orexin levels may also be evaluated.[6]

Paroxysmal movement disorders
- *Tics* are involuntary, repetitive movements or vocalizations that can be simple or complex. They often occur in childhood, may fluctuate in frequency, and can be misdiagnosed as seizures. Key features include an urge to perform the tic and some ability to suppress it.[6]
- *Stereotypies* are repetitive movements or postures, ranging from simple to complex, seen in both typical individuals and those with disorders. They differ from epileptic automatisms, which typically involve impaired awareness and occur with specific types of seizures.[6]
- *Paroxysmal kinesigenic dyskinesia* is a movement disorder marked by short episodes of abnormal movements, often triggered by sudden, ordinary actions such as standing.[3,6,15] However, these seizure-like episodes do not show any epileptiform EEG finding.[3,6,15] Patients may experience a sensation before an attack.[6] This condition can occur randomly or run in families and may be associated with epilepsy. It usually begins in childhood or adolescence and often responds positively to low doses of carbamazepine. Recognizing that movement acts as a trigger is crucial for diagnosis.[6]
- *Paroxysmal non-kinesigenic dyskinesia* is a movement disorder with mixed symptoms lasting minutes to hours. Awareness remains intact.

It is triggered by stress, alcohol, or caffeine, often starts in early childhood, and may be inherited.[6]
- *Paroxysmal exercise-induced dyskinesia* is a genetically diverse condition lasting up to 30 minutes, where exercise triggers muscle stiffness (dystonia) or irregular twisting movements (choreoathetosis), often affecting lower limbs, and can be inherited or random.[6]
- *Benign paroxysmal tonic upgaze* usually starts in infancy, characterized by extended periods of gazing upwards that can last from hours to days. It may cause ataxia and is worsened by illness, typically resolving within a few years, though it can result in developmental issues for many.[6]
- *Episodic ataxias* are uncommon dominant genetic disorders, classified as EA1 and EA2. EA1, linked to *KCNA1* mutations, causes brief ataxic or clumsiness episodes, while EA2, associated with *CACNA1A* variants, leads to longer ataxic or clumsy periods. Both can be effectively treated with acetazolamide.[6]
- *Alternating hemiplegia of childhood* is a rare disorder that begins in infancy, characterized by recurrent temporary paralysis, weakness on both sides of the body, and developmental impairment. Other signs include rapid eye movements, skin discoloration, agitation, eye misalignment, changes in automatic body functions, muscle tension or spasms, and involuntary movements between episodes.[6]
- *Hyperekplexia* features an exaggerated startle reflex and is associated with genetic variants that disrupt the inhibitory glycinergic pathway. Symptoms start in infancy, presenting as muscle stiffness and noticeable startles in response to touch or sound. Severe reactions can result in cessation of breathing (apnea) and skin discoloration (cyanosis). Although symptoms usually diminish after infancy, some adults may still experience heightened startle responses.[6]
- *Opsoclonus-myoclonus syndrome* is an autoimmune neurological disorder characterized by lack of coordination (ataxia), erratic eye movements, and myoclonus, often associated with neuroblastoma or viral infections. Symptoms can mimic epilepsy but have distinct movement patterns.[6]

Migraine-associated disorders
- *Migraine with visual aura* is common and often coexists with epilepsy.[6] Visual auras typically feature positive and negative phenomena in one visual field. Symptoms such as visual disturbances, sensory changes, and transient cognitive impairment may resemble seizure manifestations.[2,7] Complex sensory perceptions can occur and may be misdiagnosed as seizures but are more likely linked to *Alice in Wonderland syndrome,* a migraine variant.[6] Unlike epilepsy, migraine episodes typically do not include a postictal state.[11]
- *Familial hemiplegic migraine,* a subtype of migraine with aura, features focal weakness and other symptoms before headaches. It is linked to genetic variants. Severe attacks can be triggered by trauma or illness.[6]
- *Benign paroxysmal torticollis* is a migraine variant seen in young children, characterized by short episodes of neck twisting accompanied by symptoms such as skin color changes and nausea, potentially resulting in migraines later.[6]
- *Benign paroxysmal vertigo* in children involves brief episodes of vertigo, often causing anxiety, nausea, and involuntary, repetitive eye movements (nystagmus). It can precede or follow episodes of twisted neck and may lead to migraines.[6]
- *Cyclical vomiting* features repeated bouts of vomiting lasting hours to days, followed by symptom-free intervals. Frequently associated with a family history of migraines, it often starts in childhood and may progress to abdominal or classic migraines. The cause is uncertain, and episodes may persist into adulthood but become less predictable.[6]

Miscellaneous events
- *Transient ischemic attacks* (TIAs), also referred to as "mini strokes," can present with sudden neurological deficits resembling seizures, such as temporary limb weakness, speech difficulties, or sensory changes.[1,7] The absence of postictal confusion and a history of cardiovascular risk factors can help differentiate TIAs from epilepsy.[1,7]
- *Benign myoclonus of infancy* and shuddering attacks are harmless, brief episodes in infants, starting around 4 months and lasting until 6–7 years of age. Triggered by activities like feeding or head movement, these

episodes involve brief jerks or shudders without distress or awareness impairment, often mistaken for seizures, and the child resumes normal activity immediately after.[6]
- *Jitteriness* in newborns is common and often temporary. It increases with stimulation but decreases when the baby is wrapped or calmed, unlike seizures. Causes may include low calcium or neonatal abstinence syndrome.[6]
- *Sandifer syndrome* affects young children with gastroesophageal reflux, often triggered by feeding. Symptoms include back arching, involuntary movement of limbs, and head tilting. Unlike seizures, treating the reflux typically resolves the symptoms.[6]
- *Non-epileptic head drops in infants*, often mistaken for seizures, involve frequent head bobs with equal fall and rise velocity, sometimes accompanied by crying. They start between 3–6 months of age and resolve by 12 months without affecting development.[6]
- *Spasmus nutans* is an eye movement disorder in infants, starting between 4–12 months of age, which involves rapid vertical and side-to-side eye movements, sometimes with head tilting or nodding. It resolves on its own, but neuroimaging is needed to rule out brain abnormalities.[6]
- *Raised intracranial pressure* can lead to abnormal posturing, resembling seizures, alongside signs of encephalopathy such as altered consciousness and abnormal reflexes.[6]
- *Paroxysmal extreme pain disorder* is a rare genetic condition that causes severe pain episodes from infancy. Symptoms include burning or stabbing pain in the perineal area, mouth, or eyes, triggered by actions like changing nappies or eating. Accompanying autonomic features can include body flushing and, in infants, bradycardia or syncope. Although often misdiagnosed as seizures, treatment with carbamazepine may alleviate symptoms.[6]
- *Spinal myoclonus* involves sudden jerks that can happen while awake or asleep, often connected to structural issues in the spine like syringomyelia. It can be segmental, affecting certain muscle areas, or propriospinal, involving the muscles along the spine, with jerks in the neck and trunk. Propriospinal myoclonus usually happens on its own or in response to triggers, while brainstem myoclonus also impacts the

face and can be triggered by sounds. Many cases of propriospinal myoclonus don't have a clear cause.[6]
- *Hypoglycemia* or low blood sugar levels can lead to confusion, sweating, and convulsions that may be mistaken for seizures. Hypoglycemia is particularly relevant in patients with diabetes or metabolic disorders and can be confirmed through blood glucose testing during the event.[7,11]
- *Neurosyphilis*, although rare, can present with neurological symptoms such as seizures or altered consciousness, often leading to misdiagnosis. Testing for syphilis is warranted in patients with unexplained seizures and a history of possible exposure.[16]
- *Encephalitis or meningitis* can cause symptoms resembling epileptic seizures, including altered mental status, motor manifestations, and fever.[2,16] These conditions are often accompanied by systemic signs and diagnostic findings on cerebrospinal fluid analysis or imaging.[2,16]
- *Paroxysmal non-kinesigenic dyskinesia* and certain post-streptococcal syndromes, including Sydenham's chorea, can present with involuntary movements and behaviors mimicking seizures. These disorders require comprehensive clinical and diagnostic evaluation to differentiate them from epilepsy.[15]
- *Gastroesophageal reflux disease* (GERD) in infants can sometimes present with arching movements and apparent distress that mimic seizure-like activity.[11] Careful clinical evaluation, including pH monitoring, can assist in differentiating these episodes from epilepsy.[11]
- *Tongue biting*, often considered a strong indicator of epileptic seizures, can occur in sleep-related facio-mandibular myoclonus.[17] This phenomenon poses a diagnostic challenge as it may closely resemble nocturnal seizures.[17] Differentiating these cases requires video-EEG and sleep studies.[17]

Diagnostic approaches to differentiate epilepsy from imitators

Video-EEG monitoring is a cornerstone in diagnosing epilepsy and distinguishing it from non-epileptic conditions.[8,18] It allows for the recording of events alongside simultaneous EEG activity, helping to confirm whether abnormal electrical discharges are present.[8,18] This approach is especially valuable for diagnosing NES and other non-epileptic events.[8]

Comprehensive clinical history and observation are vital in differentiating epilepsy from its imitators.[1,2] Key elements include the presence of triggers, duration of the event, post-event behavior, and patient-reported symptoms.[1,2] A meticulous review of these factors can often reveal patterns consistent with non-epileptic events.

Advanced imaging, such as MRI or CT scans, and specific laboratory tests can help rule out structural brain abnormalities or underlying metabolic conditions that may present as seizures.[6,18] In cases like neurosyphilis, serological testing plays a critical role.[16] Some of these tests may not be available or accessible in LMICs. If identifying some of these imitators relies on these tests, misdiagnosing can be an issue in LMICs. Clinicians work with what they have and if these tests are not available, most people end up with a wrong epilepsy diagnosis and the unintended consequences of such a diagnosis.

Challenges in pediatric and adult populations

The presentation of epilepsy imitators can vary significantly between pediatric and adult patients. Children may show unique non-epileptic events such as breath-holding spells or shuddering attacks, often mistaken for seizures.[5,9] Adults, on the other hand, may face diagnostic challenges with conditions like syncope and NES.[3] Tailored diagnostic approaches are essential to address the differences in symptoms and triggers between these age groups.[3,5]

Conclusion

Accurate differentiation between epilepsy and its imitators is crucial to ensure appropriate treatment and avoid unnecessary interventions. The use of thorough clinical evaluation, video-EEG monitoring, and additional diagnostic tools can significantly enhance diagnostic accuracy. Continued research and education are necessary to improve clinicians' ability to distinguish epilepsy from its numerous imitators, ultimately leading to better patient care and outcomes.[2,3,15] Unfortunately, most of these diagnostic tools are not available to all populations in need. Thorough history-taking remains the key to proper diagnosis because it can be used by a clinician; however, there is a training gap in epilepsy from diagnosis to management.

References:

1. Xu, Y., Nguyen, D., Mohamed, A., Carcel, C., Li, Q., Kutlubaev, M. A., ... & Hackett, M. L. (2016). Frequency of a false positive diagnosis of epilepsy: a systematic review of observational studies. *Seizure*, *41*, 167-174. https://doi.org/10.1016/j.seizure.2016.08.005
2. International League Against Epilesy. (2022). Epilepsy imitators. https://www.epilepsydiagnosis.org/epilepsy-imitators.html
3. Brodtkorb, E. (2013). Common imitators of epilepsy. *Acta neurologica scandinavica*, *127*, 5-10. https://doi.org/10.1111/ane.12043
4. Ristić, A. J., Alexopoulos, A. V., So, N., Wong, C., & Najm, I. M. (2012). Parietal lobe epilepsy: The great imitator among focal epilepsies. *Epileptic Disorders*, *14*(1), 22-31. https://doi.org/10.1684/epd.2012.0484
5. Samia, P., & Wilmshurst, J. M. (2020). Common childhood epilepsy mimics. *Clinical Child Neurology*, 743-765. https://doi.org/10.1007/978-3-319-43153-6_23
6. International League Against Epilepsy. (2024). Diagnostic Manual. https://www.epilepsydiagnosis.org/index.html
7. Azar, N. J. (n.a). Imitators of Epilepsy. https://pdfs.semanticscholar.org/319b/2e6b317c46943b3e54fc8c3e3284e67c934c.pdf
8. Ueda, R., Shimizu-Motohashi, Y., Sugai, K., Takeshita, E., Ishiyama, A., Saito, T., ... & Sasaki, M. (2018). Seizure imitators monitored using video-EEG in children with intellectual disabilities. *Epilepsy & Behavior*, *84*, 122-126. https://doi.org/10.1016/j.yebeh.2018.05.006
9. Chen, L., Knight E.M., Tuxhorn, I., Shahid, A. & Lüders, H.O. (2015). Paroxysmal non-epileptic events in infants and toddlers: a phenomenologic analysis. *Psychiatry & Clinical Neurosciences, 69*(6):351–9. https://doi.org/10.1111/pcn.12245
10. Kodankandath, T.V., Theodore, D. & Samanta, D. (2024). Generalized Tonic-Clonic Seizure. [In: StatPearls [Internet]. Treasure Island (FL): StatPearls Publishing; Available from: https://www.ncbi.nlm.nih.gov/books/NBK554496/
11. Panayiotopoulos, C. P. (2010). Imitators of epileptic seizures. In *a clinical guide to epileptic syndromes and their treatment* (pp. 97-134). London: Springer London. https://doi.org/10.1007/978-1-84628-644-5_4
12. Lennox, W.G. (1960). Epilepsy and related disorders. Boston: Little Brown & Co.
13. Serino, D. & Fusco, L. (2015). Epileptic hypnagogic jerks mimicking repetitive sleep starts. *Sleep Medicine, 8*:1014–6. https://doi.org/10.1016/j.sleep.2015.04.015
14. Sharma, D., Murki, S. & Pratap, O.T. (2014). Benign sleep myoclonus in neonate: A diagnostic dilemma for neonatologist. *BMJ Journals*, https://doi.org/10.1136/bcr-2014-206626
15. Peila, E., Mortara, P., Cicerale, A. & Pinessi, L. (2015). Paroxysmal non-kinesigenic dyskinesia, post-streptococcal syndromes and psychogenic movement disorders: a diagnostic challenge. *BMJ Journals*. https://doi.org/10.1136/bcr-2014-207449
16. Kumari, S., Hayton, T., Jumaa, P., & McCorry, D. (2015). 'The great imitator': Neurosyphilis and new-onset refractory status epilepticus (NORSE) syndrome. *Epilepsy & Behavior Case Reports*, *3*, 33-35. https://doi.org/10.1016/j.ebcr.2015.02.001

17. Zhang, S., Aung, T., Lv, Z., Zhao, X., Wang, P., Shi, T., ... & Jin, B. (2020). Epilepsy imitator: tongue biting caused by sleep-related facio-mandibular myoclonus. *Seizure*, *81*, 186-191. https://doi.org/10.1016/j.seizure.2020.08.018
18. Depositario-Cabacar, D. F. T., & Azar, N. J. (2017). Imitators of Epilepsy. *Epilepsy Board Review: A Comprehensive Guide*, 167-170. https://doi.org/10.1007/978-1-4939-6774-2_12

CHAPTER 5 – SEIZURE TRIGGERS

More than one factor can trigger epileptic seizures in patients with photic or pattern sensitivity. ………….. Patients with pure photosensitive seizures should avoid the factors that provoke seizures.
Zeynep Vildan Okudan & Çiğdem Özkara[1]

Introduction

Epileptic seizures occur unprovoked but there are some things that trigger seizures in different people. Every person living with the condition of epilepsy needs to know what triggers their seizures to help self-manage their condition.[2] Seizure triggers range from flashing lights (also called photosensitive epilepsy), lack of sleep, menstrual cycle, eating, stress, hot baths, non-adherence to medication, thinking, reading, somatosensory effects, being startled, music, orgasm, over-exertion, lying or attempting to lie, certain sounds or noises, certain pictures, excitement, anxiety, drug and alcohol abuse, heights, certain smells, large bodies of water… the list is inexhaustible.[3,4] Seizure triggers are person-specific, therefore it is not advisable to tell PWE to avoid all these triggers. While not all seizure triggers may be listed here due to limited research, they can still significantly impact individuals with epilepsy. While the ideal way to prevent seizures triggered by various factors is to avoid those triggers, some are unavoidable. In this chapter, I will cover some triggers and possible ways to self-manage specific seizure triggers if they can be avoided or managed.

Photosensitive epilepsy

In 1997, four people were hospitalized after watching a cartoon called *Pocket Monsters* in Japan.[5] All four people had seizures at a specific time of the film when certain colors and frequencies were shown, leading to a conclusion that rapid color changes trigger photosensitive seizures.[5] Two of the people had a diagnosis of epilepsy prior to the incident, but the other two experienced their first seizures watching that film.[5] Photosensitive seizures affect up to 10% of PWE, and the incidence is higher in women and children.[6] Watching television

(TV) and playing video games have also been reported to trigger seizures under the photosensitive category.[6,7]

Self-management of TV-induced seizures include watching TV from at least 2 meters away from the TV and using a remote control to change channels.[1] People with photosensitive epilepsy induced by video games should limit the time they spend playing.[1] All people with photosensitive epilepsy will benefit from wearing blue lens and polarized glasses.[1,6] These self-management techniques will help minimize the effect of the triggers and the impacted people can also still enjoy watching TV and playing video games. Certain movies can be avoided if potential triggers are flagged. Sometimes, like in my personal lived experience, there is no actual seizure, but I just feel some electrical impulses in the brain. I therefore avoid anything that makes me feel that way in case it progresses to a seizure.

Lack of sleep

Lack of sleep is the most significant epilepsy trigger, and impacts most seizure types; however, seizures also disturb sleep quality for those seizures that occur during sleep.[8] The relationship between epilepsy and sleep is complicated, because seizures disrupt sleep and the lack of quality sleep triggers seizures.[9] Lack of sleep has been observed to trigger seizures in at least 30% of PWE.[10] According to Reddy et al.,[8] at least 25% of PWE experience seizures exclusively at night. Irregular bedtime and wake-up times increase the likelihood of seizures.[11] Addressing sleep disorders could lead to better management of seizures.[12] Self-management includes optimizing sleep and resolving sleep issues.[9,13]

Catamenial epilepsy

Seizures in some women are triggered by their menstrual cycle.[10] This is known as catamenial epilepsy and impacts almost 40% of women with epilepsy.[14] The term catamenial epilepsy refers to the regular pattern of seizure worsening that aligns with specific times in the menstrual cycle among women who have epilepsy.[15] Early astrologers wrote about the relationship between epilepsy and the moon, and early writings show that a PWE was described as someone afflicted by the moon disease.[30] In Zimbabwe, I have heard people saying *mwedzi mutete* (crescent moon) when describing or dismissing actions of someone with epilepsy or any other neurological disorders and mental illness. Among the Shona people of Zimbabwe, *mwedzi mutete* is seen as a sign of misfortune with a belief linking it to spiritual attacks and an increase in mental disorders.[16] *Mwedzi mutete* is a source of stigma as people with neurological, brain, and mental illness are usually dismissed, and their actions are attributed to *mwedzi mutete*. When someone has a seizure, people just say, *mwedzi mutete ka mazuva ano*, meaning the moon is still crescent shaped, therefore it is expected that this person will have seizures. Scientifically, catamenial epilepsy is due to changes in levels of estrogen and progesterone. The higher levels of estrogen relative to progesterone during certain periods of the menstrual cycle have been linked to increased seizure frequency.[14,15,17] Estrogen generally promotes seizure activity and progesterone inhibits seizure activity.[18] There are no self-management techniques for catamenial epilepsy, but some clinicians have tried to manage impacted women with hormonal therapy.[18] These hormonal interventions are said to be complicated and have undesirable side effects.[18] More details on catamenial epilepsy are covered in Chapter 13.

Eating and chewing

Some studies have shown that eating can trigger seizures in some people.[19] Factors contributing to the eating seizure triggers include dietary habits (carbohydrate-dense food), chewing, eating behaviors, genetics, and ethnicity.[6,19] Chewing accounts for about 98% of people with eating-induced seizures.[6] Studies suggest that the most impacted ethnic group are South Asians.[19] The stimuli for eating seizure triggers include taste, chewing, swallowing, hunger, and appetite.[6,19] People whose seizures are triggered by eating can manage their condition by adjusting how they consume food. Self-management techniques include using a straw for drinks, taking smaller bites, and avoiding overeating.[7]

Stress

Stress was found to trigger seizures in some PWE.[20,21] PWE self-report that stress is the most common trigger for their seizures.[10,21,22,23]

However, studies have not confirmed this to be universally true, but indeed, stress triggers seizures in some PWE.[21,23] Other studies revealed elevated stress levels and stressful events were linked to an increase in seizure frequency.[10,24] Animal studies have confirmed the role of stress in triggering seizures.[23] Self-management is complicated because epilepsy can also cause stress, and the stress will trigger more seizures leading to a complicated two-way relationship.[23,24] People should seek professional help whether the stress triggers seizures or not.

Hot water epilepsy and bathing seizures

In certain PWE, exposure or contact with water can trigger seizures.[1,6,25] The hot water epilepsy (HWE) was observed after hot water was poured on the body.[1,7,25] Higher prevalence has been reported in southern India where certain rituals are performed with the pouring of hot water (40–50 °C) on the head.[1,6] Factors like water temperature and quantity, particularly when poured over the head, are crucial in precipitating HWE.[6] These water triggers have been found to be common in people with certain genes, and there is a higher incidence in males.[6] People impacted by HWE experience 1–4 seizures per month if exposed to hot water.[26] Bathing seizures are almost similar to HWE. Bathing seizures are triggered by activities such as taking a bath or shower at normal body temperature.[1,2] The bathing seizures can also be triggered by exiting bath water and are usually focal.[1] Self-management of HWE includes reducing water temperature when bathing or showering.[6,7]

Non-adherence to AEDs

Some people take medication haphazardly. Medicines (AEDs) should not be taken at one's own discretion, because non-compliance to medication can result in serious seizures. Adjusting doses at home is also discouraged as that can trigger seizures. It is highly discouraged to withdraw oneself from medication as the consequences can be fatal. More details on the importance of adherence to medication is covered in Chapter 6.

Thinking

Noogenic epilepsy is a rare epilepsy that is more common in males.[1,6] Thinking epilepsy is triggered by activities such as performing calculations, solving a Rubik's cube, engaging in deep thought, decision-making, abstract reasoning, playing chess or cards, and drawing sophisticated designs or patterns.[1,6] Complicated mathematical calculations account for 72% of these seizures.[6] The seizures triggered by thinking usually start in adolescence.[1,27] Another variation of thinking-induced seizures are praxis-induced seizures.[6] These seizures can be induced by the mental process of solving sophisticated geometrical problems and decision-making.[6] Self-management of these triggers is almost impossible because it is often difficult to limit exposure to these triggers.[1,6,27]

Reading

Reading has been observed to trigger focal seizures in certain people. It was observed that the trigger was higher in patients reading loudly compared with people reading silently.[28] Reading epilepsy in uncommon and affected people experience jaw jerks.[1,28] The trigger usually starts in teenage years to early adulthood after the acquisition of reading skills, and is more common in males than females.[1,27] Though the process behind reading epilepsy is not fully understood, it is believed the visual and psychological demands of reading precipitate the seizures.[1]

Somatosensory

Somatosensory stimuli seizure triggers occur when certain areas of the body are stimulated, such as skin friction, pricking, touching or tapping, brushing teeth, or external ear canal stimulation.[1,7] Rubbing epilepsy occurs when touched or tapped on the skin. The trigger is increased by touching the head and back.[7] Toothbrush epilepsy occurs when brushing teeth. Auricular epilepsy is triggered by touching the ear. These somatosensory triggers are common in children with developmental delays.[7]

Startle

Startle-induced seizures are often provoked by sudden sensory inputs, typically sounds.[6,7] The seizures are focal and brief, with a duration of less than 30 seconds.[6,7] If the person is standing, they will likely fall with the seizure.[7] The trigger affects both males and females equally and has a low prevalence.[7]

Music

Musicogenic seizures are triggered by music.[6,7] They can be triggered even if music is played while the person is asleep. Some reports also indicate some people can be triggered just by thinking about music.[7] Some people are triggered by a specific song.[7] Seizures can be triggered by a diverse array of musical and sound stimuli, including different genres, artists, instruments, emotional tones, and listening durations, as well as various sounds like machinery, church bells, and telephones, or even by thinking about a specific song or melody.[1] Literature on this trigger is limited. Most musicogenic seizures can be self-managed by either avoiding or changing the triggering music, especially if there is a lag before the onset of the seizure or if the music is very particular.[1,7]

Orgasm

Orgasm-induced seizures are more common in women.[7] The seizures can occur a few minutes after orgasm or even after a few hours.[7] Seizures triggered by orgasm are reported as rare and literature on this area is limited.[29] However, the actual frequency of this trigger might be higher than reported in studies, as individuals might be hesitant to admit it out of embarrassment.[29] Achieving sexual climax or orgasm may activate sensitized neurons across various brain centers, leading to seizures.[1] For those affected by this trigger, their sexual lives may be negatively impacted as they are scared to reach a climax and have a seizure. Their spouses could end up frustrated leading to marital conflicts.[29] Avoiding this seizure trigger could mean the end of a marriage or sexual relationship.

Over-exertion and other

Over-exertion triggers seizures in at least 18% of PWE.[10] Lying or attempting to lie can also trigger seizures for a rare epilepsy named Pinocchio syndrome.[1] Certain sounds or noise, certain pictures or patterns,[27] excitement, anxiety, drug and alcohol abuse, heights, certain smells, and large bodies of water, have all been reported to trigger seizures in certain PWE.

Discovering the precise environmental triggers involves conducting thorough and in-depth interviews with the PWE.[6] When one knows what triggers their seizures, they are encouraged to avoid those triggers to minimize their chances of having an epileptic seizure. Regarding unavoidable triggers like the menstrual cycle, the person should ensure they are at a safe place during such a period to avoid unnecessary accidents. The key takeaway from this chapter is understanding that there are numerous seizure triggers and that it is crucial for each person to be aware of and understand their own triggers if they have them. While this chapter does not cover every possible trigger, recognizing what specifically triggers your seizures is important, and you should take necessary precautions to steer clear of those triggers if possible.

Table 3 shows warning signs of a seizure, the actual seizure and the post-ictal period. It must be noted that not all of these will appear in every seizure. A few of the listed may occur in an individual at any given time, hence it is critical to know what to expect during a seizure.

Table 3: Seizure warnings, symptoms, after-seizure

Warning signs			
Sensory		**Emotional**	**Physical**
Déjà vu	Visual loss/blurring	Fear	Dizziness
Jamais vu	Racing thoughts	Panic	Headache
Smell	Stomach feelings	Pleasant	Light-
Sound	Strange feeling	feeling	headedness
Taste	Tingling feeling		Nausea
			Numbness
Seizure symptoms			
Sensory	**Emotional**	**Physical**	
Black out	Fear	Chewing	Shaking
Confusion	Panic	movements	Staring
Deafness/sounds		Convulsions	Stiffening
Electric shock		Difficulty talking	Swallowing
feeling		Drooling	Sweating
Loss of		Eyelid fluttering	Teeth
consciousness		Eyes rolling up	Tongue biting
Smell		Falling	Tremors
Spacing out		Foot stomping	Twitching
Out of body		Hand waving	movements
experience		Inability to move	Difficulty in
Visual loss or		Incontinence	breathing
blurring		Lip smacking	Heart racing
		Making sounds	
		clenching/grinding	
After-seizure symptoms (post-ictal)			
Sensory	**Emotional**	**Physical**	
Memory loss	Confusion	Bruising and	Nausea
Writing difficulty	Depression	injuries	Pain
	Fear	Difficulty talking	Thirst
	Frustration	Sleeping	Weakness
	Shame/embarrassment	Exhaustion	Urge to urinate
		Headache	or defecate

Some people do not get warning signs, but others are lucky to have them. When a person gets warning signs, they should alert those close by so that they are able to assist during the seizure. It is also a chance to move to a safe place if the warning sign gives you enough time to do so.

References:

1. Okudan, Z. V., & Özkara, Ç. (2018). Reflex epilepsy: Triggers and management strategies. *Neuropsychiatric Disease and Treatment*, *14*, 327–337. https://doi.org/10.2147/NDT.S107669
2. Nguyen DK, Rouleau I, Sénéchal G, et al. (2015). X-linked focal epilepsy with reflex bathing seizures: Characterization of a distinct epileptic syndrome. *Epilepsia, 56*:1098–108. http://dx.doi.org/10.1111/epi.13042
3. Ighodaro ET, Maini K, Arya K, Sharma S. (2023). Focal Onset Seizure. StatPearls Publishing. Treasure Island (FL). https://pubmed.ncbi.nlm.nih.gov/29763181
4. Kodankandath TV, Theodore D, Samanta D. (2024). Generalized Tonic-Clonic Seizure. [In: StatPearls [Internet]. Treasure Island (FL): StatPearls Publishing; Available from: https://www.ncbi.nlm.nih.gov/books/NBK554496/
5. Ishida S, Yamashita Y, Matsuishi T, Ohshima M, Ohshima H, Kato H, Maeda H. (1998). Photosensitive seizures provoked while viewing "pocket monsters," a made-for-television animation program in Japan. *Epilepsia, 39*(12):1340-4. https://doi.org/10.1111/j.1528-1157.1998.tb01334.x
6. Hanif S, Musick ST. (2021). Reflex Epilepsy. *Aging and Disease, 12*(4):1010-1020. https://doi.org/10.14336%2FAD.2021.0216
7. Italiano, D., Ferlazzo, E., Gasparini, S., Spina, E., Mondello, S., Labate, A., et al. (2014). Generalized versus partial reflex seizures: A review. *Seizure, 23*:512-520. https://doi.org/10.1016/j.seizure.2014.03.014
8. Reddy, D.S., Chuang, S., Hunn, D., Crepea, A.Z., Magant, R. (2016). Neuroendocrine aspects of improving sleep in epilepsy. *Science Direct, 147*, 32-41. https://doi.org/10.1016/j.eplepsyres.2018.08.013
9. Gibbon FM, Maccormac E, & Gringras P. (2019). Sleep and epilepsy: Unfortunate bedfellows. *Archives of Disease in Childhood, 104*(2):189-192. https://doi.org/10.1136/archdischild-2017-313421
10. Ge, A., Gutierrez, E.G., Wook, L.S., Shah, S., Carmenate, Y., Collard, M., Crone, N.E., & Krauss, G.L. (2022). Seizure triggers identified postictally using a smart watch reporting system. *Epilepsy & Behavior, 126*:108472. https://doi.org/10.1016/j.yebeh.2021.108472
11. Stirling, R.E., Hidajat, C.M., Grayden, D.B., D'Souza, W.J., Naim-Feil, J., Dell, K.L., Schneider, L.D., Nurse, E., Freestone, D., Cook, M.J., & Karoly, P.J. (2023). Sleep and seizure risk in epilepsy: bed and wake times are more important than sleep duration. *Brain, 146*(7):2803-2813. https://doi.org/10.1093/brain/awac476
12. Kotagal, P. & Yardi, N. (2008). The relationship between sleep and epilepsy. *Seminars in Pediatric Neurology,15*(2):42-9. https://doi.org/10.1016/j.spen.2008.03.007
13. Liu, W.K., Kothare, S. & Jain, S. (2023). Sleep and Epilepsy. *Seminars in Pediatric Neurology, 48*:101087. https://doi.org/10.1016/j.spen.2023.101087
14. Penovich, P.E. & Helmers, S. (2008). Catamenial epilepsy. *International Review of Neurobiology, 83*:79-90. https://doi.org/10.1016/s0074-7742(08)00004-4

15. Verrotti, A., Laus, M., Coppola, G., Parisi, P., Mohn, A. & Chiarelli, F. (2010). Catamenial epilepsy: Hormonal aspects. *Gynecological Endocrinology, 26*(11):783-90. https://doi.org/10.3109/09513590.2010.490606
16. Musoni, P., Mamvuto, A., & Machingura, F. (2020). Religious artefacts, practices and symbols in the Johane Masowe Chishanu yeNyenyedzi Church in Zimbabwe: Interpreting the visual narratives. *Studia Historiae Ecclesiasticae, 46*(1), 1-17. https://doi.org/10.25159/2412-4265/6588
17. Taubøll, E., Sveberg, L. & Svalheim, S. (2015). Interactions between hormones and epilepsy. *Seizure, 28*:3-11. https://doi.org/10.1016/j.seizure.2015.02.012
18. Alshakhouri, M., Sharpe, C., Bergin, P., & Sumner, R. L. (2024). Female sex steroids and epilepsy: Part 2. A practical and human focus on catamenial epilepsy. *Epilepsia, 65*(3), 569-582. https://doi.org/10.1111/epi.17820
19. Girges, C., Vijiaratnam, N., Wirth, T., Tjoakarfa, C., Idaszak, J. & Seneviratne, U. (2020). Seizures triggered by eating - A rare form of reflex epilepsy: A systematic review. *Seizure, 83*:21-31. https://doi.org/10.1016/j.seizure.2020.09.013
20. Espinosa-Garcia, C.; Zeleke, H.; Rojas, A. (2021). Impact of Stress on Epilepsy: Focus on Neuroinflammation—A Mini Review. *International Journal of Molecular Sciences. 22(*4061):1-25. https://doi.org/10.1016/j.seizure.2020.09.013
21. Novakova, B., Harris, P.R., Ponnusamy, A. and Reuber, M. (2013). The role of stress as a trigger for epileptic seizures: A narrative review of evidence from human and animal studies. *Epilepsia, 54*(11):1866–1876, https://doi:10.1111/epi.12377
22. Novakova, B., Harris, P.R., Rawlings, G.H., Reuber, M. (2019). Coping with stress: A pilot study of a self-help stress management intervention for patients with epileptic or psychogenic nonepileptic seizures, *Epilepsy & Behavior, 94*, 169-177, https://doi.org/10.1016/j.yebeh.2019.03.002.
23. Novakova, B., Harris, P.R., Ponnusamy, A., Reuber, M. (2013). The role of stress as a trigger for epileptic seizures: A narrative review of evidence from human and animal studies. *Epilepsia, 54*(11), 1866-1876. https://doi.org/10.1111/epi.12377
24. Temkin, N.R., Davis, G.R. (1984). Stress as a risk factor for seizures among adults with epilepsy. *Epilepsia, 25*(4), 450-456. https://doi.org/10.1111/j.1528-1157.1984.tb03442.x
25. Peron, A., Baratang, N.V., Canevini, M.P., Campeau, P.M. & Vignoli, A. (2018). Hot water epilepsy and SYN1 variants. *Epilepsia, 59*(11). 2162-2163. https://doi:10.1111/epi.14572
26. Gururaj, G., & Satishchandra, P. (1992). Correlates of hot water epilepsy in rural south India: a descriptive study. *Neuroepidemiology, 11*:173-179. https://doi.org/10.1159/000110929
27. Ferlazzo, E., Zifkin, B.G., Andermann, E. & Andermann, F. (2005) Cortical triggers in generalized reflex seizures and epilepsies. *Brain 128:*700–710. https://doi.org/10.1093/brain/awh446
28. Salek-Haddadi, A., Mayer, T., Hamandi, K., Symms, M., Josephs, O., Fluegel, D., Woermann, F., Richardson, M.P., Noppeney, U., Wolf, P. & Koepp, M.J. (2009). Imaging seizure activity: a combined EEG/EMG-fMRI study in reading epilepsy. *Epilepsia. 50*(2):256-64. https://doi.org/10.1111/j.1528-1167.2008.01737.x
29. Ozkara, C., Ozdemir, S., Yilmaz, A., Uzan, M., Yeni, N., Ozmen, M. (2006). Orgasm-induced seizures: A study of six patients *Epilepsia, 47*, 2193-2197. https://doi.org/10.1111/j.1528-1167.2006.00648.x
30. Temkin, O. (1971). *The Falling Sickness: A history of epilepsy from the Greeks to the beginnings of modern neurology.* The John Hopkins University Press: Baltimore and London.

Chapter 6 – Epilepsy Treatment Options

The object of treatment is to prevent the occurrence of seizures by maintaining an effective dose of one or more anti-epileptic drugs.
John Martin[1]

Introduction

This chapter covers scientific treatment options for epilepsy. Different communities around the world have diverse beliefs about the causes of epilepsy, influencing their treatment choices. This chapter focuses on scientific treatments, while non-scientific options will be covered in the next chapter on complementary and alternative medicine (CAM). Though AEDs are the first-line treatment, surgery, vagus nerve stimulation, and ketogenic diet may be considered if medicines fail. While epilepsy surgery could benefit many who don't respond to medication, it's often inaccessible in LMICs.[2] Other options like vagus nerve stimulation[3] and a ketogenic diet[4] may help some patients. This chapter covers three specific treatment options: pharmacotherapy, surgery, and ketogenic diet.

PHARMACOTHERAPY: ANTI-EPILEPSY DRUGS

Epilepsy is typically managed, not cured, with medication. AEDs are the primary treatment for epilepsy, enabling up to 70% of patients to lead normal lives.[5,6,7] About 30–40% of PWE have drug-resistant forms and will continue experiencing seizures even if they are on AEDs.[8,9,10,20] Before 1993, the only available AEDs were older medications like phenobarbital, phenytoin, primidone, carbamazepine, sodium valproate, and ethosuximide that were developed in the early 20th century.[9,20] These older AEDs are associated with more side effects, possibly because they have been used in clinical practice for a longer period compared to the newer ones.[9,20]

Since the 1990s, more AEDs have been introduced, bringing the total to more than 30 in clinical use.[10,11] The rise in AED options allows clinicians to better tailor treatments, enhancing effectiveness and minimizing side effects.[10] Newer AEDs work through advanced mechanisms of action, improving efficacy, while reducing side effects.[9,20] While newer AEDs have not been proven more effective than older ones, studies show that they offer a broader spectrum of activity, fewer drug interactions, an improved side-effect profile, and are better tolerated.[9,20] Some clinicians still prefer the old AEDs because of proven efficacy, cost, or availability. With numerous options available, selecting the right treatment requires an in-depth understanding of how each drug fits specific seizure types for personalized care.

In LMICs, most PWE are treated by nurses because there are few or no doctors at their local level and sometimes no neurologist in the whole country. Though general practitioners and nurses play a key role in epilepsy care, most of them have limited knowledge on the newer AEDs.[9,20] In the US, most PWE are managed by primary care physicians, many of whom lack confidence in treating epilepsy.[9,20] Nearly half of these PWE seen by nurses or primary care doctors continue to experience seizures, side effects, and polytherapy.[9,20] Initially used as add-ons, newer AEDs like lamotrigine, levetiracetam, and topiramate are now preferred as monotherapies due to their unique mechanisms, fewer side effects, and reduced drug interactions.[11] Some of these newer AEDs include brivaracetam, cannabidiol, cenobamate, clobazam, divalproex, eslicarbazepine, felbamate, gabapentin, lacosamide, lamotrigine, levetiracetam, lorazepam, midazolam, oxcarbazepine, perampanel, pregabalin, tiagabine, topiramate, vigabatrin, and zonisamide.

Epilepsy is a syndrome of seizures with a variety of symptoms, needing tailored management approaches. Selection of the AED is based on seizure type, epilepsy syndrome, potential drug side effects, age, sex, co-morbidities, drug interactions, and availability.[6,9,11,20] Even in consideration of all these factors, the ideal treatment for individual epilepsy patients remains unclear.[11] Clinicians may know the correct AED for a seizure type or epilepsy syndrome, but the specific AED may be unavailable in that country or too expensive for the patient. In LMICs, AED options are limited, leading some countries to create treatment protocols based on available drugs rather than the best treatment option.

Monotherapy is preferred for most patients to minimize side effects, though some may need polytherapy if their seizures cannot be controlled on one AED. Polytherapy increases the risk of side effects, sometimes without improving seizure control. In a 30-year longitudinal study in Scotland with 1,795 PWE, 87% achieved seizure control with one AED, and 3% became seizure-free after switching. Of the remaining 180 participants who did not respond to monotherapy, only 12% (22 people) and 4% (7 people) benefited from two and three AEDs, respectively, with additional AEDs offering limited improvement.[8] Polytherapy may not benefit the patient as anticipated by the clinician. The goal of treatment is to prevent seizures by maintaining an effective AED dose.[1]

AEDs can have serious side effects but shouldn't be stopped abruptly. Withdrawal from AEDs should strictly be under the supervision of a doctor. These medications can have serious interactions with other AEDs and other drugs as well. Key risks for PWE include status epilepticus, sudden unexpected/unexplained death in epilepsy (SUDEP), trauma from seizures, and suicide. Consistent AED availability is crucial for effective seizure management.

Drug choice

Table 4 summarizes the findings concerning drug choice based on unique patient specifications from a study conducted in 2016 seeking expert opinion from 42 epilepsy-specialized physicians in the US.[91] The findings were confirmed by a similar study in South Korea in 2020.[5]

Table 4: Drug choice

Medicine	Situation
Sodium valproate	Genetically mediated generalized epilepsies, except in women of childbearing age
Ethosuximide	Absence seizures
Levetiracetam	Genetic generalized tonic-clonic and myoclonic seizures Initial treatment of focal seizures The elderly Patients with liver issues, or have undergone organ transplantation
Lamotrigine	Initial treatment of focal seizures The elderly Epilepsy patients with depression
Oxcarbazepine	Initial treatment of focal seizures

Compiled from information extracted from Byun et al.[5] and Shih et al.[91]

All available drugs are not covered in the study shown in Table 4. Most LMICs will have the older drugs and a few of the newer ones. Older drugs have been tried and tested for a longer time, and most clinicians will have a better understanding on how these drugs work and possible side effects. Though newer drugs are said to have fewer side effects, they have not been in use for a long time and more side effects could be discovered as their use becomes widespread.

Table 5 summarizes all the drugs recommended by the International League Against Epilepsy for each seizure type and epilepsy syndrome. I created the table from information extracted from the Epilepsy Foundation.[12]

Table 5: Seizure medication list

Seizure type or epilepsy syndrome	Medication
Unknown onset	Midazolam nasal spray

Tonic-clonic seizures	Carbamazepine Clobazam Diazepam Felbamate Lamotrigine	Levetiracetam Lorazepam Midazolam nasal Oxcarbazepine Perampanel	Phenobarbital Phenytoin Primidone Topiramate Valproic acid
Tonic seizures	Lorazepam Phenobarbital	Midazolam nasal spray	
Focal aware onset seizure	Brivaracetam Carbamazepine Cenobamate Clobazam Diazepam Divalproex sodium Eslicarbazepine acetate Felbamate	Gabapentin Lacosamide Lamotrigine Levetiracetam Lorazepam Midazolam nasal Oxcarbazepine Perampanel	Phenobarbital Phenytoin Pregabalin Tiagabine Topiramate Valproic Acid Vigabatrin Zonisamide
Secondarily generalized or bilateral tonic-clonic seizures	Brivaracetam Carbamazepine Clobazam Eslicarbazepine Acetate Felbamate Lacosamide	Lamotrigine Levetiracetam Lorazepam Midazolam nasal Oxcarbazepine Perampanel	Phenobarbital Phenytoin Topiramate Valproic acid Vigabatrin Zonisamide
Refractory seizures	Clobazam Felbamate Lamotrigine Lorazepam	Phenobarbital Phenytoin Topiramate	Valproic acid Vigabatrin Zonisamide
Myoclonic seizures	Clobazam Clonazepam Diazepam	Levetiracetam Lorazepam Midazolam nasal	Primidone Valproic acid

Febrile seizures	Lorazepam Midazolam		
Focal impaired awareness or complex partial seizures	Brivaracetam Carbamazepine Clobazam Diazepam Eslicarbazepine Acetate Felbamate Gabapentin Lacosamide	Lamotrigine Levetiracetam Lorazepam Midazolam nasal Oxcarbazepine Perampanel Phenobarbital	Phenytoin Pregabalin Tiagabine Topiramate Valproic acid Vigabatrin Zonisamide
Clonic seizures	Lorazepam	Midazolam	Phenobarbital
Atypical absence seizures	Clobazam Ethosuximide	Lorazepam	Midazolam
Atonic seizures	Clobazam Diazepam	Felbamate Lorazepam	Midazolam
Absence seizures	Clobazam Clonazepam Diazepam	Divalproex Sodium Ethosuximide	Lorazepam Midazolam
Temporal lobe epilepsy	Brivaracetam Carbamazepine Eslicarbazepine Acetate Felbamate Lacosamide Lamotrigine	Levetiracetam Lorazepam Oxcarbazepine Perampanel Phenobarbital	Phenytoin Topiramate Valproic acid Vigabatrin Zonisamide
Reflex epilepsies	Lorazepam		
Ring chromosome 20 syndrome	Lorazepam		
Rasmussen's syndrome	Lorazepam Phenobarbital		

Lennox–Gastaut syndrome	Clobazam Clonazepam Diazepam Felbamate	Fenfluramine Lamotrigine Lorazepam Phenobarbital	Rufinamide Topiramate Valproic acid
Juvenile myoclonic epilepsy	Lamotrigine Levetiracetam	Lorazepam Primidone	Valproic acid
Infantile spasms/West's syndrome	Lorazepam	Vigabatrin	
Hypothalamic hamartoma	Lorazepam		
Dravet syndrome	Fenfluramine	Lorazepam	Stiripentol
Childhood and juvenile absence epilepsy	Ethosuximide	Lorazepam	
Seizure clusters	Diazepam nasal spray		
Prolonged seizures of various types	Diazepam nasal spray		
Developmental/epileptic encephalopathy with spike wave activation in sleep (DEE-SWAS)	Lorazepam		
Benign Rolandic epilepsy	Lorazepam		

Extracted from the Epilepsy Foundation[12]

Emergency medications

Emergency AEDs are used in emergency situations and do not replace daily AEDs.[13] These AEDs can be administered through the nose, by mouth, under the tongue, inside the cheek, or rectally depending on circumstances.[13] Benzodiazepines (diazepam, lorazepam, midazolam) are used in emergency situations as they are fast acting. The use of personal emergency medicines in epilepsy is not widespread in LMICs. These medications are normally administered when the patient reaches the emergency rooms. However, in countries with adequate resources, these medications are used for emergencies at the time of need when the seizure happens.

Pharmacokinetics

Interactions between anti-epileptic drugs are complex and may enhance toxicity without a corresponding increase in anti-epileptic effect.
John Martin[1]

For a good understanding of this section, it may be necessary to define a few terms. I will consider what the body does to the drug (pharmacokinetics) and what the drug does to the body (pharmacodynamics). Pharmacokinetics refers to the processes by which drugs are absorbed, distributed, metabolized, and eliminated in the body, directly influencing the effectiveness of treatment.[14] Each stage plays a crucial role in the clinical effectiveness and safety profile of AEDs. Understanding these processes is essential as they determine the drug's concentration in the bloodstream and ultimately its therapeutic (healing) effects and side effects.[10] Factors such as age, weight, genetic variations, and the presence of coexisting conditions can affect the pharmacokinetics of AEDs.[6,15] For example, older patients or those with liver or kidney impairment may experience altered drug metabolism, necessitating dose adjustments.[5,16]

When a drug is administered, it must be within the therapeutic level to obtain the desired effects. It must be noted that a single dose of drug will undergo the process of absorption, distribution, metabolism, and elimination. Depending on the drug, the timing of this process varies. Figure 3 shows what happens to a single dose given by mouth.

Figure 3: Pharmacokinetics illustrated

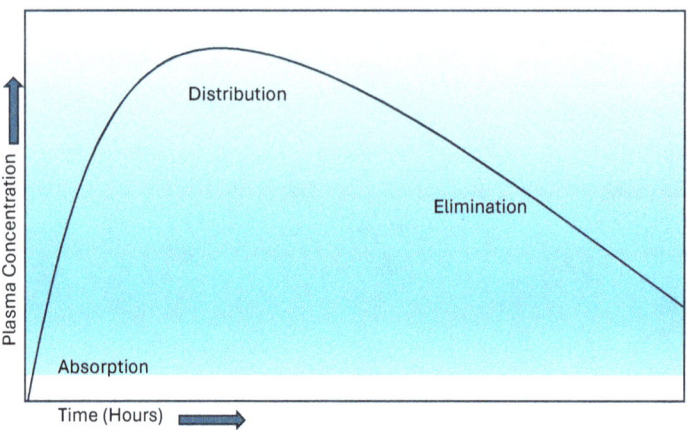

Absorption

Absorption is the process by which a drug enters the bloodstream after administration. When a drug is taken into the body, it is absorbed. The rate and extent of absorption can be influenced by factors such as the drug's formulation (tablet, capsule, injection), route of administration (intravenous, intramuscular, swallowed, under the tongue), and the environment in the stomach and intestines.[11,17] For instance, drugs taken by mouth must pass through the digestive system before reaching blood circulation, with factors like the concentration of stomach acid and food intake affecting absorption.[7,18] Immediate-release formulations, like emergency medicines, are normally absorbed rapidly, while extended-release forms will maintain steady blood levels over time.[10]

A patient might be taking their AED as prescribed but still experience seizures. This is not about DRE, but about the drug's formulation, which impacts its bioavailability. Bioavailability is a measure of the extent and rate at which an active drug or metabolite enters blood circulation, thereby becoming available for the body to use.[19] For example, a phenobarbitone tablet manufactured by Company A is absorbed differently from one manufactured by Company B. Though they are both tablets, their bioavailability is different because each manufacturer uses other ingredients besides the active ingredient to make the tablets, called excipients. These excipients impact drug absorption. Therefore, switching brands of the same medication can result in breakthrough seizures due to inconsistencies in absorption. All things being equal, it is advisable to maintain one brand. Should circumstances force one to change brands, precautions should be taken as breakthrough seizures are likely to occur. If a patient tells the pharmacist they want a particular brand, please never think that the patient is just being difficult. If possible, give the patient the brand they normally take. The issue of brands also spills over to medical insurance companies, where they insist clients get a generic (no trade name) drug. The generic brand may not work for that client and their doctor may insist on a trademarked brand.[13] Sharing medications is discouraged because treatment plans between PWE. Even when the medication is the same, differences in formulation affects absorption.

Antacids containing calcium interfere with phenytoin, phenobarbitone, carbamazepine and gabapentin by reducing stomach acid and creating insoluble compounds that hinder absorption.[14] Absorption interactions are less in newer AEDs. The implications of absorption on treatment are significant. Poor or variable absorption can lead to fluctuations in plasma drug levels, which may reduce efficacy or increase the risk of adverse effects. Ensuring consistent absorption is essential for maintaining therapeutic drug concentrations and avoiding breakthrough seizures.[9,20,21]

Distribution

Distribution involves the movement of the drug from the bloodstream into body tissues, including the brain, the site of action for AEDs. Distribution is affected by several factors, including drug-related and body-related factors. Drug-related factors include lipid solubility (lipophilic or highly soluble in fats) and molecular size. Body-related factors include plasma binding proteins, liver disease, cardiac problems, and pregnancy.[22,23] Drugs typically bind to proteins within the plasma. Some drugs are highly protein bound whereas others do not bind strongly. The drug that is left unbound to protein is responsible for the therapeutic effect or the toxic effect of a drug. When two drugs are administered at the same time, and are both highly protein bound, they will be competing for a limited number of binding sites. This can create toxic effects due to too much unbound drug circulating in the body. Therefore, before two drugs are administered, this must be considered as it might produce unanticipated results. For drugs with no proper documentation, as you will see in the next chapter on CAM, this is a real problem. Drugs that bind extensively to plasma proteins, like phenytoin, have a reduced free fraction available for therapeutic action.[6] Equally, highly lipophilic drugs, such as diazepam, can cross the blood-brain barrier more easily, leading to faster onset of action.[5,24]

Clinicians should understand these dynamics as they affect people taking multiple drugs.[16] The concept of distribution is important as it affects the effectiveness of a drug and possible interactions with other medicines. AEDs with high protein binding can be displaced by other medications, increasing the concentration of the free, active drug and raising the risk of toxicity.[15,25] Clinicians should monitor and adjust medications to avert all types of risks attributable to interactions, particularly for people on polypharmacy.

Metabolism

During metabolism, primarily occurring in the liver, the body chemically changes the drugs into metabolites. These metabolites can be active or inactive. However, some drugs are excreted through the kidneys unchanged. Most AEDs undergo chemical changes in the liver through the isoenzyme system called cytochrome P450 (CYP). CYP plays a pivotal role in drug interactions.[6,22] The enzymes predominantly responsible for AED metabolism are CYP2C9, CYP2C19, and CYP3A.[6,22] Other AEDs like valproic acid (valproate), lorazepam and lamotrigine are metabolized via the enzyme uridine diphosphate glucuronosyltransferase (UGT). The CYP isoenzyme system and interactions will be explained in detail under the pharmacodynamics section. Common AEDs exhibit varied pharmacokinetic profiles.

Understanding metabolic pathways is important in clinical practice, because they have a bearing on dosage, potential drug–drug interactions, and the selection of AEDs for patients with liver disease.[12,26] Personalized treatment plans can be designed to achieve the best outcome, that is, effective, with minimal side effects, and a high possibility of adherence to treatment.[7,15] Understanding these facts is crucial for optimizing treatment, as poorly managed pharmacokinetic interactions can result in suboptimal drug levels and increased seizure frequency.[9,20,27] People experiencing interactions, side effects, and poor seizure control may end up frustrated and stop medication, therefore impacting adherence and seizure control. That is the reason clinicians must come up with personalized treatment plans to increase the chances of success. There is no one-size-fits-all in epilepsy management.

Elimination

The process of removal of the drug and its products from the body is called elimination. This is the final stage of pharmacokinetics, and primarily happens through the kidneys. The rate of elimination affects the drug's half-life (the time the drug takes from dosing until the serum level drops by 50%) and, consequently, dosing frequency.[10,24] It is therefore preeminent that before the drug is eliminated, another dose be introduced to maintain drug levels at therapeutic levels. To maintain serum levels within the therapeutic range, multiple doses of the drug must be given depending on the half-life. The plasma concentration increases and decreases until the minimum and maximum plasma concentrations remain constant (steady state). The steady state is reached after about five half-lives. At this stage, the serum levels are maintained at a therapeutic level without going under (sub-therapeutic) or above (toxic). This is illustrated in Figure 4. AEDs such as gabapentin are excreted unchanged in the urine, making their clearance dependent on renal function.[22,23] Reduced renal function, common in older adults or patients with kidney disease, can lead to drug accumulation and increased risk of toxicity.[5,25] Monitoring kidney function is crucial for adjusting doses of AEDs excreted through urine to prevent toxic buildup.[16,21] This is especially important for patients on long-term therapy or those with coexisting renal conditions, as impaired elimination can significantly alter drug levels and impact overall seizure management.[13,18]

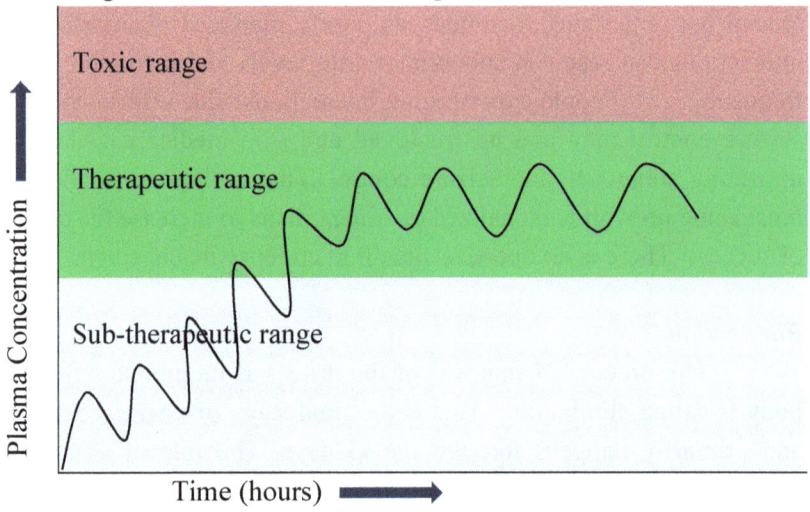

Figure 4: An illustration of drug level maintenance in the blood

The main reason I am trying to explain this in laymen's terms is because many people take their drugs anyhow, without knowing what effect this will have on seizure control. It is a bit technical, but if you take your time to understand, you will get value from this. This applies to any medication one may be taking and not only AEDs. To maintain the plasma concentration within the therapeutic range, a drug must be taken as frequently as prescribed. The understanding of these pharmacokinetic processes ensures clinicians make informed decisions regarding drug choice, dose, and the management of potential side effects, leading to more effective and individualized treatment for PWE.[8,10,12]

Some drugs like phenobarbitone have a long half-life and must be taken once daily, meaning every 24 hours. For those drugs that must be taken twice a day, like *carbamazepine* and sodium valproate, they are to be taken every 12 hours, while gabapentin is taken three times a day, amounting to a dose every 8 hours. The aim of taking any drug is to ensure the plasma concentration of that drug remains in the therapeutic range to derive the benefit of taking it. This maintenance of plasma concentration in the therapeutic range can be affected by many things, such as not adhering to the stated dose, not adhering to the prescribed frequency of taking that drug, and drug interactions. Taking drugs more frequently than prescribed can result in toxicity, and this can be fatal.

Pharmacodynamics of AEDs

Pharmacodynamics involves the mechanism of action by which a drug produces its effects. For example, how AEDs work to prevent seizures. Pharmacodynamic effects encompass the therapeutic and adverse impacts of a drug on the brain and other bodily systems.[14] Every drug taken has a specific site of action and this site of action can be the heart, the central nervous system (as in AEDs), or any other part. Most AEDs function by supporting neuronal membranes or regulating neurotransmitter activity to reduce responsiveness in the brain.[6,7] A key component affecting AED pharmacodynamics is the CYP enzyme system, which is responsible for metabolizing the drug and thus impacts its effectiveness.

The cytochrome P450 (CYP) isoenzyme system

The CYP enzyme system is a group of enzymes found primarily in the liver. CYP is responsible for the chemical modification (oxidative metabolism) of many AEDs. These enzymes are classified into different forms of the same enzyme called isoenzymes. Each isoenzyme has specific roles in drug metabolism.[10,22] Variations in the activity of these isoenzymes can influence the concentration of drugs, impacting their therapeutic and adverse effects.

CYP3A4 is one of the most important isoenzymes in the liver, metabolizing approximately 50% of clinically used drugs, including several AEDs like carbamazepine.[5,21] This enzyme's activity can be induced (stimulated) or inhibited (suppressed) by various substances, causing significant drug interactions. For example, phenobarbitol induces CYP3A4, therefore increasing the metabolism of co-administered drugs, potentially lowering their effectiveness.[17,18] Conversely, valproate inhibits CYP3A4 activity, leading to higher levels of certain AEDs and an increased risk of toxicity.[7,10]

CYP2C9 and CYP2C19: CYP2C9 and CYP2C19 are other isoenzymes important in the metabolism of AEDs. CYP2C9 breaks down drugs like phenytoin and valproate.[6,24] Other variants in the

CYP2C9 gene can increase or reduce metabolism, calling for dose adjustments to maintain therapeutic levels.[27,28] CYP2C19 metabolizes drugs such as clobazam and is subject to genetic variations leading to poor or ultra-rapid metabolism.[11,26] These genetic differences affect the effectiveness of a drug and its safety, and are why it is critical to have individualized treatment approaches.[10,25]

CYP1A2 and other isoenzymes: CYP1A2 is a less common isoenzyme contributing to the metabolism of certain AEDs, such as lamotrigine.[16,22] For example, smoking induces CYP1A2, leading to a decrease in the blood levels of lamotrigine, potentially compromising its effectiveness.[6,15] Other isoenzymes, including CYP2D6, may play minor roles but are essential when considering polypharmacy where interactions could change metabolic pathways.[9,20,23]

Clinicians need to understand these enzymes for managing potential drug interactions and personalizing treatment strategies. Genetic testing for CYP variants, especially for CYP2C9 and CYP2C19, could help clinicians predict possible patient responses to specific AEDs. The test results can be used to inform therapy choices to improve treatment outcomes.[18,25] This tailored pharmacotherapy ensures improved seizure control with fewer side effects.[7,11] More importantly, the tailored approach could help the management of multiple conditions needing polypharmacy. Polypharmacy cannot be avoided in such situations, but clinicians will be better equipped to make better decisions on the choices of AEDs to use so that interactions may be minimized.[8,12,22] These tests are good in an ideal world, but most PWE live in communities where these tests may never be available. If clinicians have in-depth knowledge of these enzymes, they can make treatment decisions based on how these enzymes generally work.

Drug interactions between AEDs

A PWE can suffer from any other condition, so the issue of drug interactions will be discussed in this section. I will look at interactions between different AEDs as well as interactions between AEDs and other medicines. As already mentioned, some of these interactions can be very complex. Before a person is commenced on any treatment, all the other drugs the person may be taking for other pre-existing conditions must be taken into consideration. If the patient is a woman of childbearing age, the contraception method used needs to be taken into consideration as well. Interactions between AEDs and other drugs are of significant concern. Knowledge of these interactions is critical, especially for patients on AED polytherapy. Interactions can impact both the pharmacokinetics and pharmacodynamics of AEDs, leading to altered therapeutic effects and possible side effects.[6,18] Drug interactions result from the induction and inhibition of enzymes. Table 6 shows the effect of older AEDs on newer AEDs when they are given concomitantly. Generally, older AEDs reduce the effectiveness of newer AEDs except for a few that are not affected.

Table 6: Effects of older AEDs on newer AEDs

	Gabapentin/pregabalin	Lamotrigine	Topiramate	Tiagabine	Levetiracetam	Zonisamide	Lacosamide
Phenytoin	None	↓	↓	↓	None	↓	None
Carbamazepine	None	↓	↓	↓	None	↓	None
Valproic acid	None	↑	None	None	None	None	None
Phenobarbitone	None	↓	↓	↓	None	↓	None
Primidone	None	↓	↓	↓	None	↓	None

This is a summary from information extracted from the chapter entitled "Anti-epileptics."[29]

Enzyme-inducing AEDs:

Enzyme-inducing AEDs, such as carbamazepine and phenytoin, increase the metabolism of other drugs, potentially decreasing their effectiveness.[9,20,21] Enzyme inducers decrease serum concentrations of other drugs metabolized by the same isoenzyme.[10,24] Enzyme-inducers enhance the activity of hepatic cytochrome P450 enzymes, accelerating the metabolism of co-administered medications, including other AEDs. The plasma concentrations of these metabolized drugs will drop, making it necessary for clinicians to adjust doses to maintain their efficacy.[10,22] For instance, when carbamazepine is combined with lamotrigine, the increased enzyme activity can lower the concentration of lamotrigine, potentially reducing its effectiveness. As a result, clinicians may need to increase the dose of lamotrigine to achieve adequate seizure control.[16,21] This enzyme induction affects all the other drugs a person may be taking, if the same isoenzyme is involved, so it is always good to determine the type of isoenzymes involved in the metabolism of all the drugs a person will be taking. This is not possible with CAM, because in most cases no one knows what they are really taking.

Enzyme-inhibiting AEDs

Enzyme inhibitors, like valproate, can slow the metabolism of co-administered drugs, raising their levels and risk of side effects.[10,28] The enzyme-inhibitors can slow down the metabolism of other medications that rely on hepatic enzyme pathways, leading to higher plasma concentrations and an increased risk of dose-dependent side effects.[10,24] An example is the interaction between valproate and lamotrigine: valproate inhibits the metabolism of lamotrigine, significantly increasing its plasma concentration. This interaction can enhance lamotrigine's anti-epileptic effects but also raises the risk of adverse effects, such as lack of balance, clumsiness, and dizziness, if not properly monitored and adjusted.[6,28]

Synergistic and antagonistic effects

AEDs can either complement (synergistic effect) or oppose (antagonistic effect) each other when used together. For example, sodium channel blockers like phenytoin and carbamazepine share similar mechanisms and may not provide additive therapeutic benefits when combined. The patient does not benefit in any way from taking both drugs. Instead, combining these drugs could increase the risk of side effects due to elevated drug levels in the blood.[11,23] On the other hand, combining AEDs with different mechanisms, such as a sodium channel blocker with a GABAergic agent like valproate, may improve seizure control with fewer side effects because of their complementary mechanisms of action.[11,23]

Management strategies

Generally, older AEDs reduce the effectiveness of newer AEDs except for a few that are not affected. Clinicians should select drug combinations that work and monitor drug levels in the blood consistently.[16,21] Drug monitoring ensures AED concentrations remain within the therapeutic range. Maintaining AED blood levels within the therapeutic range helps reduce breakthrough seizures and the risk of toxicity.[16,21] Additionally, clinicians must inform PWE to watch out for possible interactions every time a new drug is introduced, or a medication is changed.[7,17]

Interactions between AEDs and other drugs

As already mentioned, a PWE can also have other medical conditions like everyone else. AEDs can interact with non-epileptic medications, which poses challenges for patients with coexisting conditions. These interactions can alter the pharmacokinetics of non-AED drugs, potentially impacting their therapeutic efficacy and safety.[17,27] When there are co-morbidities, the interactions become more complex. I will now look at interactions between AEDs and some common drugs used in hypertension and other conditions. All possible interactions are beyond the scope of this book, so I will just cover a few.

Cardiovascular medications

Several drugs for high blood pressure (antihypertensives) interact with AEDs. Lipophilic beta-receptor antagonists (propranolol and metoprolol) are extensively metabolized by several isoenzymes of the CYP system. For these drugs to be effective in reducing blood pressure, larger doses will have to be administered, otherwise normal doses will just be wasted away. Calcium channel antagonists (nifedipine, felodipine, amlodipine, nicardipine, and nimodipine) are extensively metabolized by CYP3A4, suggesting that if they are taken at the same time as some enzyme-inducers, they may be ineffective. If you have high blood pressure and are on these drugs, and your blood pressure does not come down, this could be the reason.

Phenytoin induces the CYP2C9 enzyme, leading to increased clearance of warfarin, a drug that prevents blood clots (anticoagulant). This interaction can reduce warfarin's anticoagulant effect, raising the risk of all medical conditions caused by blood clots (thromboembolic events). To minimize the risk of thromboembolic events, it is recommended clinicians monitor the international normalized ratio (INR) closely to be ready to adjust warfarin doses as needed when used with phenytoin.[5,9,20] Careful consideration must be made before prescribing any drug to a person taking AEDs. Table 7 summarizes some of the interactions one may expect when taking enzyme-inducing AEDs and other medicines.

Anti-inflammatory drugs

Valproate inhibits the metabolism of drugs metabolized via glucuronidation, such as aspirin. This interaction can increase the plasma levels of valproate, heightening the risk of dose-dependent toxicities like tremor, sedation, or encephalopathy.[11,13] Proper dose adjustments and patient monitoring are advised when these drugs are taken together.

Psychotropic medications

The interaction between AEDs and drugs acting on the brain to alter mood, behavior, thoughts, and perception (psychotropic drugs) is important to discuss particularly for epilepsy patients who also have psychiatric conditions. Enzyme-inducing AEDs like carbamazepine can decrease the effectiveness of psychotropic drugs, such as certain antipsychotics and antidepressants, by speeding up their metabolism. This can reduce the effectiveness of these psychotropic drugs and may require an adjustment of their doses.[18,25] Conversely, some psychotropic medications inhibit AED metabolism, potentially raising plasma levels and increasing the risk of side effects.[7,24]

Antibiotics and antifungals

Some antibiotics (e.g., erythromycin) and antifungals (e.g., fluconazole) inhibit hepatic enzyme activity, slowing down the metabolism of AEDs like carbamazepine and phenytoin. This can result in elevated levels of AEDs in the blood. This could lead to toxic effects, presenting as dizziness, nausea, or loss of balance. Clinicians should be cautious and adjust AED doses, if necessary, when these interactions occur.[6,27]

Oral contraceptives

Enzyme-inducing AEDs, including phenytoin and carbamazepine, can significantly increase the metabolism of oral contraceptives. When this happens, the level of oral contraceptives in the blood is reduced, decreasing their effectiveness and increasing the risk of unplanned pregnancies. When treating women of childbearing age taking these AEDs, clinicians should counsel these women to use additional or alternative contraceptive methods to avoid potential treatment failures.[16,28] Falling pregnant while on AEDs has its own challenges as will be discussed in detail in Chapter 13.

Table 7: Interactions between enzyme-inducing AEDs and other drugs

AED	Interactions
Carbamazepine (CBZ)	· Reduces plasma concentration of mebendazole · Reduces bioavailability of praziquantel · Alcohol worsens central nervous system effects of CBZ · Isoniazid, clarithromycin, erythromycin cause elevations in serum concentration of CBZ · Increase risk of isoniazid-induced hepatotoxicity · Diminishes warfarin activity through increased metabolism · Antidepressants antagonize CBZ activity by lowering seizure threshold · Ketoconazole & fluconazole increase plasma concentration of CBZ · Chloroquine & mefloquine lower seizure threshold by antagonizing CBZ · Metronidazole & CBZ taken together may result in severe side effects · Haloperidol increases serum concentration of CBZ · Reduces plasma concentration of antipsychotics · Ritonavir, nelfinavir & lopinavir may increase plasma concentration of CBZ to toxic levels · Verapamil inhibits CBZ metabolism · Reduces blood ciclosporin concentration · Increased clearance of corticosteroids resulting in reduced efficacy · Acetazolamide increases CBZ serum concentration · Induces symptomatic hyponatremia when taken with hydrochlorothiazide or frusemide · Risk of neurotoxicity when used with metoclopramide · Cimetidine increases CBZ plasma concentration · Increases theophylline elimination · Vitamin B3 increases CBZ plasma concentration · Serum concentration reduced by phenobarbital · Interactions with phenytoin are complex and variable

- Serum concentration increased by valproic acid
- Decreases plasma concentration of itraconazole
- Reduces plasma concentration of HIV protease inhibitors
- May reduce effects of nifedipine
- Affects the threshold for use of antidote in treatment of paracetamol (acetaminophen) poisoning
- Increases clearance of corticosteroids

Phenobarbital (PHB)	<ul><li>Diminishes *warfarin* activity through increased metabolism</li><li>Reduces plasma concentration of antipsychotics</li><li>Reduces blood ciclosporin concentration</li><li>Chloramphenicol increases serum concentration of PHB</li><li>Enhances metabolism of doxycycline</li><li>Antidepressants lower seizure threshold in people taking PHB.</li><li>Valproate increases plasma PHB concentration by up to 48%</li><li>PHB increases clearance of valproate</li><li>Vigabatrin lowers plasma concentration of PHB in some patients</li><li>Reduces serum concentration of CBZ</li><li>Reduces gastrointestinal absorption of griseofulvin</li><li>Decreases plasma concentration of itraconazole</li><li>Metronidazole treatment failure in people on PHB</li><li>Reduces plasma concentration of HIV protease inhibitors</li><li>Reduces plasma concentration of some beta-blockers</li><li>May reduce effects of nifedipine</li><li>Increases clearance of verapamil</li><li>Reduces plasma protein binding of verapamil</li><li>Frusemide increases PHB plasma concentration for patients taking PHB and another AED</li><li>Increases theophylline elimination</li><li>Influenza vaccination causes prolonged rises in serum concentration of PHB</li><li>Vitamin B6 reduces serum PHB concentration</li><li>Folic acid and folinic acid reduce plasma concentration of PHB</li><li>Affects the threshold for use of antidote in treatment of paracetamol poisoning</li><li>Reduces efficacy of corticosteroids</li></ul>

Phenytoin (PHT)	- Reduces plasma concentration of mebendazole
- Reduces bioavailability of praziquantel
- Reduces plasma concentration of antipsychotics
- Reduces blood ciclosporin concentration
- Reduces diuretic effect of frusemide
- Chloramphenicol increases serum concentration of PHT
- Enhances metabolism of doxycycline
- Isoniazide raises PHT concentration leading to toxicity
- Nitrofurantoin reduces PHT serum concentration leading to loss of seizure control
- Rifampicin reduces plasma concentration of PHT
- Cotrimoxazole inhibits PHT metabolism leading to toxicity
- Antidepressants and antipsychotics lower seizure threshold
- Imipramine increases PHT plasma concentration
- Interactions with CBZ are complex and variable
- Decreases plasma concentration of itraconazole
- Increases metabolism of metronidazole
- Reduces plasma concentration of HIV protease inhibitors
- May reduce effects of nifedipine
- Reduces verapamil plasma concentration
- Increases clearance of theophylline
- Affects the threshold for use of antidote in treatment of paracetamol poisoning
- Interactions with CBZ are complex and variable
- Reduces plasma concentration of ethosuximide
- Interactions with valproate are complex and variable
- Decreases plasma concentration of ketoconazole & itraconazole
- Antimalarials may antagonize PHT by lowering seizure threshold
- Complex and variable interactions associated with cancer chemotherapy
- Decreased PHT serum concentration when taken with any of the following antiretrovirals: zidovudine, nelfinavir, acyclovir, ritonavir, lopinavir

- Efavirenz inhibits PHT clearance
- Diazepam & chlordiazepoxide increase PHT plasma concentration
- Nifedipine increases PHT serum concentration
- Increases digoxin clearance
- Reduces efficacy of corticosteroids
- Cimetidine increases chances of PHT toxicity
- Vitamin B6, folic acid & folinic acid reduce serum PHT concentration resulting in increased seizure frequency

This is a summary from information extracted from the chapter entitled "Anti-epileptics."[29]

Clinical implications and recommendations

Newer AEDs like levetiracetam are less affected by metabolic enzyme interactions. If a clinician decides to put anyone on polytherapy for valid reasons, these newer AEDs make good options for combining with other AEDs.[24] AEDs, especially the enzyme-inducing ones, interact with many groups of drugs, leaving room for a limited number of drugs that can be used for other conditions when a person is also taking AEDs. Even when presenting at a local clinic with a cold, remember to mention that you are also taking AEDs and specify the type you are taking. Ask the clinician to check for possible interactions between the AED and the new medicine they intend giving you.

The presence of complex drug interactions emphasizes the importance of personalized epilepsy treatment. Clinicians should perform comprehensive medication reviews, including over the counter and herbal products, to assess the potential for drug interactions. Regular monitoring of drug plasma levels, patient education, and adherence to treatment are essential for minimizing the risks associated with AED interactions.[15,30] Choosing AEDs with minimal interaction potential and adjusting treatment plans based on interaction profiles can enhance the safety and efficacy of epilepsy management.[12,23] Overall, awareness of drug interactions and proactive management can lead to better treatment outcomes and improved quality of life for individuals with epilepsy.

Side effects of AEDs

All medicines, including AEDs, have side effects. Side effects of a drug are those unintended effects of the drug. The side effects of AEDs are well documented, but do not happen to everyone and when they occur, the severity differs from person to person due to factors like dosage, treatment duration, and patient-specific characteristics such as age and co-morbid conditions.[6,18] Even though AEDs are central to the treatment of epilepsy, effectively reducing seizure frequency and severity for 70% of PWE, these drugs have a variety of side effects that can impact treatment adherence and overall quality of life. Understanding the range and nature of these side effects is essential for clinicians and patients alike. In this section, I will cover the common side effects of AEDs. As already mentioned, these side effects will not happen to everyone taking these drugs.

Common side effects:

Central nervous system:

Most AEDs induce central nervous system (CNS) side effects, which can impact the mental and physical abilities of someone taking them. For example, drugs such as phenytoin, carbamazepine, phenobarbitone, and topiramate cause drowsiness, dizziness, and issues with coordination in most people.[11,17] People on lamotrigine or levetiracetam may become irritable and experience mood changes. These side effects impact social interactions and mental health.[18] Cognitive impairments such as attention deficits and memory issues are also notable side effects, particularly with topiramate, which is known for its impact on word retrieval and for slowing down the brain's processing speed.[17]

Gastrointestinal disturbances:

Gastrointestinal disturbances are a commonly reported side effect of AEDs. Medications such as valproate and carbamazepine can cause nausea, vomiting, and abdominal pain. These effects can sometimes lead to poor adherence.[9,15,20] While these side effects are less severe than CNS impacts, they can still affect a person's willingness to continue treatment, especially if they are chronic.

Dermatological reactions:

Common skin-related side effects include rashes and hypersensitivity reactions and can be concerning especially if they become severe. Lamotrigine is linked with a risk of serious skin conditions such as Stevens–Johnson syndrome, which requires immediate medical intervention.[6,27] Phenytoin or carbamazepine can also cause skin reactions in people with certain genetic markers.[5,6] These skin reactions make genetic screening a necessity in some patient populations to mitigate risks.

Weight changes:

AEDs can influence body weight in various ways. For example, valproate causes weight gain. People using valproate for a long time could end up with metabolic syndrome.[22,23] People with pre-existing conditions like obesity or diabetes may feel the greatest impact. On the other hand, topiramate is associated with weight loss that could be beneficial to people already struggling with obesity. However, it could also lead to unintentional undernutrition if not monitored.[17,23] Most AEDs cause weight gain. Topiramate may not be the best alternative for the seizure type. Some clinicians prescribe the most effective AED and add topiramate to counteract the weight gain. This resulting polypharmacy may not be ideal for most PWE due to other associated side effects.

Serious and long-term side effects

Hepatotoxicity:

Long-term use of AEDs can lead to significant health challenges. Valproate and carbamazepine are known for the potential to cause severe liver damage, making it necessary to have liver function tests.[10,26] Liver enzyme elevations may not show any symptoms initially but can progress to more severe liver dysfunction if not caught early.[26]

Hematological effects:

Carbamazepine and phenytoin are associated with blood-related (hematological) side effects, such as anemia or leukopenia. People taking these AEDs will need constant monitoring of their count to catch these side effects early.[5,25] Zonisamide can cause an imbalance in the body's acid-base regulation, a condition called metabolic acidosis that may lead to fatigue and confusion, especially in people with pre-existing kidney issues.[25]

Bone health:

Long-term use of AEDs, particularly older drugs like phenytoin and phenobarbital, can cause bone weakness, increasing the risk of fractures and osteoporosis over time.[7,21] These AEDs quicken vitamin D metabolism, reducing calcium absorption, which leads to bone health issues. Though newer AEDs like levetiracetam seem more favorable towards bone health, long-term use can still have skeletal impacts, making it necessary to monitor bone density, especially in older adults and those with pre-existing risk factors for osteoporosis.[7,21]

Teratogenic effects:

Medicines that can cause malformations or abnormalities in the fetus are called teratogens. AEDs that cross the placenta could have teratogenic effects. Teratogenic risks are a significant concern when treating women of childbearing age. Valproate is well known for causing abnormalities present at birth (congenital malformations) and developmental disorders in children exposed to it in the womb.[13,28] Women of childbearing age taking valproate will need counseling and education before they decide to become pregnant. If they decide to get pregnant, it is advised to find an alternative AED beforehand.[28] Though lamotrigine and levetiracetam are considered safer options, they are not entirely free of risks.[18,28] There is always a risk to the unborn baby when taking AEDs.

Psychiatric and behavioral effects:

Mood swings, depression, and anxiety have been observed with levetiracetam and zonisamide.[6,24] These side effects present treatment challenges, especially for people already known to have mood disorders. Levetiracetam increases the risk of irritability and aggression, making it a less suitable option for some individuals.[25] Valproate has mood-stabilizing properties that could benefit people with co-morbid bipolar disorder.[24] The psychiatric side effects of AEDs require careful monitoring, especially during the initial stages of treatment, and may require constant dose adjustments.[16,24]

Individualized responses to AEDs:

Factors like genetics, age, and co-morbidities cause people to experience side effects differently. Some people will never report certain side effects, yet others experience severe forms of those side effects. Genetic differences can affect metabolism of AEDs, influencing both efficacy and side effects.[12,17] For example, these genetic variations influence the metabolism of phenytoin that could lead to toxic effects.[12] Personalized treatment plans that consider all factors are crucial for minimizing side effects and improving treatment outcomes.[10,11]

Impact on pharmacotherapy in epilepsy treatment

The effect of a drug is related to its concentration at the site of action. The site of action in many cases is not accessible for sampling drug concentrations. The easier route is to measure the concentration in the blood or plasma, saliva, urine or any other easily sampled fluids. There is a known association between the drug concentration in the plasma and concentration at the receptor site where the drug generates its therapeutic effect. Any change in plasma concentration is translated to a change in drug concentration at the site of action whether negative or positive. This might not be true for all drugs, but this is the general assumption I will work with in this book. At the site of action, the drug must bind to the receptor for it to have an effect.

Importance of adherence to AEDs

Adherence to treatment means taking the AED at the prescribed dose, at the right time, and at the correct frequency with no gaps. Adherence is the cornerstone to achieving optimal seizure control and epilepsy management. However, adherence can be challenging due to factors such as complex medication schedules, side effects, socioeconomic barriers, and psychological issues.[30] Poor adherence could lead to increased seizure frequency, increased risk of status epilepticus, and poor quality of life, plus the possibility of more severe long-term outcomes, including SUDEP.[6,21] Consistent medication intake helps maintain therapeutic drug levels, reduces the risk of breakthrough seizures, and improves overall patient outcomes.[8,15] Poor adherence remains a significant challenge in epilepsy management, with substantial consequences that can affect both the individual and broader healthcare systems. I will discuss some of the consequences in the following subsections.

Consequences of non-adherence to AEDs

Increased seizure frequency: Non-adherence to AEDs can result in drug levels that remain below therapeutic ranges, leading to an increased frequency of seizures.[17,22] Recurring seizures not only disrupt daily life but can also exacerbate the underlying condition, causing neuronal damage and contributing to the progression of epilepsy.[10,25] Poor adherence can also cause toxic levels of the drug in the body, especially when people increase doses or take extra doses. Studies have shown that individuals who fail to adhere to prescribed medication regimens are at a higher risk of emergency room visits and hospital admissions due to uncontrolled seizures.[5,23]

Status epilepticus: One of the most severe consequences of non-adherence is the increased risk of status epilepticus (SE), a prolonged seizure lasting more than 5 minutes or a series of seizures without regaining consciousness between episodes.[7,21] When someone goes into SE, they need immediate medical intervention, because SE can cause brain damage or even death.[16,24] The risk of SE is higher in people who do not consistently take their AEDs as prescribed.[9,12,20] SE is covered in detail in Chapter 9.

Reduced quality of life: Non-adherence to medication affects the person's quality of life and mental health. Frequent and uncontrolled seizures can lead to injuries, intellectual decline, and psychosocial challenges, such as anxiety and depression.[6,17] The stigma associated with poorly managed epilepsy can worsen mental health issues, contributing to social isolation and reduced participation in work or school activities.[11,26]

Impact on treatment outcomes: Poor adherence derails treatment plans and impacts the overall effectiveness of AED therapy. Poor adherence may influence clinicians to incorrectly assume treatment resistance, causing unnecessary changes to the treatment protocol. These changes could lead to an increased risk of adverse side effects without addressing the root cause of poor seizure control.[10,27] Even with the changes, the person may remain non-adherent to treatment causing further frustration to all involved in the management of the condition. Poor adherence can result in higher healthcare costs due to additional testing, hospitalizations, and the use of more expensive treatment options.[28,30]

Economic and healthcare system burden: The economic impact of non-adherence does not only affect the person who does not adhere to treatment guidelines but puts the burden on the economy and healthcare system. This burden includes increased emergency visits, hospitalization, and the need for more intensive treatment contributing to the financial strain on healthcare systems.[21,25] Studies have demonstrated that improving medication adherence could significantly reduce these costs by minimizing the incidence of seizures and related complications.[8,18]

The role of clinicians in adherence

Patients often struggle with adherence due to side effects, fear of stigma, and forgetfulness, among other reasons.[16] To combat this, healthcare providers should focus on strategies such as patient education, simplified dosing regimens, and continuous counseling. Studies have shown that involving patients in their treatment plans, regular follow-ups, and providing clear information about the importance of adherence can significantly improve outcomes.[28,30] Clinicians play a pivotal role in encouraging adherence by customizing treatment plans to fit individual lifestyles and regularly reviewing patients' progress. Collaborative approaches that include caregivers and patient support groups can also contribute to better medication management and adherence.[12,13] Through such efforts, adherence rates can improve, ensuring effective seizure control and an enhanced quality of life for PWE.[8,10]

In summary, adherence to AEDs is crucial for effective seizure control and preventing complications. Patients who do not adhere to their medication regimens face a higher risk of recurrent seizures, SE, diminished quality of life, and increased healthcare costs.[12,15,22] Addressing the barriers to adherence can significantly improve outcomes and reduce the burden on healthcare systems.[5,10]

Conclusion

Most PWE (approximately 70%) respond well to AEDs and become seizure-free. An in-depth understanding of pharmacokinetics and pharmacodynamics is critical in pharmacotherapy to increase chances of seizure control with minimal side effects. Managing side effects is a critical component of epilepsy treatment. Clinicians must weigh the benefits of seizure control against the potential side effects when choosing AEDs. Ongoing monitoring, patient education, and individualized treatment approaches are essential to ensure optimal therapeutic outcomes and adherence.[13,30] Understanding the diverse side effects associated with AEDs enables more informed decision-making and helps maintain patient quality of life throughout treatment.

As mentioned in the introduction of this chapter, some PWE (approximately 30%) will not gain seizure control with AEDs, even if put on polytherapy. Drug-resistant epilepsy is defined as the inability to achieve sustained seizure freedom after trying two suitable and well-tolerated anti-epileptic drug regimens whether as monotherapy or polytherapy.[31] This is a working definition, which means that our understanding of DRE can change as clinicians obtain more information. People with DRE have more options like surgery or a ketogenic diet, as will be discussed in the next sections. The important thing is to work with the health team so that all options are explored without giving up.

EPILEPSY SURGERY

Introduction

Epilepsy surgery is an important treatment option particularly for people with focal epilepsy that is drug resistant. For eligible people, surgery is the most effective path to seizure control, with the potential to dramatically improve cognition, behavior, and quality of life.[32,33] The old treatment protocols considered surgery to be an option of last resort due to its invasive nature and associated risks. Improved outcomes as a result of advancements in imaging and surgical techniques have made epilepsy surgery gain recognition, making it a critical intervention method that can be used earlier for eligible patients.[34,35] Studies show that early referral and surgery offer better long-term results.[36] The studies emphasize the importance for early referral for evaluation and timely intervention to prevent the cumulative burden of uncontrolled seizures and improve outcomes.[36]

Eligibility and patient selection for epilepsy surgery

Not everyone with epilepsy is a suitable candidate for epilepsy surgery. To maximize the benefits of epilepsy surgery, careful selection and assessment of candidates are essential. Eligible candidates have focal DRE, where seizure frequency and severity persist despite adequate medication trials. Current guidelines recommend a systematic approach to identifying candidates earlier because delays could cause cognitive decline that cannot be fixed by surgery.[37,38] Also, early intervention could help avoid psychosocial difficulties in patients with longstanding epilepsy.[37,38] Underutilization of epilepsy surgery remains a concern, due to certain barriers ranging from a lack of specialist referrals to patient misconceptions about the safety and effectiveness of the procedure. Scholars have identified a big gap between those who qualify and those who undergo surgery, stressing the need for targeted education to address these challenges.[39,40]

Presurgical evaluation

The success of epilepsy surgery heavily relies on presurgical evaluation to localize the seizure origin and to assess its removability.

This evaluation includes a combination of clinical history, neuropsychological testing, and neuroimaging, such as MRI, PET, and single photon emission computed tomography (SPECT), to understand structural and functional aspects of the epileptic focus.[35,41] The emergence of these advanced neuroimaging tests has made it possible for previously excluded people to now qualify for surgery, especially those with MRI-negative epilepsy.[42,43] Also, implant-based monitoring with stereo electroencephalography (SEEG) or subdural grid placement can be used for complicated cases to locate the epileptogenic zone with higher accuracy.[34] All these tests, including clinical judgment, help in identifying the exact epileptogenic area with precision.[44] This means even though a lot of equipment is needed, qualified clinicians able to interpret the results and make a clinical judgment are vital.

It is hoped that new technologies, such as network connectivity models and the examination of physical wiring of the brain (connectomics), could enhance presurgical planning. For instance, connectivity studies have suggested that certain structural networks associated with epilepsy may predict surgical outcomes.[45,46] However, further research is still ongoing to determine how they can be used in clinical settings.[47] These advanced technologies are not available in most LMICs, and this useful procedure remains out of reach for many eligible PWE.

Types of epilepsy surgery

Epilepsy surgery includes various approaches, customized for each person's seizure cause and location in the brain. Surgery aimed at removing a part of the body (resective surgeries), such as lobectomy (removal of a portion of the brain, e.g., temporal lobectomy, frontal lobectomy), lesionectomy (removal of a lesion, e.g., tumor, scar tissue), and tailored resections (e.g., occipital resections), aim to remove the brain tissue responsible for generating seizures.[33,48] Temporal lobectomy is one of the most studied forms of epilepsy surgery and shows significant success rates.[33,48] Positive outcomes have been associated with lesionectomy, a procedure used to remove identified lesions, like epilepsy-associated tumors believed to be the cause of seizures.[49]

In cases where resective surgery is not feasible, non-resective options should be considered. An alternative could be neurostimulation therapies. These therapies include vagus nerve stimulation (VNS) and responsive neurostimulation (RNS). These provide therapeutic benefits by regulating neuronal activity without removing brain tissue, thus posing less risk for functional impairment.[50,51] Other approaches, such as corpus callosotomy, are useful in patients with generalized or multifocal epilepsy, particularly when drop attacks are present. Hemispherectomy (removal of half of the brain), although drastic, remains an effective option for patients with extensive unilateral epileptic zones, often in children with severe developmental epileptic encephalopathies.[52]

New techniques like laser interstitial thermal therapy (LITT) and focused ultrasound provide innovative, minimally invasive options for targeting and eliminating small areas of seizure activity. LITT, guided by MRI, selectively removes epileptogenic tissue, offering a safe and effective option for patients unable to undergo open resection.[47]

Surgical outcomes and prognostic factors

The outcome of epilepsy surgery varies, but most people experience a reduction in seizures with many people becoming completely seizure-free.[32,53] Outcomes depend on seizure type, location, and underlying pathology. For example, temporal lobe epilepsy surgery has high success rates, with approximately 70% of patients achieving seizure freedom in the short term after surgery. Long-term studies show that living seizure-free contributes to cognitive and psychosocial improvements, highlighting the life-changing opportunities offered by surgery.[32,53]

Specific factors contribute to epilepsy surgical outcomes, including the duration of time the person has had epilepsy before surgery, the completeness of the resection, and patient age.[54,55] Younger patients and those with a shorter duration of epilepsy tend to experience better outcomes. Prolonged seizures are associated with structural and functional brain changes that complicate surgical treatment.[54,55] The cause of the epilepsy also contributes to surgical outcomes; for example, outcomes are typically more favorable in cases involving identifiable lesions or tumors.[49,56]

Pediatric epilepsy surgery

Pediatric patients represent a unique population in epilepsy surgery, with notable benefits from early intervention. Early surgery can prevent developmental delays and improve cognitive outcomes, making it a key treatment option for children with drug-resistant focal epilepsy.[52,57] Children who could benefit from surgery include those with genetic epilepsies and structural lesions. Studies have demonstrated better developmental trajectories and quality of life for children who undergo surgery early.[58]

Barriers to epilepsy surgery

Rathore et al.[59] list the barriers to epilepsy surgery as follows:
- Large population with high epilepsy burden
- Widespread poverty
- High rate of illiteracy and lack of public awareness
- Social stigma, superstition, and lack of faith in modern medicine
- Lack of epilepsy training in undergraduate and post-graduate curricula
- Misguided fears about risks of epilepsy surgery
- Inadequate, unequal, and inefficient healthcare facilities
- Lack of trained professionals and infrastructure to establish comprehensive epilepsy care programs
- Little inclination among trained personnel to initiate epilepsy surgery programs.[59]

In addition to the barriers listed above, several studies focused on epilepsy surgery have identified other barriers, which will be discussed in more detail here.

Limited awareness and knowledge: One of the primary barriers to epilepsy surgery is lack of awareness among both patients and healthcare providers. Research shows that many healthcare providers, including general neurologists, do not fully understand the indications for and benefits of epilepsy surgery, contributing to delays in referrals for surgical evaluation.[39,40] Some clinicians still hold on to the old mentality that surgery is only a last resort for "severe" cases. This contributes to surgical evaluation delays, compromising outcomes.[36,38] Additionally, patients and families often have limited knowledge about surgical options and may not be informed about the safety and efficacy of modern epilepsy surgeries.[36,39]

Stigma and psychological barriers: Epilepsy is frequently associated with significant social stigma, as detailed in Chapter 14. Fear of being stigmatized can discourage people from seeking surgical interventions for epilepsy. Both patients and their families may fear social exclusion or discrimination if the epilepsy diagnosis becomes more public through the surgical process.[39] Cultural beliefs may contribute to families resisting surgical recommendations, believing that epilepsy can only be managed through non-invasive methods.[55] The fear of possible complications and impacts on personality or cognition can hinder people from considering surgery even when it is recommended by medical professionals.[48]

Economic and geographic limitations: Financial and geographic factors pose additional challenges to accessing epilepsy surgery, particularly in LMICs. Surgery requires specialized facilities, equipment, and expertise, often concentrated in urban centers or high-resource regions. Many patients in LMICs must travel significant distances, sometimes thousands of miles, to reach epilepsy surgery centers, incurring prohibitive travel, accommodation, and procedural costs.[60] Even in high-income countries, insurance coverage for epilepsy surgery and related pre-surgical evaluations can vary widely, leaving some patients unable to afford the necessary assessments and treatments.[47] Efforts in countries such as India and Georgia demonstrate that establishing low-cost, accessible epilepsy surgery programs can help address these barriers. To expand epilepsy surgery access in resource-limited settings, it is critical to develop cost-effective surgical protocols and increase the training of local clinicians.[59,61]

Lack of surgical infrastructure and trained professionals: Surgical infrastructure is essential for epilepsy surgery but often limited in availability. Many regions lack adequate facilities, equipment, and, crucially, trained personnel to perform epilepsy surgery and conduct pre-surgical evaluations.[47] For example, in sub-Saharan Africa, epilepsy surgery is only available at two institutions in South Africa, limiting accessibility both geographically and economically.[2] The specialized training required for epileptologists, neurosurgeons, and neuroimaging specialists involved in epilepsy surgery makes it hard to scale up programs, particularly in areas with limited access to advanced neurological training programs.[60,61] These limitations create a bottleneck effect where eligible patients face long waiting lists or are unable to access surgery at all. Being on the waiting list for too long may steal the potential benefit of surgery. There is a need for more epilepsy centers with adequately trained personnel to close this gap.

Systemic delays and referral gaps: Studies indicate that many patients who could benefit from epilepsy surgery remain in the care of general neurologists or primary care physicians. These clinicians may not be aware of the referral criteria, leading to delays that can negatively impact long-term outcomes.[38] People need to be referred to these specialist services, however, if clinicians are not even aware who to refer, that can contribute to delays. These referral delays result in a lengthy pre-surgical process.[36] This referral gap highlights the need for clear, accessible guidelines to facilitate timely and appropriate referrals for epilepsy surgery.[39]

Addressing barriers to improve access

Addressing these barriers to epilepsy surgery requires a multifaceted approach that includes increasing awareness, reducing stigma, and expanding surgical infrastructure. Education campaigns aimed at healthcare providers can improve understanding of surgical options and encourage earlier referrals. Public health initiatives that inform patients and families about epilepsy surgery could reduce stigma and misconceptions, enabling more patients to consider surgery as a viable treatment option.[40]

Despite the proven benefits of epilepsy surgery for drug-resistant patients, numerous barriers prevent eligible individuals from accessing this potentially life-changing intervention. These barriers range from logistical and structural issues within healthcare systems to social and psychological obstacles affecting both patients and healthcare providers. Recognizing and addressing these barriers is essential to improving access to epilepsy surgery and ensuring optimal patient outcomes.

Conclusion

Epilepsy surgery offers a life-altering option for patients with DRE, with evidence supporting its efficacy in achieving seizure control and improving quality of life. However, surgery remains underutilized. Timely referrals, improved patient selection, and expansion of surgical programs could unlock the full potential of epilepsy surgery. With further advancements in research and technology, epilepsy surgery could become a critical component of comprehensive epilepsy care.[32,51]

In regions with limited resources, strategies such as telemedicine consultations, low-cost surgical centers, and collaborations with international epilepsy organizations can help bridge the access gap.[60,61] Such approaches, combined with supportive policy changes and funding for epilepsy care infrastructure, could significantly increase the number of patients who benefit from epilepsy surgery, enhancing outcomes and quality of life for many with DRE.

KETOGENIC DIET IN EPILEPSY TREATMENT

Introduction

The ketogenic diet (KD) offers a non-pharmacological and non-surgical option for managing epilepsy, particularly for DRE. Ketogenic diets are high-fat, low-carbohydrate, and moderate-protein diets that shifts the body's primary energy source from glucose to ketone bodies, which may have antiseizure effects.[62] Since their development in the early 20th century, KDs have remained significant in epilepsy treatment and have regained popularity as an alternative for managing DRE.[63,64]

Historical background

During the 1920s, researchers found that fasting reduced seizure frequency in children. The apparent success of fasting in lessening incidence of seizures prompted physicians to create a diet that mimicked fasting's biochemical effects, providing a sustainable, non-invasive seizure management option.[62] This marked the beginning of the KD. As AEDs became popular, KD and other dietary treatment options lost popularity, but never disappeared. The KD regained popularity around the 1990s, to address an increase in DRE, becoming a key treatment option for managing epilepsy that is unresponsive to pharmacological treatments.[63,64]

Ketosis and brain metabolism

It is critical to understand how the KD generates the antiseizure effects. It works by changing the way the brain uses energy. This diet influences brain metabolism, neurotransmission, and neuronal stability. The KD induces ketosis by lowering carbohydrate intake, which limits glucose and forces the body to metabolize fats. The breakdown of fats produces ketone bodies, including beta-hydroxybutyrate (BHB) and acetoacetate, which cross the blood-brain barrier and serve as alternative energy sources for neurons. Studies have shown that ketones have neuroprotective effects that stabilize brain energy levels and lower neuron activity, resulting in lower seizure incidence.[65,66]

Antiseizure effects of ketone bodies

Ketones enhance neurotransmitters, especially gamma-aminobutyric acid (GABA), which has a calming effect on the brain.[66,68] Increased GABA activity stabilizes brain networks, preventing seizure spread. Ketone bodies also reduce reactive oxygen species, which have been linked to neuronal damage in epilepsy.[66,68] The ketogenic diet also has anti-inflammatory effects that may help managing epilepsy, because inflammation is a known factor in seizure disorders.[62,65] These effects are particularly relevant for children with epilepsy, who may benefit developmentally and neurologically from a ketogenic diet's neuroprotective properties.

Types of ketogenic diet

Over time, variations of the classical ketogenic diet have been developed, to allow for flexibility while maintaining efficacy. Here are some of the variations:

Classical ketogenic diet: The classical ketogenic diet uses a 4:1 ratio of fats to carbohydrates and proteins, requiring careful calculation of food intake to achieve sustained ketosis. This version is most widely used and requires close monitoring to maintain ketosis and manage any side effects.[69,70] This diet requires accurate meal planning and adherence to maintain ketosis.

Modified Atkins diet (MAD): This option allows more carbohydrates, making it less restrictive, increasing flexibility and adherence. Studies suggest that MAD can achieve similar levels of seizure control as the classical diet.[71,72]

Low glycemic index treatment (LGIT): LGIT allows low-glycemic carbohydrates, which do not significantly raise blood sugar. The diet offers more dietary choices while still reducing seizure frequency. LGIT is particularly useful for patients who have difficulty with strict KD adherence.[71]

Comparative studies show that the different variations all offer similar levels of seizure control.[73,74] It is recommended to tailor the diet to suit individual needs to increase levels of adherence without compromising effectiveness.

Efficacy in pediatric epilepsy

The effectiveness of the KD in childhood epilepsy has been well documented, especially in children with DRE. Studies demonstrate that there is a reduction in seizure frequency in children with DRE on the KD. For example, a meta-analysis reported significant seizure reduction in over 50% of children on the KD, with some achieving complete seizure control.[75,76] Childhood epilepsy syndromes like Dravet and Lennox–Gastaut syndromes respond favorably to the KD.[77,78] These syndromes often show resistance to medications, making the KD a valuable alternative.[77,78] Starting the KD early has been seen to likely improve developmental outcomes and reduce the need for multiple medications.[79,80] Some research indicates that the KD may benefit cognitive development in children with epilepsy. Improvements in behavior, attention, and memory have been observed, likely due to reduced seizure frequency and reduced exposure to medications.[79,80]

Efficacy in adult epilepsy

While KD research has mainly focused on children, it has been shown to manage DRE in adults in the few studies that have been carried out.[79,80]. Several trials have demonstrated the KD's effectiveness in adults with refractory epilepsy, although long-term adherence and tolerance can be more challenging.[79,80] For adults, adapting and adhering to the diet pose the greatest challenge; however, when adherence is possible, the KD provides a viable treatment option. For better tolerance, the personalized treatment plan can incorporate elements of the other variations of the KD to see what works best for the individual.[81] The KD may be particularly beneficial for adults with specific neurological conditions, such as mitochondrial disorders, where metabolic adjustments may aid seizure control. These conditions often benefit from the KD's neuroprotective and metabolic effects.[81]

Safety, tolerability, and side effects

Just like any other treatment plan, the KD's effectiveness also comes with potential side effects and safety considerations, especially in long-term usage. Common adverse effects include gastrointestinal discomfort (nausea, constipation), metabolic issues (excess acid in the body, low blood sugar), and nutrient deficiencies due to the restrictive nature of the KD.[62,82] Managing these side effects is crucial for adherence. To improve coping with the diet and increase adherence, fat ratios can be adjusted, dietary supplements can be introduced, and regular monitoring should be implemented. Dietitians and clinicians form part of the healthcare team supporting families through the management of side effects and dietary adjustments.[83,84] If a child is on a long-term KD, it is of paramount importance to consider issues around growth, bone health, and cholesterol levels.[79,85] Monitoring and adjusting the diet over time helps address these concerns while sustaining the antiseizure benefits.[79,85]

Benefits of the ketogenic diet

In addition to seizure control, a ketogenic diet may offer cognitive and quality of life improvements.

- Some studies suggest that the KD enhances cognitive performance and behavior, particularly in children who have experienced developmental delays.[79,86]
- Reductions in seizures may enable better social interaction and learning.[79,86] Improved seizure control is associated with better quality of life, social functioning, and overall psychological well-being for both children and adults on the KD.
- Patients report fewer hospitalizations and less reliance on medications.[87,88]
- The KD may also improve mood regulation and reduce behavioral problems, enhancing patients' psychosocial adjustment and overall quality of life.[79,86]
- Emerging evidence links the KD's effects on epilepsy with changes in the gut microbiota. Studies indicate that the KD potentially promotes beneficial bacterial populations that influence neurotransmitter production and reduce neuroinflammation. These changes may play a role in the KD's antiseizure effects.[67,89]
- Research into gut–brain interactions suggests that microbiota shifts induced by the KD could contribute to seizure reduction by decreasing inflammatory responses and enhancing brain health.[89]

Guidelines for clinical implementation

Implementing a ketogenic diet as a treatment for epilepsy requires careful planning, and several medical experts and family support. Medical experts include neurologists and dieticians at the minimum. The neurologist will monitor treatment, while the dietician creates the meal plans, and the family ensures adherence to the diet. The KD initiation starts with an overall health check then a slow introduction of dietary adjustments, while monitoring ketones frequently. This phased approach allows for safe ketone level achievement while monitoring patient responses.[82,90] The dietician also addresses all nutrient needs, which is vital for both short-term success and long-term adherence.[82] Regular monitoring and dietary adjustments based on patient tolerance and clinical response ensure the best possible outcome for patients on the KD.[90]

Barriers to adherence and broader use

While the KD offers substantial benefits, challenges remain in its broader application and long-term use. People with limited resources may not be able to adhere to the diet because the foods required may not be a staple food in that community. The restrictiveness of a KD, along with costs and cultural dietary preferences, can limit broader implementation. Developing more accessible dietary modifications remains an area of interest.[62,88] Research is exploring KDs' potential applications in other neurological disorders, such as Alzheimer's and Parkinson's, which may benefit from their metabolic effects.[68,81]

Conclusion

The ketogenic diet continues to demonstrate significant efficacy in the management of DRE, offering seizure reduction and, in some cases, complete seizure control for both pediatric and adult patients. Although its exact mechanisms remain an area of active research, evidence supports the roles of ketone bodies, metabolic modulation, and changes in gut microbiota as contributing factors to its anticonvulsant properties.[62,65,66,67] The diet's long-term effects also show potential benefits on cognition and behavior, which may improve overall quality of life in individuals with refractory epilepsy.[79,85] However, the diet's stringent nature poses challenges related to adherence, potential side effects, and the need for close medical and nutritional supervision.[70,90] Variants such as the modified Atkins and low-glycemic index diets offer more flexible options with favorable outcomes, thus broadening dietary choices for patients. Future directions should include refining dietary protocols to enhance both efficacy and tolerability, alongside research into personalized approaches based on genetic and metabolic profiles. The KD, therefore remains a valuable and evolving treatment for epilepsy that warrants continued exploration and clinical application. Ongoing research aims to refine KD protocols for enhanced efficacy and tolerability. Additionally, studies are focused on elucidating the underlying mechanisms of KDs' antiseizure effects and optimizing individualized treatment plans.

References:

1. Martin, J. et al eds. 2009. *British National Formulary. 62nd ed.* London: Pharmaceutical Press. 252-268.
2. World Health Organization. (2004). *Epilepsy in the WHO Africa Region: Bridging the Gap: The Global Campaign Against Epilepsy "Out of the Shadows."* Geneva: World Health Organization. https://www.ibe-epilepsy.org/downloads/EPILEPSY%20AFRICAN%20Report.pdf
3. Garcia-March, G., Bordes, V., Talamantes, F., Masbout, G., Roldan, P., & Barcia-Salorio, J. L. (1999). Vagus nerve stimulation for the control of medically resistant epilepsy, *Epilepsia, 40*/2: 89-90.
4. Charlie Foundation. (2012). Ketogenic Diet. http://www.charliefoundation.org/faq/ketogenic-diet.html
5. Byun, J-I., Kim, D.W., Kim, K.T., Yang, K.I., Lee, S.T., ... Cho, Y.W. (2020). Treatment of epilepsy in adults: Expert opinion in South Korea. *Epilepsy & Behavior*, 105, https://doi.org/10.1016/j.yebeh.2020.106942
6. Kanner, A.M., & Bicchi, M.M. (2022). Antiseizure medications for adults with epilepsy: A review. *JAMA,* 327(13), 1269–1281. https://doi:10.1001/jama.2022.3880
7. International League Against Epilepsy. (2024). Medical therapies for epilepsy. *ILAE*, https://www.ilae.org/patient-care/medical-therapies
8. Chen, Z., Brodie, M.J., Liew, D., & Kwan, P. (2018). Treatment outcomes in patients with newly diagnosed epilepsy treated with established and new antiepileptic drugs: A 30-year longitudinal cohort study. *Journal of American Medical Association*, 75/3: 279-286. https://jamanetwork.com/journals/jamaneurology/article-abstract/2666189
9. Schmidt, D. (2009). Drug treatment of epilepsy: options and limitations. *Epilepsy & Behavior*, 15(1), 56-65. https://doi.org/10.1016/j.yebeh.2009.02.030
10. Perucca, E. (2021). The pharmacological treatment of epilepsy: Recent advances and future perspectives. *Acta Epileptologica, 3*(1), 22. https://doi.org/10.1186/s42494-021-00055-z
11. Kim, H., Kim, D.W., Lee, S.T., Byun, J.I., Seo, J.G., No, Y.J., Kang, K.W., Kim, D., Kim, K.T., Cho, Y.W., & Yang, K.I. (2020). Antiepileptic drug selection according to seizure

type in adult patients with epilepsy. *Journal of Clinical Neurology, 16*(4):547-555. https://doi.org/10.3988/jcn.2020.16.4.547
12. Epilepsy Foundation. (2024). Seizure medication list, https://www.epilepsy.com/tools-resources/seizure-medication-list?q=/tools-resources/seizure-medication-list%3Fq%3D/tools-resources/seizure-medication-list%3Ff%5B0%5D%3Dused_to_treat%3A35716&f%5B0%5D=used_to_treat%3A30
13. Melinosky, C. (2023). Epilepsy drugs to treat seizures. *WebMD*. https://www.epilepsy.com/tools-resources/seizure-medication-list?q=/tools-resources/seizure-medication-list%3Fq%3D/tools-resources/seizure-medication-list%3Ff%5B0%5D%3Dused_to_treat%3A35716&f%5B0%5D=used_to_treat%3A30
14. Mifsud, J. et al 2012. "VIREPA Course on Clinical Pharmacology and Pharmacotherapy: Clinical Pharmacokinetics of AEDs." Stockholm: International League Against Epilepsy.
15. Perucca, P., Scheffer, I. E., & Kiley, M. (2018). The management of epilepsy in children and adults. *Medical Journal of Australia, 208*(5), 226-233. https://doi.org/10.5694/mja17.00951
16. Swiss League Against Epilepsy. (2023). Epilepsy medication. *SLAE*, https://www.epi.ch/en/what-you-need-to-know-about-epilepsy-medicines/
17. Liu, G., Slater, N., & Perkins, A. (2017). Epilepsy: Treatment options. *American Family Physician, 96*(2), 87-96. https://www.aafp.org/pubs/afp/issues/2017/0715/p87.html
18. Glauser, T., Ben-Menachem, E., Bourgeois, B., Cnaan, A., Guerreiro, C., Kälviäinen, R., ... & ILAE Subcommission on AED Guidelines. (2013). Updated ILAE evidence review of antiepileptic drug efficacy and effectiveness as initial monotherapy for epileptic seizures and syndromes. *Epilepsia, 54*(3), 551-563. https://doi.org/10.1111/epi.12074
19. Chapereka, R. 2013. Interview with Ruth Chapereka, a pharmacist. Harare, Zimbabwe. [20 June 2013].
20. LaRoche, S.M., & Helmers, S.L. The new antiepileptic drugs: Scientific review. *JAMA*. 2004;291(5):605–614. https://doi:10.1001/jama.291.5.605
21. Laxer, K. D., Trinka, E., Hirsch, L. J., Cendes, F., Langfitt, J., Delanty, N., ... & Benbadis, S. R. (2014). The consequences of refractory epilepsy and its treatment. *Epilepsy & Behavior, 37*, 59-70. https://doi.org/10.1016/j.yebeh.2014.05.031
22. Shih, J. J., Whitlock, J. B., Chimato, N., Vargas, E., Karceski, S. C., & Frank, R. D. (2017). Epilepsy treatment in adults and adolescents: Expert opinion, 2016. *Epilepsy & Behavior, 69*, 186-222. https://doi.org/10.1016/j.yebeh.2016.11.018
23. Im, K., Lee, S.A., Kim, J.H., Kim, D.W., Lee, S.K., Seo, D.W., Ji Woong Lee, J.W. (2021). Long-term efficacy and safety of perampanel as a first add-on therapy in patients with focal epilepsy: Three-year extension study, *Epilepsy & Behavior, 125*, https://doi.org/10.1016/j.yebeh.2021.108407
24. Hirsch, M., Hintz, M., Specht, A., Schulze-Bonhage, A. (2018). Tolerability, efficacy and retention rate of Brivaracetam in patients previously treated with Levetiracetam: A monocenter retrospective outcome analysis, *European Journal of Epilepsy, 61*: 98-103. https://doi.org/10.1016/j.seizure.2018.07.017
25. Fattorusso, A., Matricardi, S., Mencaroni, E., Dell'Isola, G.B., Cara, G.D., Striano, P., Verrotti, A. (2021). The pharmacoresistant epilepsy: An overview on existent and new emerging therapies, *Frontiers in Neurology, 12*, https://doi.org/10.3389/fneur.2021.674483
26. Gao, L., Lu, Q., Wang, Z., Yue, W., Wang, G., Shao, X., Guo, Y., Yi, Y., Hong, Z., Jiang, Y., Xiao, B., Cui, G., Gao, F., Hu, J., Liang, J., Zhang, M. & Wang, Y. (2023). Efficacy and safety of perampanel as early add-on therapy in Chinese patients with focal-onset seizures: A multicenter, open-label, single-arm study. *Frontiers in Neurology, 30*, 1-13. https://doi.org/10.3389/fneur.2023.1236046

27. Schmidt, D. (2002). The clinical impact of new antiepileptic drugs after a decade of use in epilepsy. *Epilepsy Research, 50*(1-2), 21-32. https://doi.org/10.1016/S0920-1211(02)00065-7
28. Kim, H., Faught, E., Thurman, D.J., Fishman, J. & Kalilani, L. (2019). Antiepileptic drug treatment patterns in women of childbearing age with epilepsy. *JAMA Neurology, 76*(7):783–790. https://doi.org/10.1001/jamaneurol.2019.0447
29. Sweetman, S.C. et al eds. 2009. "Antiepileptics" in: *Martindale: The Complete Drug Reference*. 36th ed. London: Pharmaceutical Press. 465-516.
30. Ferrari, C.M.M., Cardoso de Sousa, R.M. and, Castro, L.H.M. (2013). Factors associated with treatment non-adherence in patients with epilepsy in Brazil, *Seizure, 22*, 384-389. http://dx.doi.org/10.1016/j.seizure.2013.02.006
31. Kwan, P., Arzimanoglou, A., Berg, A. T., Brodie, M. J., Allen Hauser, W., Mathern, G., ... & French, J. (2010). Definition of drug resistant epilepsy: Consensus proposal by the ad hoc Task Force of the ILAE Commission on Therapeutic Strategies. *Epilepsia, 51*(6):1069–1077. https://doi.org/10.1111/j.1528-1167.2009.02397.x
32. Ryvlin, P., Cross, J. H., & Rheims, S. (2014). Epilepsy surgery in children and adults. *The Lancet Neurology, 13*(11), 1114-1126. https://www.thelancet.com/journals/laneur/article/PIIS1474-4422(14)70156-5/abstract
33. Spencer, S., & Huh, L. (2008). Outcomes of epilepsy surgery in adults and children. *The Lancet Neurology, 7*(6), 525-537. http://doi.org/10.1016/s1474-4422(08)70109-1
34. Jobst, B. C., & Cascino, G. D. (2015). Resective epilepsy surgery for drug-resistant focal epilepsy: A review. *JAMA, 313*(3), 285-293. https://doi.org/10.1001/jama.2014.17426
35. Noachtar, S., & Borggraefe, I. (2009). Epilepsy surgery: A critical review. *Epilepsy & Behavior, 15*(1), 66-72. https://doi.org/10.1016/j.yebeh.2009.02.028
36. Jehi, L., Jette, N., Kwon, C. S., Josephson, C. B., Burneo, J. G., Cendes, F., ... & Wiebe, S. (2022). Timing of referral to evaluate for epilepsy surgery: Expert Consensus Recommendations from the Surgical Therapies Commission of the International League Against Epilepsy. *Epilepsia, 63*(10), 2491-2506. https://doi.org/10.1111/epi.17350
37. Vakharia, V. N., Duncan, J. S., Witt, J. A., Elger, C. E., Staba, R., & Engel Jr, J. (2018). Getting the best outcomes from epilepsy surgery. *Annals of Neurology, 83*(4), 676-690.
38. Baud, M. O., Perneger, T., Rácz, A., Pensel, M. C., Elger, C., Rydenhag, B., ... & Seeck, M. (2018). European trends in epilepsy surgery. *Neurology, 91*(2), e96-e106. https://doi.org/10.1212/WNL.0000000000005776
39. Samanta, D., Ostendorf, A. P., Willis, E., Singh, R., Gedela, S., Arya, R., & Perry, M. S. (2021). Underutilization of epilepsy surgery: Part I: A scoping review of barriers. *Epilepsy & Behavior, 117*. https://doi.org/10.1016/j.yebeh.2021.107837
40. Engel, J. (2019). Evolution of concepts in epilepsy surgery. *Epileptic Disorders, 5*(5), 391-409. https://doi.org/10.1684/epd.2019.1091
41. Kovac, S., Vakharia, V. N., Scott, C., & Diehl, B. (2017). Invasive epilepsy surgery evaluation. *Seizure, 44*, 125-136. https://doi.org/10.1016/j.seizure.2016.10.016
42. Baumgartner, C., Koren, J. P., Britto-Arias, M., Zoche, L., & Pirker, S. (2019). Presurgical epilepsy evaluation and epilepsy surgery. *F1000Research, 8*. https://doi.org/10.12688/f1000research.17714.1
43. Zijlmans, M., Zweiphenning, W., & van Klink, N. (2019). Changing concepts in presurgical assessment for epilepsy surgery. *Nature Reviews Neurology, 15*(10), 594-606. https://doi.org/10.1038/
44. West, S., Nevitt, S. J., Cotton, J., Gandhi, S., Weston, J., Sudan, A., ... & Newton, R. (2019). Surgery for epilepsy. *Cochrane Database of Systematic Reviews*, (6). https://doi.org/10.1002%2F14651858.CD010541.pub3

45. Hebbink, J., Meijer, H., Huiskamp, G., van Gils, S., & Leijten, F. (2017). Phenomenological network models: Lessons for epilepsy surgery. *Epilepsia, 58*(10), e147-e151. https://doi.org/10.1111/epi.13861
46. Taylor, P. N., Sinha, N., Wang, Y., Vos, S. B., de Tisi, J., Miserocchi, A., ... & Duncan, J. S. (2018). The impact of epilepsy surgery on the structural connectome and its relation to outcome. *NeuroImage: Clinical, 18*, 202-214. https://doi.org/10.1016/j.nicl.2018.01.028
47. Dorfer, C., Rydenhag, B., Baltuch, G., Buch, V., Blount, J., Bollo, R., ... & Cukiert, A. (2020). How technology is driving the landscape of epilepsy surgery. *Epilepsia, 61*(5), 841-855. https://doi.org/10.1111/epi.16489
48. Engel Jr, J. (2018). The current place of epilepsy surgery. *Current opinion in neurology, 31*(2), 192-197. https://doi.org/10.1097/WCO.0000000000000528
49. Pelliccia, V., Deleo, F., Gozzo, F., Sartori, I., Mai, R., Cossu, M., & Tassi, L. (2017). Early and late epilepsy surgery in focal epilepsies associated with long-term epilepsy-associated tumors. *Journal of Neurosurgery, 127*(5), 1147-1152. https://doi.org/10.3171/2016.9.JNS161176
50. Englot, D. J., Birk, H., & Chang, E. F. (2017). Seizure outcomes in nonresective epilepsy surgery: an update. *Neurosurgical Review, 40*, 181-194. https://doi.org/10.1007/s10143-016-0725-8
51. Englot, D. J. (2018). A modern epilepsy surgery treatment algorithm: Incorporating traditional and emerging technologies. *Epilepsy & Behavior*,
52. Cross, J. H., Reilly, C., Delicado, E. G., Smith, M. L., & Malmgren, K. (2022). Epilepsy surgery for children and adolescents: Evidence-based but underused. *The Lancet Child & Adolescent Health, 6*(7), 484-494. https://www.sciencedirect.com/science/article/pii/S2352464222000980
53. Bell, G. S., De Tisi, J., Gonzalez-Fraile, J. C., Peacock, J. L., McEvoy, A. W., Harkness, W. F., ... & Duncan, J. S. (2017). Factors affecting seizure outcome after epilepsy surgery: an observational series. *Journal of Neurology, Neurosurgery & Psychiatry, 88*(11). https://discovery.ucl.ac.uk/id/eprint/1572331/17/De%20Tisi_Epilepsy%20surgery%20for%20JNNP.pdf
54. Bjellvi, J., Olsson, I., Malmgren, K., & Wilbe Ramsay, K. (2019). Epilepsy duration and seizure outcome in epilepsy surgery: A systematic review and meta-analysis. *Neurology, 93*(2), e159-e166. https://doi.org/10.1212/WNL.0000000000007753
55. Rathore, C., & Radhakrishnan, K. (2017). Epidemiology of epilepsy surgery in India. *Neurology India, 65*(Suppl 1), S52-S59. https://doi.org/10.4103/neuroindia.NI_924_16
56. Mohan, M., Keller, S., Nicolson, A., Biswas, S., Smith, D., Osman Farah, J., ... & Wieshmann, U. (2018). The long-term outcomes of epilepsy surgery. *PloS one, 13*(5). https://doi.org/10.1371/journal.pone.0196274
57. Braun, K. P., & Cross, J. H. (2018). Pediatric epilepsy surgery: the earlier the better. *Expert Review of Neurotherapeutics, 18*(4), 261-263. https://doi.org/10.1080/14737175.2018.1455503
58. Stevelink, R., Sanders, M. W., Tuinman, M. P., Brilstra, E. H., Koeleman, B. P., Jansen, F. E., & Braun, K. P. (2018). Epilepsy surgery for patients with genetic refractory epilepsy: a systematic review. *Epileptic Disorders, 20*(2), 99-115. https://doi.org/10.1684/epd.2018.0959
59. Rathore, C., Rao, M.B. and Radhakrishnan, K. (2014). National epilepsy surgery program: realistic goals & pragmatic solutions. *Neurology India.* 62: 124-129
60. Jukkarwala, A., Baheti, N. N., Dhakoji, A., Salgotra, B., Menon, G., Gupta, A., ... & Rathore, C. (2019). Establishment of low-cost epilepsy surgery centers in resource poor setting. *Seizure, 69*, 245-250. https://doi.org/10.1016/j.seizure.2019.05.007

61. Dugladze, T., Bäuerle, P., Kasradze, S., Lomidze, G., Gzirishvili, N., Tsikarishvili, V., ... & Gloveli, T. (2020). Initiating a new national epilepsy surgery program: Experiences gathered in Georgia. *Epilepsy & Behavior, 111*. https://doi.org/10.1016/j.yebeh.2020.107259
62. Elia, M., Klepper, J., Leiendecker, B., & Hartmann, H. (2017). Ketogenic diets in the treatment of epilepsy. *Current Pharmaceutical Design, 23*(37), 5691-5701. https://doi.org/10.2174/1381612823666170809101517
63. Ułamek-Kozioł, M., Czuczwar, S. J., Januszewski, S., & Pluta, R. (2019). Ketogenic diet and epilepsy. *Nutrients, 11*(10), 2510. https://doi.org/10.3390/nu11102510
64. Haridas, B., & Kossoff, E. H. (2022). Dietary treatments for epilepsy. *Neurologic Clinics, 40*(4), 785-797. https://doi.org/10.1016/j.ncl.2022.03.009
65. Boison, D. (2017). New insights into the mechanisms of the ketogenic diet. *Current Opinion in Neurology, 30*(2), 187–192. https://doi.org/10.1097/WCO.0000000000000432
66. Simeone, T.A., Simeone, K.A., Stafstrom, C.E. & Rho, J.M. (2018). Do ketone bodies mediate the anti-seizure effects of the ketogenic diet? *Neuropharmacology 133*, 233–241. https://doi.org/10.1016/j.neuropharm.2018.01.011
67. Lindefeldt, M., Eng, A., Darban, H., Bjerkner, A., Zetterström, C.K., Allander, T., Andersson, B., Borenstein, E., Dahlin, M. & Prast-Nielsen, S. (2019) The ketogenic diet influences taxonomic and functional composition of the gut microbiota in children with severe epilepsy. *NPJ Biofilms Microbiomes 5*,5. https://doi.org/10.1038/s41522-018-0073-2
68. D'Andrea Meira, I., Romão, T. T., Pires do Prado, H. J., Krüger, L. T., Pires, M. E. P., & da Conceição, P. O. (2019). Ketogenic diet and epilepsy: what we know so far. *Frontiers in Neuroscience, 13*, 5. https://doi.org/10.3389/fnins.2019.00005
69. Hee Seo, J., Mock Lee, Y., Soo Lee, J., Chul Kang, H., & Dong Kim, H. (2007). Efficacy and tolerability of the ketogenic diet according to lipid: nonlipid ratios—comparison of 3: 1 with 4: 1 diet. Epilepsia, 48(4), 801-805.. https://doi.org/10.1111/j.1528-1167.2007.01025.x
70. Zupec-Kania, B.A. & Spellman, E. (2008) An overview of the ketogenic diet for pediatric epilepsy. *Nutrition in Clinical Practice, 23*, 589–596. https://doi.org/10.1177/0884533608326138
71. Miranda, M.J., Turner, Z. & Magrath, G. (2012) Alternative diets to the classical ketogenic diet--can we be more liberal? *Epilepsy Research, 100*(3), 278–285. https://doi.org/10.1016/j.eplepsyres.2012.06.007
72. Kossoff, E. H., Dorward, J. L., Turner, Z., & Pyzik, P. L. (2011). Prospective study of the modified atkins diet in combination with a ketogenic liquid supplement during the initial month. *Journal of Child Neurology, 26*(2), 147-151.. https://doi.org/10.1177/0883073810375718
73. Martin, K., Jackson, C. F., Levy, R. G., & Cooper, P. N. (2016). Ketogenic diet and other dietary treatments for epilepsy. *Cochrane Database of Systematic Reviews, (2)*. https://doi.org/10.1002/14651858.CD001903.pub3
74. Rezaei, S., Abdurahman, A. A., Saghazadeh, A., Badv, R. S., & Mahmoudi, M. (2019). Short-term and long-term efficacy of classical ketogenic diet and modified Atkins diet in children and adolescents with epilepsy: a systematic review and meta-analysis. *Nutritional Neuroscience, 22*(5), 317-334. https://doi.org/10.1080/1028415X.2017.1387721
75. Sourbron, J., Klinkenberg, S., van Kuijk, S. M., Lagae, L., Lambrechts, D., Braakman, H. M., & Majoie, M. (2020). Ketogenic diet for the treatment of pediatric epilepsy: review and meta-analysis. *Child's Nervous System, 36*, 1099-1109. https://doi.org/10.1007/s00381-020-04578-7

76. Henderson, C.B., Filloux, F.M., Alder, S.C., Lyon, J.L. & Caplin, D.A. (2006). Efficacy of the ketogenic diet as a treatment option for epilepsy: Meta-analysis. *Journal of Child Neurology, 21*, 193–198. https://doi.org/10.2310/7010.2006.00044
77. Neal, E. G., Chaffe, H., Schwartz, R. H., Lawson, M. S., Edwards, N., Fitzsimmons, G., ... & Cross, J. H. (2008). The ketogenic diet for the treatment of childhood epilepsy: a randomised controlled trial. *The Lancet Neurology, 7*(6), 500-506. https://doi.org/10.1016/S1474-4422(08)70092-9
78. Martin-McGill, K. J., Bresnahan, R., Levy, R. G., & Cooper, P. N. (2020). Ketogenic diets for drug-resistant epilepsy. *Cochrane Database of Systematic Reviews, (6)*. https://doi.org/10.1002/14651858.CD001903.pub4
79. IJff, D. M., Postulart, D., Lambrechts, D. A., Majoie, M. H., de Kinderen, R. J., Hendriksen, J. G., ... & Aldenkamp, A. P. (2016). Cognitive and behavioral impact of the ketogenic diet in children and adolescents with refractory epilepsy: a randomized controlled trial. *Epilepsy & Behavior, 60*, 153-157. https://doi.org/10.1016/j.yebeh.2016.04.033
80. Lambrechts, D. A., De Kinderen, R. J. A., Vles, J. S. H., De Louw, A. J. A., Aldenkamp, A. P., & Majoie, H. J. M. (2017). A randomized controlled trial of the ketogenic diet in refractory childhood epilepsy. *Acta Neurologica Scandinavica, 135*(2), 231-239. https://doi.org/10.1111/ane.12592
81. Paleologou, E., Ismayilova, N., & Kinali, M. (2017). Use of the ketogenic diet to treat intractable epilepsy in mitochondrial disorders. *Journal of Clinical Medicine, 6*(6), 56. https://doi.org/10.3390/jcm6060056
82. Roehl, K., & Sewak, S. L. (2017). Practice paper of the academy of nutrition and dietetics: classic and modified ketogenic diets for treatment of epilepsy. *Journal of the Academy of Nutrition and Dietetics, 117*(8), 1279-1292. https://doi.org/10.1016/j.jand.2017.06.006
83. Levy, R.G., Cooper, P.N., Giri, P. & Weston, J. (2012). Ketogenic diet and other dietary treatments for epilepsy. *Cochrane Database of Systematic Reviews*. https://doi.org/10.1002/14651858.CD001903.pub2
84. Cicek, E., & Sanlier, N. (2023). The place of a ketogenic diet in the treatment of resistant epilepsy: a comprehensive review. *Nutritional Neuroscience, 26*(9), 828-841. https://doi.org/10.1080/1028415X.2022.2095819
85. van Berkel, A.A., IJff, D.M. & Verkuyl, J.M. (2018). Cognitive benefits of the ketogenic diet in patients with epilepsy: A systematic overview. *Epilepsy & Behavior, 87*, 69–77. https://doi.org/10.1016/j.yebeh.2018.06.004
86. Lambrechts, D. A. J. E., Bovens, M. J. M., De la Parra, N. M., Hendriksen, J. G. M., Aldenkamp, A. P., & Majoie, M. J. M. (2013). Ketogenic diet effects on cognition, mood, and psychosocial adjustment in children. *Acta Neurologica Scandinavica, 127*(2), 103-108. https://doi.org/10.1111/j.1600-0404.2012.01686.x
87. Wijnen, B. F., de Kinderen, R. J., Lambrechts, D. A., Postulart, D., Aldenkamp, A. P., Majoie, M. H., & Evers, S. M. (2017). Long-term clinical outcomes and economic evaluation of the ketogenic diet versus care as usual in children and adolescents with intractable epilepsy. *Epilepsy Research, 132*, 91-99. https://doi.org/10.1016/j.eplepsyres.2017.03.002
88. Verrotti, A., Iapadre, G., Di Francesco, L., Zagaroli, L., & Farello, G. (2020). Diet in the treatment of epilepsy: what we know so far. *Nutrients, 12*(9), 2645. https://doi.org/10.3390/nu12092645
89. Xie, G., Zhou, Q., Qiu, C. Z., Dai, W. K., Wang, H. P., Li, Y. H., ... & Wang, W. J. (2017). Ketogenic diet poses a significant effect on imbalanced gut microbiota in infants with refractory epilepsy. *World Journal of Gastroenterology, 23*(33), 6164–6171. https://doi.org/10.3748/wjg.v23.i33.6164

90. Kossoff, E. H., Zupec-Kania, B. A., Auvin, S., Ballaban-Gil, K. R., Christina Bergqvist, A. G., Blackford, R., ... & Practice Committee of the Child Neurology Society. (2018). Optimal clinical management of children receiving dietary therapies for epilepsy: Updated recommendations of the International Ketogenic Diet Study Group. *Epilepsia Open, 3*(2), 175-192. https://doi.org/10.1002/epi4.12225
91. Shih, J. J., Whitlock, J. B., Chimato, N., Vargas, E., Karceski, S. C., & Frank, R. D. (2017). Epilepsy treatment in adults and adolescents: expert opinion, 2016. *Epilepsy & Behavior, 69*, 186-222. https://doi.org/10.1016/j.yebeh.2016.11.018

CHAPTER 7 – COMPLEMENTARY AND ALTERNATIVE MEDICINE

Now, the aggressive marketers are coming to the people. Pushed by a passion to make profit, they sell these products claiming they cure any condition. The herbs are said to be both safe and effective. Desperate to be seizure-free, several people have bought and consumed these products.
Clotilda Chinyanya

Medieval treatments for epilepsy ranged from rational methods like diet and drugs to superstitious and magical practices involving amulets, lunar phases, and human or animal substances. Some extreme rituals, labeled as "sacred medicine," included using frog liver, dog bile, and even urine from a seizure witness.
Owsei Temkin[52]

Introduction

Complementary and alternative medicine (CAM) includes various practices and treatments used alongside or instead of conventional medical approaches. In epilepsy management, CAM is popular in different cultures and regions due to various reasons such as availability, the need for holistic treatment, and traditional beliefs.[1,2] Even in Medieval times, things like a dog's bile, human blood, and human urine were given to PWE to treat epilepsy.[52] In the pursuit of seizure freedom, some people are willing to try any alternative that offers hope of relief. The loss of control associated with seizures can have psychosocial consequences.[3] This chapter will explore the types of CAM therapies commonly used in epilepsy, the potential risks and drug interactions associated with CAM, and the regulatory landscape that influences its use, ultimately highlighting the critical role of clinicians in navigating CAM for epilepsy patients.

CAM encompasses a wide range of practices and therapies that exist outside of conventional medical approaches.[1,4] For individuals with epilepsy, the use of CAM has gained considerable interest, driven by both dissatisfaction with the limitations of AEDs and a growing preference for natural and holistic health approaches.[5,6,7] As discussed previously, at least 30% of PWE do not respond to AED treatment, causing some of them to seek alternative treatment options. Also, AEDs cause several side effects, sometimes with no seizure control, and most AEDs interact with other drugs a person may be taking for co-morbidities.[8,9,10]

The appeal of CAM in epilepsy is not only rooted in the hope for better seizure control but also in the perception of holistic benefits.[11,12,13] CAM practices encompass a diverse array of interventions, including herbal remedies, dietary supplements, mind–body practices, acupuncture, and special diets.[1,4,14] Herbal medicine is the most popular form of CAM and has been used purportedly to cure a number of ailments from the beginning of the human species.[12]

These therapies align with a broader cultural trend toward natural and integrative health solutions. Within CAM, therapies such as cannabidiol (CBD) and the ketogenic diet have received significant attention due to emerging evidence suggesting possible benefits in seizure reduction.[2,15,16] However, while some CAM therapies are backed by promising data, like the KD and CBD, many others lack sufficient scientific validation, making it difficult for patients and clinicians to weigh the risks and benefits accurately.[17,18,19]

Types of CAM used in epilepsy
Ayurveda

Ayurveda, the world's oldest medical system that originated in India, is said to have been used for many ailments, including epilepsy, since 12,000 B.C.[20] Ayurveda describes epilepsy as *Apasmara*, meaning loss of consciousness.[13] The focal-aware seizures, referred to as *Apasmara Poorva Roopa*, include symptoms like hearing sounds, sensing darkness, delusions, and dreamlike states. *Apasmara* involves falling, shaking, eye rolling, teeth grinding, and foaming at the mouth.[13] Epilepsy is categorized into four types based on *dosha* (humors) imbalances and is considered a chronic, severe disease with various causes.[13] Treatment focuses on correcting these factors, dietary management, and avoiding hazardous situations. In Ayurvedic medicine, epilepsy is understood as shown in Figure 5.

Figure 5: Ayurveda systems of the body

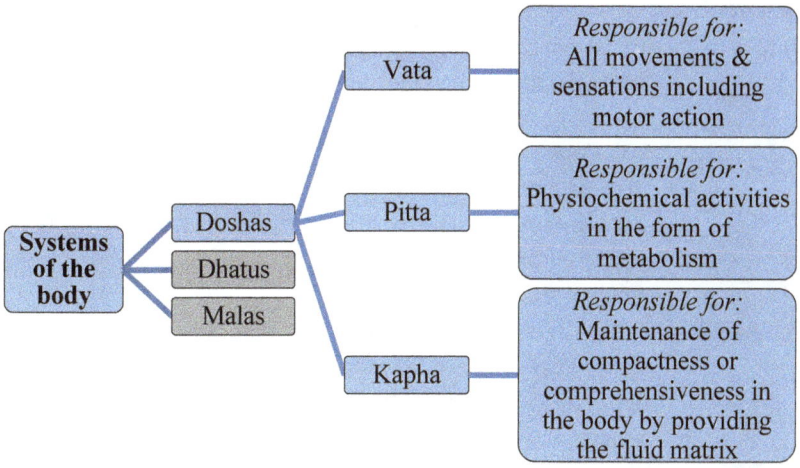

Extracted from information in an article by Manyam[13]

The three *doshas* are Vata, Pitta, and Kapha.[21,22] In Ayurveda, everyone has these three *doshas*, but in different combinations.[22] The combination determines who someone is, but can also fluctuate based on several factors, including nutrition, surroundings, stage in life, climate, and time of the year.[22] A disturbance in any *dosha* can result in illness.[13,22] In Ayurvedic medicine, epilepsy is believed to originate from *Vata*, as this is the system responsible for neurology.[13] Other *doshas* are also involved as they help describe the different aspects and presentations of epilepsy.[13,20] The types of epilepsy are determined by the *doshas*, for example, a disturbance in the *Vata* leads to *Vatika* epilepsy. The summary of epilepsy types, presentation, treatment, and prognosis are shown in Table 8.

Table 8: Types of epilepsy in Ayurveda

Type of epilepsy	Presentation	Treatment	Prognosis
Vatika	Recurrent seizures featuring irrepressible crying, blackout, quivering, teeth grinding, delusions, extreme anxiety, distress, phobias, fury, exhilaration, and hyperventilation. A headache follows the attack.	Enema	Treatable with difficulty
Pattika	Nervousness, feeling extremely hot or thirsty, aura followed by seizures complemented by groaning and foaming at the mouth (yellow froth) and hitting oneself to the ground. The patient scratches the ground and has delusions of horrific things.	Purging	Treatable with difficulty
Kaphaja	The seizure is preceded by an aura where the patient sees all objects as white and feels cold. During the seizure the patient falls and produces whitish froth at the mouth. The seizure is protracted with delayed recovery.	Emesis	Treatable with difficulty
Tri-doshic or Sannipatika	A combination of all three. It presents with symptoms associated with the other three at the same time.	Incurable	Very poor

Extracted from information in articles by Manyam[13] and Brown[20]

In Ayurveda, the type of epilepsy determines the treatment, though all options seem to be focused on cleansing the gut. They also recognize a category of incurable epilepsy. In Ayurvedic medicine, the aim is to treat the whole person (body, mind, spirit), but the doctor must address the *doshas* first.[13] This is the reason they will cleanse the system before the introduction of individualized medicine to treat the condition.[13] Treatment comprises herbs, spices, diet, minerals (silver, mercury, lead), yoga, and positive living.[20]

Herbal medicine

Herbal treatments have been explored for their potential to alleviate seizure activity and improve overall neurological health. Among the most studied is *Cannabis sativa*, particularly cannabidiol (CBD), which is recognized for its antiseizure properties due to its interaction with endocannabinoid receptors and modulation of synaptic transmission.[5,14,23] Research has shown that CBD can be effective in reducing seizure frequency, especially in DRE like Dravet syndrome.[5,14,23]

Bacopa monnieri, commonly used in Ayurvedic medicine, is believed to enhance cognitive function and has antioxidant effects that may protect neurons and reduce seizure activity.[27] While some herbs show some antiseizure properties, they also pose risks of seizure-inducing effects as well as interacting with AEDs. For instance, *Ginkgo biloba* has been associated with an increased risk of seizures, by lowering seizure threshold.[6,23,28]

Several herbal extracts, such as those from valerian and passion flower, have traditionally been used in epilepsy treatment.[6,28,29] The use of herbal extracts should be carefully managed to avoid toxic reactions or interference with conventional treatment.[5,23] While these remedies show promise, careful consideration of dosages and potential interactions with AEDs is necessary. CBD has the most evidence in managing certain epilepsy syndromes.[23] Other herbs lack consistent clinical backing.

Most herbs are distributed through social network marketing. They are readily available and aggressively marketed, therefore there is a need to give guidance to PWE to help them decide whether these herbs are worth trying. Desperate to be seizure-free, several people have bought these products. I want to explore the effectiveness of these products so that PWE can make an informed decision on whether to buy.

Dietary supplements in epilepsy management

Magnesium is an essential mineral that plays a role in brain activity and nerve transmission. Magnesium deficiency has been linked to increased chances of seizures in PWE, suggesting that taking magnesium as a supplement could help individuals with epilepsy.[6,16,23] However, while certain findings indicate potential antiseizure effects, extreme caution should be exercised because too much magnesium can cause gastrointestinal effects and even toxicity in high doses.[6,16,23]

Various vitamins have been studied for their role in seizure control. For example, vitamin B6 (pyridoxine) deficiency is known to cause seizures in rare cases, so taking a vitamin B6 supplement can help.[15,16] It is important to note that not all PWE have this pyridoxine-dependent epilepsy, therefore indiscriminately taking vitamin B6 might not benefit everyone with epilepsy. Other minerals, such as zinc and selenium, are critical in maintaining normal neurological functions. However, their effectiveness as supplements in epilepsy has not been proved.[2,24] Vitamin B6, magnesium, and folic acid are sometimes used in epilepsy management, given their neurological roles.[6,25] In general, care should be exercised when taking supplements because taking them in excess could lead to toxicity or interact negatively with AEDs.[9,24]

The ketogenic diet, high in fats and low in carbs, has shown efficacy in reducing seizures, especially in pediatric cases. This requires supplements to offset potential deficiencies.[25] More on the KD is explained in Chapter 6.

Omega-3 fatty acids, found in fish oil, are known for their anti-inflammatory and brain-protecting properties. Some studies show that taking omega-3 supplements could reduce seizure frequency and improve overall brain health.[16,26] However, clinical results have not confirmed this theory. Side effects of excessive intake include potential blood-thinning effects, which may pose risks, especially for those on anticoagulants[26] (medicines that prevent clot formation, e.g., warfarin).

Amino acids such as taurine and L-glutamine play a critical role in brain signaling and could help in managing seizures.[4,23] Taurine, for example, may regulate the stimulatory-suppressive balance in the brain.[28] However, the effectiveness and safety of amino acid supplements have not been adequately proved in large-scale clinical trials.[23]

Probiotics - Emerging studies seek to explore the relationship between gut health and brain function. This is called the gut–brain axis. The gut–brain axis is being studied for its role in seizure activity. Though initial findings show promise, there is no adequate evidence for standard recommendations.[2,15]

A well-balanced diet rich in essential nutrients is crucial for overall brain health and may complement epilepsy management.[4,25] Dietary patterns like the ketogenic diet emphasize the importance of macronutrient distribution for seizure control.[25,26] However, arbitrary use of dietary supplements without expert supervision can disturb nutritional balance and negatively impact health.[25,26]

Risks and interactions

While dietary supplements can benefit individuals taking them, they are also associated with significant risks, especially when used together with AEDs. Possible interactions with AEDs could alter their effectiveness, even leading to toxicity in some cases.[6,9,23] St. John's wort, for example, can lower blood levels of certain AEDs, reducing their effectiveness.[5,6,9] Additionally, contaminants in unregulated supplements, such as heavy metals, can have toxic effects on the brain.[6,9]

Consideration for clinicians

Clinicians should assess the potential benefits and risks of dietary supplements for patients with epilepsy, ensuring their safe integration into treatment plans.[4,16,23] This includes a thorough review of current medications, dietary habits, and any supplements being taken.[2,24,26] Patient education is essential to highlight the importance of evidence-based use of supplements and avoid unsupervised, potentially harmful practices.[23,24,26] If you're taking dietary supplements, be sure to inform your doctor so they can provide appropriate guidance.

Acupuncture and traditional Chinese medicine

Acupuncture and traditional Chinese medicine (TCM) are among the most prominent forms of CAM used in epilepsy management.

Acupuncture involves inserting fine needles into specific body points to balance energy flow.[30,31] It is believed to regulate brain chemical transmitter levels and support internal production of a pain-relieving compound.[30,31] Through the regulation of neural activity, acupuncture is believed to influence seizure frequency.[30,31] While it is accepted in Eastern medicine to control seizures, there is no scientific evidence supporting its effectiveness in epilepsy management.[30,31] TCM often includes herbal remedies aimed at enhancing *qi* (vital energy) balance. Certain traditional formulas, such as *Dingxian Wan*, have historical use for seizure reduction. However, the safety and efficacy of TCM need more rigorous examination to establish reliable clinical recommendations.[23,30]

Mind–body techniques

Mind–body techniques, like meditation, yoga, and guided imagery, draw attention to the relationship between mental states and physical health. These approaches can help reduce stress and anxiety. Some people have seizures triggered by stress and anxiety, so it is believed by reducing these triggers, seizure frequency will be lowered as well.[1,26] Research indicates that mindfulness practices can have a positive impact on patients with epilepsy, potentially enhancing quality of life and psychological resilience. Yoga has been associated with reduced seizure activity in some cases through mechanisms of the parasympathetic nervous system, which regulates involuntary functions like respiration rate, blood pressure, and digestion to name a few.[25,26]

Biofeedback and neurofeedback

Biofeedback and neurofeedback are techniques used to train individuals to control specific processes in the body by providing real-time feedback as things happen.[2,16] Biofeedback includes observing and managing functions of the body like muscle tension. Neurofeedback specifically focuses on brainwave activity.[16] The individual will be better equipped to gain control over some voluntary processes that could trigger seizures.[2,16] Some evidence, though little, is available to support the effectiveness of neurofeedback in the reduction of seizure frequency, especially for people with DRE.[2,16] The actual mechanism may involve the regulation of neural pathways linked to seizure onset and control.[26]

Homeopathy and naturopathy

Homeopathy, developed in the 18th century by Samuel Hahnemann, a German physician, is founded on the principle that "like cures like."[15,19] It is believed substances causing symptoms in healthy individuals can be administered in highly diluted forms to treat similar symptoms. Scientific validation of the effectiveness of homeopathy in treating epilepsy is limited.[15,19] Naturopathy uses natural remedies, including dietary supplements, vitamins, and lifestyle changes, to support overall health and potentially mitigate seizure triggers.[32] As covered earlier, it has been scientifically proven that some natural supplements can interact with AEDs, putting people at risk of adverse effects or altered AED efficacy. For instance, St. John's wort, a common supplement used for mood regulation, can significantly decrease the effectiveness of AEDs through cytochrome P450 enzyme induction.[6,33]

Chiropractic and osteopathic medicine

Chiropractic and osteopathic procedures have been linked to seizure control, maybe because they focus on spinal alignment and its impact on the nervous system. There is minimal evidence confirming that spinal manipulation as done during chiropractic adjustments contributes to a reduction in seizure frequency.[20,28,34] Osteopathic medicine focuses on musculoskeletal treatment, which includes cranial techniques aimed at improving cerebrospinal fluid flow and overall neurological health.[16,32,35]

Aromatherapy

Aromatherapy utilizes essential oils such as lavender and chamomile. These oils are associated with reducing stress through their calming properties. The reduction in stress could help with seizure management.[13,14,36] These oils are thought to act on the body system responsible for regulating emotions and stress. Some studies suggest consistent use of specific essential oils could decrease the possibility of seizures in some people.[22,23,37]

Music therapy

Music therapy uses stimuli created by certain rhythms and harmonies to regulate brain wave activity and emotional states. Certain studies have suggested listening to Mozart's compositions might reduce seizure frequency, but evidence is inconsistent.[25] Certain types of music, especially those with rhythmic patterns like the brain's natural waves, may help in seizure management.[17,38,39] Music therapy can also reduce anxiety and improve quality of life, making it a valuable complement to more traditional treatment approaches.[11,26,40]

Religious and spiritual practices in epilepsy management

Religious and spiritual practices have long been integral to managing chronic illnesses like epilepsy. While modern medicine is key for seizure control, many individuals and communities combine spiritual practices to enhance well-being and coping. In some cases, these spiritual practices can also impact adherence negatively, however. Though not a replacement for medical care, spiritual practices are important in addressing the psychological and social aspects of epilepsy, and clinicians should acknowledge people as spiritual beings and take what they believe into consideration when creating a treatment plan.

Prayer and faith healing

Some PWE incorporate prayer and faith healing into their conventional treatment. In many cultures, prayer is used to seek help from a higher power, which can result in improved seizure control or overall well-being.[31,41] Faith healing is popular especially where access to medical care is limited or where spiritual beliefs are deeply intertwined with health practices.[4,31] Faith-based approaches work best when combined with conventional medicine, where faith supports the emotional side, giving people a sense of empowerment.[1]

Meditation and contemplative prayer

Meditation and contemplative prayer reduce seizures by promoting relaxation and reducing stress.[29,32] Studies have shown that these practices have an effect on regulating brain activity, leading to seizure management.[25,26] Techniques such as mindfulness meditation help improve self-awareness and calm the nervous system, making them useful as part of a broader treatment plan for epilepsy.[1] While there is inadequate clinical evidence, many PWE have self-reported an improvement in their quality of life when including meditation as part of their treatment plan.[19]

Rituals and ceremonial practices

In some communities and cultures, certain rituals and ceremonies play a pivotal role in how epilepsy is perceived and managed.[12,31] These rituals could include chants, dances, or herbal applications all performed with the belief individuals will be protected and spiritually cleansed.[12,40] These practices can strengthen social bonds and provide psychological benefits to individuals and their families.[31] However, the effectiveness of these rituals from a medical perspective remains a topic for further study.[32,42]

Support from religious communities

Different religious communities provide psychosocial benefits to those living with epilepsy.[3,35] The collective backing of a community provides a sense of belonging, reduces stigma, and promotes positive mental health.[43] Studies have shown that individuals who feel supported by their religious groups report lower levels of anxiety and depression.[3,35] Moreover, religious leaders often play a role in educating communities about epilepsy, helping to dispel myths and encourage treatment adherence.[11,31] This is not universal because some religions alienate PWE or consider them people who need to be "fixed" (see Chapter 11).

Spiritual counseling and pastoral care

Spiritual counseling and pastoral care are integral for many patients who seek guidance beyond the medical sphere. These services offer emotional and spiritual support, helping individuals navigate the complexities of chronic illness.[34,38] Pastoral counselors are trained to work alongside medical professionals to provide holistic care that addresses both spiritual and psychological needs.[1] This integrated approach can aid in enhancing patients' adherence to medical regimens and overall coping strategies.[2,35]

Holistic integrative approaches

Holistic approaches that integrate spiritual and medical practices are increasingly popular among PWE.[4,26] These methods combine traditional spiritual practices with modern medical treatment to support overall well-being.[4,44] An example includes combining prayer or meditation with lifestyle modifications such as dietary adjustments and regular exercise, aimed at reducing seizure frequency.[29,41] Studies have indicated that when patients engage in comprehensive care that includes both spiritual and medical elements, there is often an improvement in their outlook and treatment adherence.[17,18]

Motivations for using CAM

Multiple factors influence the use of CAM. Some of the factors include cultural beliefs, dissatisfaction with conventional treatments, and personal preference for natural therapies.[38,42,45] Cultural and societal factors are key drivers in the adoption of CAM, as people from various cultural backgrounds find comfort integrating traditional and natural remedies into their care.[9,24,36] Additionally, the cost and accessibility of AEDs, particularly in low-resource settings, drive some patients to seek alternative treatments as a more affordable option.[31,40] Many people, especially in LMICs, still use CAM as their first line of addressing any health issues.[12] People have genuine reasons for resorting to CAM and I discuss a few of the reasons in the following sub-sections.

Drug-resistant epilepsy

As previously mentioned, seizures of 30% of PWE do not respond to AEDs, meaning they have DRE. People with DRE are likely to resort to CAM. No one would want to continue having seizures, so if the conventional medicines fail, people naturally try other things.

Side effects of AEDs

AEDs have undesirable side effects and herbal medicines are said to have "no side effects." Whether this is true will be discussed in this chapter. Logically, a person would want a product with no side effects. If people are convinced that a product has no side effects, it would be sound to try it.

Accessibility and affordability

In regions with limited access to AEDs, CAM becomes an affordable alternative, often available through traditional practitioners.[7,46] Payment methods for the herbal medicines, especially those that come from traditional herbalists, witchdoctors or "prophets" seem more comfortable because livestock is accepted as a form of payment in LMICs. The sad thing is that many have ended up with empty kraals, yet their condition persists.[53]

Supernatural beliefs

In certain communities, as discussed in earlier chapters, it is generally believed epilepsy is a spiritual condition or witchcraft-induced, and cannot be treated with conventional medicines. According to Mugumbate and Mushonga,[11] what people understand to be the cause of epilepsy is what leads them to seek "traditional methods where ancestors are consulted by a traditional healer" as a treatment option. A supernatural condition needs a spiritual cure. According to the World Health Organization (WHO),[7] in Senegal, it takes an average of 13.4 years for a PWE to visit a healthcare center.[53] The same average could be applied to many African countries. PWE in Buhera (Zimbabwe) only sought medical treatment after an average of 5 years from the first time they had seizures.[11] Before seeking medical attention, they will be trying different methods of treatment dependent on their beliefs.[11,53]

Clinician training gap

Some clinicians are not immune to the prevailing beliefs on the condition of epilepsy. There is also a training gap on the condition causing many failing to give proper counseling to newly diagnosed patients, which in my view is the greatest contributor to people resorting to CAM. From observation, I have witnessed healthcare workers refer PWE to herbalists, witchdoctors or prophets. Society regards healthcare workers as opinion leaders on health issues, so if a clinician tells me to try CAM, I am likely to try it.

Unavailability of AEDs

Someone may be truly committed to adhere and comply to treatment regimens, but most of the health centers in most LMICs do not usually have stock.[7] At times they only have one type, usually phenobarbitone, and those on other medicines are given the available medicine out of the healthcare worker's ignorance because they think any AED will work for any type of epilepsy. When someone starts having seizures because they cannot access medicines from the local clinic, they are likely to resort to CAM.

Distance from medical facilities

Many people, especially in the rural areas, live far away from the nearest health center and would need to board a bus to go there, yet the witch doctor, prophet, or herbalist will be in their neighborhood. Out of desperation, the first port of call will be the witch doctor's practice and depending on the beliefs of the affected people, they may never go to a healthcare facility.

Seizure control and quality of life

Some patients report better mood, reduced anxiety, and improved seizure control with CAM, though self-reports lack objective validation.[4,41] Through the power of word of mouth or social media, people provide reviews for the CAM they have used. Using these reviews, others make decisions to try CAM with the hope of getting similar results as shared by the reviewers.

Cultural health practices

Many traditional cultures integrate CAM into daily healthcare, increasing its popularity among communities with strong cultural ties.[11,35]

Natural product perception

The belief that natural remedies are inherently safer or more effective fuels CAM's popularity despite limited evidence.[11]

Risks associated with CAM in epilepsy

Evidence suggests most patients never disclose their use of CAM to their doctor.[5] They will attend all review sessions with their doctor and never tell them they are also taking other things besides the drugs they have been prescribed. This situation makes it very difficult to tell why someone continues to have seizures or why they present with certain side effects that may not be associated with the prescription drug. The doctor may be forced to change the drug to another one or even to increase the dose depending on the presentation, yet these anomalies will be coming from taking CAM. To emphasize this point, Sweetman *et al.* report the case of a 55-year-old man who was on phenytoin and valproate treatment. The man died while taking over-the-counter supplements, such as vitamins and herbal products, including *Ginkgo biloba* extract, without his doctor's knowledge.[47] Post-mortem analysis revealed that the levels of both AEDs in his system were below therapeutic range. While the exact cause of death was uncertain, the authors theorized that *G. biloba* might have induced hepatic enzymes, leading to increased drug clearance.[47]

Are these herbs as "clean" as people would want us to believe?

Many herbs contain seizure-inducing neurotoxins, may be contaminated with heavy metals like lead or arsenic, or include hidden conventional drugs. They can also alter how anti-epileptic drugs are absorbed, metabolized, or excreted, potentially reducing their effectiveness.
Samuels, et al.[5]

After a detailed study on pharmacokinetics and pharmacodynamics in the previous chapter, this statement makes a lot of sense, does it not? CAM therapies can pose significant safety concerns, particularly when they are used concurrently with AEDs. Some herbal and dietary supplements can interact with AEDs, either enhancing or diminishing their effects and potentially leading to an increase in seizure frequency.[20,23,34] Additionally, the fluctuation, inconsistency, and unpredictability in the quality and potency of CAM products presents a safety issue, as contamination, dilution, and inconsistent active ingredient concentrations are common.[25,30,41] Chronic exposure to heavy metal contaminants, for example, can result in damage to the nervous system, which is particularly concerning for epilepsy patients.[9] Due to these concerns, understanding the safety profile, efficacy, and potential interactions of each CAM intervention is crucial for safe incorporation into epilepsy care.[28,43]

Studies have shown that ephedra, herbal caffeine, Creatine, St. John's wort (SJW), and *G. biloba* were responsible for inducing seizures in people taking them for weight loss or athletic performance at the recommended doses.[5,6,23] These elements lower seizure threshold, inadvertently worsening epilepsy.[5,23] SJW is a herbal remedy that has been used for centuries for treatment of mild depression and wounds. Research has shown that SJW interacts with many drugs including AEDs by induction of several drug-metabolizing enzymes, thereby reducing the effectiveness of these AEDs (phenobarbitone, carbamazepine, and phenytoin) leading to possible seizures.[33] Grapefruit juice increases the bioavailability of carbamazepine by inhibiting CYP3A4 enzymes in the gut wall and liver.[8] Valerian and kava, for example, may increase sedation, potentially interacting with AEDs and impairing cognitive function.[23]

The following essential oils are strong seizure inducers: *Eucalyptus, fennel, hyssop, pennyroyal, rosemary, sage, savin, tansy, thuja, turpentine, and wormwood due to their content of highly reactive monoterpene ketones, such as camphor, pinocamphone, thujone, cineole, pulegone, sabinylacetate, and fenchone.*[14]

Other herbs, shankhapusphi, star anise, star fruit, evening primrose oil and starflower (borage) have all been associated with inducing seizures.[5]

Another problem is that often, no one really knows what active ingredients could be contained in the herbal medicines they could be taking. Most conventional medicines are extracted from plants, so if someone is taking adequate doses of a conventional drug, and they are also given herbs from which that same drug is extracted from, there is a risk of over-dosage. Moreover, the interactions of conventional AEDs are well known and documented, but with CAM, these interactions are unknown. If they were known and publicized, people could be advised not to mix a particular CAM with a particular AED.

Herbal medicines pose a health threat in that no two plants contain the same active ingredients in the same quantities.[20] Many factors influence these variations like weather conditions or where the plant was picked from (near a river, at the bottom or top of a mountain, etc.). The season of picking also affects the quality of the plant in terms of the active ingredient and the type of soil plays an important part.

Regulation of CAM for epilepsy

Given these complex dynamics, the regulation of CAM presents its own set of challenges. Regulatory frameworks for CAM vary widely across regions, with some countries offering minimal oversight of CAM products compared with the stringent controls applied to pharmaceuticals.[37,46,48] For example, the US treats CAM as dietary supplements, whereas Europe has stricter oversight.[37,46] In some countries, there is not even a label or container to talk about. The CAM is dispensed in any packaging, including newspapers, leaves, cotton, gourds, or empty cooking oil bottles. The dose can be described in terms of a pinch or a drop. Lack of standardized manufacturing and labeling protocols can lead to inconsistencies in potency and safety.[31]

This disparity in regulation raises concerns about product quality, labeling, and safety standards, making it difficult for both patients and healthcare providers to navigate the CAM landscape effectively.[35,49] In many cases, CAM products are marketed as dietary supplements rather than medicines, resulting in reduced regulatory scrutiny and leaving patients at risk of using potentially unsafe or ineffective therapies.[44,50] Patients often perceive CAM as safe due to its "natural" label, underscoring the need for regulatory bodies to address misconceptions and ensure transparent labeling.[46]

CAM and drug interactions

As already discussed in the previous chapter, drug interactions occur in any of the following forms:
- One drug can weaken the other—the CAM can weaken the AED or vice versa through enzyme induction or inhibition. For example, SJW induces enzyme activity, reducing AED effectiveness and increasing seizure risk.[5,8,33] Also, grapefruit juice inhibits enzyme CYP3A4, potentially increasing the effects of certain AEDs.[8,23]
- One drug can cause an increase in blood concentration of the other drug resulting in a high possibility of toxic effects of the drug whose levels have been raised, whether AED or CAM or both drugs, leading to undesirable effects.

- CAM practices like Ayurveda and TCM emphasize multiple active ingredients, which may interact unpredictably with conventional drugs.[33]

In summary combining drugs carries with it risk of interactions: some may be minor, but others can be dangerous and even life-threatening.

Do not buy stories of people who claim that nutritional supplements have no effect on conventional medicines. I discussed the risks of interactions caused by vitamin B6, folic acid and folinic acid, meaning supplements can cause interactions. As discussed, grapefruit juice causes serious interactions, so it is not as easy as people make it look.

The greatest danger of CAM is that many times, no one knows what they are really taking. The modern packages that are being used now may not list everything contained in that product. At times they just list the "major" ingredient(s) they want to profile and ignore other things that may be contained in that preparation, whether intentional or out of ignorance. The person taking the product is at a great risk from side effects that they never anticipated.

The role of the clinician in CAM

The role of clinicians in guiding patients through CAM use in epilepsy is paramount. As CAM continues to grow in popularity, it is essential that healthcare providers engage patients in open discussions regarding their CAM use, potential risks, and known evidence.[39] Clinicians can encourage open discussions about CAM to avoid hidden risks, particularly with potentially interacting supplements.[1,50] By fostering a non-judgmental approach, clinicians can encourage honest communication, which is critical for managing potential adverse effects and avoiding hidden interactions between CAM and AEDs.[51] For CAM therapies with some evidence of efficacy, such as the ketogenic diet or CBD, clinicians may play a key role in ensuring that these interventions are used safely and in conjunction with conventional epilepsy treatments.[17,25,26] Furthermore, educating patients on the limitations and risks associated with unproven CAM therapies can promote informed decision-making and reinforce trust between patients and providers.[3,6] Regular assessments to monitor potential adverse effects from CAM are essential, especially when combined with AEDs.[50] Where evidence supports it, clinicians might consider recommending specific CAM interventions, such as CBD for treatment-resistant epilepsy, within a conventional plan.[2] Clinicians should respect patient beliefs about CAM, promoting a collaborative approach to epilepsy management.[2,16]

Conclusion

In summary, CAM in epilepsy presents both opportunities and challenges, with a variety of therapies that appeal to patients for their perceived benefits in seizure control and quality of life. However, the integration of CAM into epilepsy management requires careful consideration of efficacy, safety, regulation, and the role of clinicians in guiding its use. I conclude this chapter by saying "It is your responsibility to take care of your health. Do not just take a product because someone says it will work. It might have worked for them, but there is no guarantee it will work for you. If you really think you are a CAM person, then be 100% CAM and avoid mixing drugs because the results can be fatal. The same applies to someone who is for AEDs, be 100% on AEDs and avoid mixing with CAM. If you need to take both, do it in liaison with your doctor." If we do this, it will be easier to manage our different conditions.

References:

1. Asadi-Pooya, A. A., Brigo, F., Lattanzi, S., Karakis, I., Asadollahi, M., Trinka, E., ... & Jusupova, A. (2021). Complementary and alternative medicine in epilepsy: A global survey of physicians' opinions. *Epilepsy & Behavior, 117*. https://doi.org/10.1016/j.yebeh.2021.107835
2. Farrukh, M. J., Makmor-Bakry, M., Hatah, E., & Tan, H. J. (2018). Use of complementary and alternative medicine and adherence to antiepileptic drug therapy among epilepsy patients: a systematic review. *Patient Preference and Adherence*, 2111-2121. https://doi.org/10.2147/PPA.S179031
3. Baker, G.A. (2002). The Psychosocial Burden of Epilepsy, *Epilepsia, 43* (Suppl. 6):26–30.
4. Mesraoua, B., Kissani, N., Deleu, D., Elsheikh, L., Ali, M., Melikyan, G., ... & Asadi-Pooya, A. A. (2021). Complementary and alternative medicine (CAM) for epilepsy treatment in the Middle East and North Africa (MENA) region. *Epilepsy Research, 170*. https://doi.org/10.1016/j.eplepsyres.2020.106538
5. Samuels, N., Finkelstein, Y., Singer, S. R., & Oberbaum, M. (2008). Herbal medicine and epilepsy: proconvulsive effects and interactions with antiepileptic drugs. *Epilepsia, 49*(3), 373-380. https:doi.org/10.1111/j.1528-1167.2007.01379.x

6. Haller, C. A., Meier, K. H., & Olson, K. R. (2005). Seizures reported in association with use of dietary supplements. *Clinical Toxicology, 43*(1), 23-30. https://doi.org/10.1081/CLT-44771
7. World Health Organization. (2004). *Epilepsy in the WHO Africa Region: Bridging the Gap: The Global Campaign Against Epilepsy "Out of the Shadows."* Geneva: World Health Organization. https://www.ibe-epilepsy.org/downloads/EPILEPSY%20AFRICAN%20Report.pdf
8. Garg, S. K., Kumar, N., Bhargava, V. K., & Prabhakar, S. K. (1998). Effect of grapefruit juice on carbamazepine bioavailability in patients with epilepsy. *Clinical Pharmacology & Therapeutics, 64*(3), 286-288. https://doi.org/10.1016/S0009-9236(98)90177-1
9. Dunbabin, D.W. (1992). Lead poisoning from Indian herbal medicine (Ayurveda), *The Medical Journal of Australia, 157*(11-12), 835-836. https://cir.nii.ac.jp/crid/1571698599960217088
10. Krishnamurthy, M.S. (2014). Epilepsy – Ayurvedic understanding and its treatment. http://easyayurveda.com/2014/04/23/epilepsy-ayurvedic-understanding-treatment/
11. Mugumbate, J. and Mushonga, J. (2013). Myths, perceptions, and incorrect knowledge surrounding epilepsy in rural Zimbabwe: A study of the villagers in Buhera District, *Epilepsy & Behavior, 27*, 144–147.
12. Carod-Artal, F.J. & V´azquez-Cabrera, C.B. (2007). An anthropological study about epilepsy in native tribes from Central and South America. *Epilepsia, 48*(5), 886–893.
13. Manyam, B.V. (1992). Epilepsy in Ancient India, *Epilepsia, 33*(3):473-175. https://doi.org/10.1111/j.1528-1157.1992.tb01694.x
14. Burkhard, P. R., Burkhardt, K., Haenggeli, C. A., & Landis, T. (1999). Plant-induced seizures: Reappearance of an old problem. *Journal of Neurology, 246*, 667-670. https://doi.org/10.1007/s004150050429
15. Zhu, Z., Mittal, R., Walser, S. A., Lehman, E., Kumar, A., Paudel, S., & Mainali, G. (2022). Complementary and alternative medicine (CAM) use in children with epilepsy. *Journal of Child Neurology, 37*(5), 334-339. https://doi.org/10.1177/08830738211069790
16. Asadi-Pooya, A. A., Homayoun, M., & Sharifi, S. (2019). Complementary and integrative medicine in epilepsy: what patients and physicians perceive. *Epilepsy & Behavior, 101*. https://doi.org/10.1016/j.yebeh.2019.106545
17. Bosak, M., & Słowik, A. (2019). Use of complementary and alternative medicine among adults with epilepsy in a university epilepsy clinic in Poland. *Epilepsy & Behavior, 98*, 40-44. https://doi.org/10.1016/j.yebeh.2019.06.004
18. Farrukh, M. J., Makmor-Bakry, M., Hatah, E., & Jan, T. H. (2021). Impact of complementary and alternative medicines on antiepileptic medication adherence among epilepsy patients. *BMC Complementary Medicine and Therapies, 21*, 1-9. https://doi.org/10.1186/s12906-021-03224-2
19. Zhu, Z., Dluzynski, D., Hammad, N., Pugalenthi, D., Walser, S. A., Mittal, R., ... & Naik, S. (2023). Use of integrative, complementary, and alternative medicine in children with epilepsy: A global scoping review. *Children, 10*(4), 713. https://doi.org/10.3390/children10040713
20. Brown, E. (2010). Ayurveda and the "Sacred Disease" : Treating epilepsy with ancient Ayurvedic wisdom. www.chopra.com/files/docs/teacherdownloads/.../Epilepsy,%20Erin%20brown.pdf
21. Wikipedia. (2024). Dosha. https://en.wikipedia.org/wiki/Dosha
22. Singh, A. (2022). Doshas in Ayurveda - Vata, Pitta and Kapha. https://www.forestessentialsindia.com/blog/doshas-in-ayurveda-vata-pitta-and-kapha.html?srsltid=AfmBOorAr7PyKybMY28EKgHio0oe0nbk0COk_xsnK2FE4M70IvMg5RoX

23. Liu, W., Ge, T., Pan, Z., Leng, Y., Lv, J., & Li, B. (2017). The effects of herbal medicine on epilepsy. *Oncotarget, 8*(29). https://doi.org/10.18632/oncotarget.16801
24. Tsvere, M., Chiweshe, M. K., & Mutanana, N. (2020). General side effects and challenges associated with anti-epilepsy medication: A review of related literature. *African Journal of Primary Health Care and Family Medicine, 12*(1), 1-5. https://doi.org/10.4102/phcfm.v12i1.2162
25. Brackney, D. E., & Brooks, J. L. (2018). Complementary and alternative medicine: The Mozart Effect on childhood epilepsy—A systematic review. *The Journal of School Nursing, 34*(1), 28-37. https://doi.org/10.1177/1059840517740940
26. Dawit, S., & Crepeau, A. Z. (2020). When drugs do not work: Alternatives to antiseizure medications. *Current Neurology and Neuroscience Reports, 20*, 1-8. https://doi.org/10.1007/s11910-020-01061-3
27. LiverTox. (2024). Clinical and Research Information on Drug-Induced Liver Injury [Internet]. Bethesda (MD): National Institute of Diabetes and Digestive and Kidney Diseases; 2012. *Bacopa Monnieri*. [Updated 2024 Apr 24]. https://www.ncbi.nlm.nih.gov/books/NBK603563/
28. Sharifi-Rad, J., Quispe, C., Herrera-Bravo, J., Martorell, M., Sharopov, F., Tumer, T. B., ... & Calina, D. (2021). A pharmacological perspective on plant-derived bioactive molecules for epilepsy. *Neurochemical Research, 46*(9), 2205-2225. https://doi.org/10.1007/s11064-021-03376-0
29. Bahr, T. A., Rodriguez, D., Beaumont, C., & Allred, K. (2019). The effects of various essential oils on epilepsy and acute seizure: a systematic review. *Evidence-Based Complementary and Alternative Medicine, 2019*(1). https://doi.org/10.1155/2019/6216745
30. Lin, C. H., & Hsieh, C. L. (2021). Chinese herbal medicine for treating epilepsy. *Frontiers in Neuroscience, 15*. https://doi.org/10.3389/fnins.2021.682821
31. Kpobi, L., Swartz, L., & Keikelame, M. J. (2018). Ghanaian traditional and faith healers' explanatory models for epilepsy. *Epilepsy & Behavior, 84*, 88-92. https://doi.org/10.1016/j.yebeh.2018.04.016
32. Auditeau, E., Moyano, L. M., Bourdy, G., Nizard, M., Jost, J., Ratsimbazafy, V., ... & Boumediene, F. (2018). Herbal medicine uses to treat people with epilepsy: A survey in rural communities of northern Peru. *Journal of Ethnopharmacology, 215*, 184-190. https://www.sciencedirect.com/science/article/pii/S0378874117342162
33. Medicines Control Agency (MCA). (2000). Committee on safety of medicines. Reminder: St John's Wort (Hypericum Perforatum) Interactions. Current problems, http://www.mhra.gov.uk/home/groups/pl-p/documents/.../con007462.pdf.
34. Mutanana, N. (2019). Challenges associated with anti-epilepsy medication and use of complementary or alternative medicines among people with epilepsy in rural communities of Zimbabwe. *Malaysian Journal of Medical and Biological Research, 6*(2), 77-84. https://www.academia.edu/download/85318294/423.pdf
35. Falcicchio, G., Negri, F., Trojano, M., & La Neve, A. (2022). On epilepsy perception: Unravelling gaps and issues. *Epilepsy & Behavior, 137*. *https://doi.org/10.1016/j.yebeh.2022.108952*
36. Nasif, M. B., Koubeissi, M., & Azar, N. J. (2021). Epilepsy–from mysticism to science. *Revue Neurologique, 177*(9), 1047-1058. https://doi.org/10.1016/j.neurol.2021.01.021
37. Stockings, E., Zagic, D., Campbell, G., Weier, M., Hall, W. D., Nielsen, S., ... & Degenhardt, L. (2018). Evidence for cannabis and cannabinoids for epilepsy: a systematic review of controlled and observational evidence. *Journal of Neurology, Neurosurgery & Psychiatry, 89*(7), 741-753. https://jnnp.bmj.com/content/89/7/741?link_id=12&can_id=a21edf2cf58c74fb33e63502

907aab7c&source=email-norml-news-of-the-week-3152018-2&email_referrer=email_318733&email_subject=norml-news-of-the-week-3152018
38. Rutebemberwa, E., Ssemugabo, C., Tweheyo, R., Turyagaruka, J., & Pariyo, G. W. (2020). Biomedical drugs and traditional treatment in care seeking pathways for adults with epilepsy in Masindi district, Western Uganda: A household survey. *BMC health services research, 20*, 1-13. https://doi.org/10.1186/s12913-019-4879-2
39. Can, V., Bulduk, M., Ayşin, N., Can, E. K., & Aydın, N. (2024). Determination of complementary and alternative medicine use frequency and related factors in children with epilepsy: A descriptive Cross-Sectional study from eastern Turkey. *Epilepsy & Behavior, 160*. https://doi.org/10.1016/j.yebeh.2024.110041
40. Birhan, Y. S. (2022). Medicinal plants utilized in the management of epilepsy in Ethiopia: ethnobotany, pharmacology and phytochemistry. *Chinese Medicine, 17*(1), 129. https://doi.org/10.1186/s13020-022-00686-5
41. Beattie, J. F., Thompson, M. D., Parks, P. H., Jacobs, R. Q., & Goyal, M. (2017). Caregiver-reported religious beliefs and complementary and alternative medicine use among children admitted to an epilepsy monitoring unit. *Epilepsy & Behavior, 69*, 139-146. https://doi.org/10.1016/j.yebeh.2017.01.026
42. M. Manchishi, S. (2018). Recent advances in antiepileptic herbal medicine. *Current Neuropharmacology, 16*(1), 79-83. https://doi.org/10.2174/1570159X15666170518151809
43. Kissani, N., Moro, M., & Arib, S. (2020). Knowledge, attitude and traditional practices towards epilepsy among relatives of PWE (patients with epilepsy) in Marrakesh, Morocco. *Epilepsy & Behavior, 111*. https://doi.org/10.1016/j.yebeh.2020.107257
44. Tan, M., & Kavurmaci, M. (2021). Complementary and alternative medicine use in Turkish patients with epilepsy. *Alternative Therapies in Health and Medicine, 27*.
45. Çarman, K. B., Gürlevik, S. L., Kaplan, E., Dinleyici, M., Yarar, C., & Arslantaş, D. (2018). The evaluation of use of complementary and alternative medicine practices in the treatment of children with chronic neurological disease. *Haydarpasa Numune Medical Journal, 58*(3), 117-121. https://doi.org.10.14744/hnhj.2018.43265
46. James, P. B., Wardle, J., Steel, A., & Adams, J. (2018). Traditional, complementary and alternative medicine use in Sub-Saharan Africa: a systematic review. *BMJ global health, 3*(5). http://dx.doi.org/10.1136/bmjgh-2018-000895
47. Sweetman, S.C. et al eds. 2009. "Antiepileptics" in: *Martindale: The Complete Drug Reference.* 36th ed. London: Pharmaceutical Press. 465-516.
48. Challal, S., Skiba, A., Langlois, M., Esguerra, C. V., Wolfender, J. L., Crawford, A. D., & Skalicka-Woźniak, K. (2023). Natural product-derived therapies for treating drug-resistant epilepsies: from ethnopharmacology to evidence-based medicine. *Journal of Ethnopharmacology, 317*. https://doi.org/10.1016/j.jep.2023.116740
49. Bogaert, B. (2024). Patient experiential knowledge and CAM: A case study of refractory epilepsy patients in France. https://www.researchgate.net/publication/381478999_Patient_experiential_knowledge_and_CAM_a_case_study_of_refractory_epilepsy_patients_in_France?enrichId=rgreq-76e0ad2be2dab134c1443f9be21a0325-XXX&enrichSource=Y292ZXJQYWdlOzM4MTQ3ODk5OTtBUzoxMTQzMTI4MTI1MjI1NDI5NEAxNzE4NjMyMzY4OTI1&el=1_x_2&_esc=publicationCoverPdf
50. Lau, B. T., Makmor-Bakry, M., Tan, H. J., Ng, S. Y., & Redzuan, A. M. (2020). Patient's Practice of Complementary and Alternative Medicine (CAM) for the Management of Epilepsy. *Journal of Advanced Pharmacy Education and Research, 10*(3-2020), 1-7.
51. Girgis, M. M. F., Fekete, K., Homoródi, N., Márton, S., Fekete, I., & Horváth, L. (2022). Use of complementary and alternative medicine among patients with epilepsy and diabetes

mellitus, focusing on the outcome of treatment. *Frontiers in Neuroscience, 15.* https://doi.org/10.3389/fnins.2021.787512
52. Temkin, O. (1971). *The Falling Sickness: A history of epilepsy from the Greeks to the beginnings of modern neurology.* The John Hopkins University Press: Baltimore and London.
53. International Bureau for Epilepsy. (2012). The dilemma of epilepsy – Personal short stories. https://www.ibe-epilepsy.org/wp-content/uploads/2012/07/IBE-Story-Book-Final.pdf

CHAPTER 8 – SUDDEN UNEXPECTED DEATH IN EPILEPSY (SUDEP)

SUDEP is the most important epilepsy-related cause of death, ranking second only to stroke among neurologic diseases in terms of potential years of life lost.
Thurman, Hesdorffer & French[2]

Young PWE face a 24- to 28-fold increased risk of SUDEP compared to the general population. However, the incidence of SUDEP varies widely across epilepsy populations.
T. Tomson, et al.[1]

Introduction

Epilepsy is a serious and often deadly condition, contradicting the belief that seizures are not life-threatening. The risk of early death is greatly increased for those who continue to have seizures without full control.[1,3] SUDEP, or sudden unexpected death in epilepsy, was formally recognized in the 1990s, and remains one of the most serious complications of epilepsy. It is particularly concerning due to its unpredictable nature. Studies estimate 1:1,000 PWE will die of SUDEP.[4] Actually, epilepsy is associated with a two- to three-fold increase in mortality compared with the general population, particularly in patients with poorly controlled seizures.[5,6] SUDEP is the most important direct epilepsy-related cause of death,[7,8] with at least 36% of deaths in epilepsy attributed to SUDEP.[9] The true figure may be nearer half of all epilepsy-related deaths, underscoring the importance of ongoing research and awareness initiatives to understand and mitigate SUDEP's risks. These low numbers could be due to under-reporting as will be covered later in this chapter. The global impact of SUDEP calls for increased awareness among clinicians, patients, and caregivers. Public health efforts are essential to promote SUDEP awareness, especially in low-resource settings where epilepsy treatment and monitoring are less accessible.[10,11] Improving education around SUDEP is necessary not only for families affected by epilepsy but also within the medical community to standardize preventive strategies and improve patient counseling. I have been treated by two specialist physicians and two neurologists in managing my seizures throughout the years, but none of them has ever discussed SUDEP with me.

Definition

What exactly is SUDEP? I will explore a few definitions for SUDEP in the literature and discuss them below. SUDEP is the sudden and unexpected, non-traumatic, and non-drowning death in individuals with epilepsy, where post mortem examination does not reveal any cause of death.[12,13] This phenomenon typically occurs in individuals with uncontrolled seizures, particularly those experiencing generalized tonic-clonic seizures.[12,13] The precise mechanisms behind SUDEP remain unclear, but it is believed to be associated with a combination of factors, including respiratory dysfunction, cardiac abnormalities, and autonomic dysregulation that may occur during or following a seizure.[13,14] SUDEP is underscored by its contribution to premature mortality in PWE, particularly among those with DRE.[6,15]

"SUDEP is an unexpected death in a person with epilepsy in whom no clear causes for death are found despite full postmortem examination."[1] In trying to make the issue of SUDEP clearer, Kloster and Engelskjøn state that it is "sudden" because it happens in a matter of minutes or hours.[16] They also say it is "unexpected" because the victims would have been in a reasonable state of health before they die.[16] What is clear from these definitions is that the PWE will not be having any signs of illness, yet they die unexpectedly. When an autopsy is conducted, nothing is detected as cause of death. SUDEP is classified into several types based on clinical findings and circumstances. Classification primarily includes the following categories:

Definite SUDEP: Defined as a sudden, unexpected, non-traumatic, and non-drowning death in a person with epilepsy, without any clear cause of death after a thorough autopsy.[14] The death typically occurs during or shortly after a seizure but without any other identifiable medical condition or injury.[14]

Probable SUDEP: This category is like definite SUDEP but lacks a post-mortem examination to confirm the absence of other causes.[12] Probable SUDEP is suspected when there is no other clear cause of death, even though autopsy results are unavailable.[12]

Possible SUDEP: This classification applies when an individual with epilepsy dies unexpectedly, but there are coexisting factors or medical conditions that might have contributed to the death, making it difficult to confirm SUDEP as the sole cause.[12]

Near-SUDEP: Refers to instances where a PWE experiences a life-threatening event resembling SUDEP, such as respiratory or cardiac arrest during a seizure, but is resuscitated successfully.[5] This category is important for studying risk factors and early interventions.

These classifications aid in understanding and studying SUDEP by recognizing cases with and without complete information on cause of death, helping researchers and clinicians improve identification and prevention efforts.

Epidemiology and incidence

SUDEP incidence is generally reported at between 1: 1,000 and 1:4,500 epilepsy patients per year, though the rate can be as high as 9:1,000 in those with DRE.[17,18] Factors such as seizure frequency, particularly generalized tonic-clonic seizures (GTCS), contribute significantly to the risk profile of SUDEP.

Specific populations face higher or lower risks based on various factors, including age, sex, and co-morbid conditions.[19,20] For example, SUDEP incidence is higher among young adults compared with children or elderly PWE. Males with both epilepsy and intellectual disabilities are also at a greater risk of SUDEP.[19,20] Such population-specific insights aid clinicians in identifying at-risk individuals and adapting preventative measures accordingly.

There are also notable differences in SUDEP rates globally. For example, incidence rates tend to be higher in countries with fewer healthcare resources, where epilepsy care is often limited.[21] These disparities highlight the need for worldwide efforts to improve epilepsy treatment and SUDEP prevention strategies across various healthcare systems.

Prevalence of SUDEP by region

The prevalence and recognition of SUDEP vary significantly across different countries and regions, often influenced by healthcare infrastructure, socioeconomic conditions, and cultural beliefs surrounding epilepsy.

North America: In the United States, SUDEP awareness has improved due to increased advocacy from epilepsy foundations and patient groups. Researchers have stressed the importance of monitoring for high-risk patients and the integration of SUDEP risk assessments into epilepsy care.[15] Despite these efforts, SUDEP rates remain high. Factors like inconsistent access to specialized epilepsy care and gaps in SUDEP counseling practices have been identified as contributing to these high rates.[22]

Europe: European countries have made notable progress in SUDEP research and awareness campaigns.[11] For example, countries such as the UK and Norway have developed national guidelines on SUDEP risk communication and risk reduction strategies, driven by collaborations between researchers and epilepsy organizations.[11] However, incidence rates vary across the continent, with some countries reporting higher rates likely due to improved case identification and reporting standards.[21]

Africa and Asia: In many African and Asian countries, SUDEP remains under-reported and less recognized. Limited access to epilepsy treatment, as well as cultural stigmas surrounding epilepsy, can hinder discussions on mortality and SUDEP.[23] Additionally, socioeconomic barriers reduce the availability of diagnostic and therapeutic options, potentially contributing to higher SUDEP risks among underserved populations.[20]

Australia and New Zealand: These countries have seen growing awareness of SUDEP, supported by regional epilepsy organizations that actively promote SUDEP education and risk reduction strategies.[10] Despite these efforts, rural areas may face limited access to specialized epilepsy care, which can impact SUDEP prevention efforts.[10]

Latin America: Like African and Asian regions, many Latin American countries face challenges with SUDEP awareness due to limited epilepsy resources and a lack of public health initiatives focused on epilepsy-related mortality.[10] Research and awareness campaigns are less common, making SUDEP a relatively unknown concern within general epilepsy care in these regions.[10]

Regional disparities in SUDEP awareness, research, and prevention reflect broader healthcare inequalities, underscoring the need for global standards and increased advocacy efforts to address SUDEP more effectively worldwide.

Pathophysiology and risk factors

SUDEP is caused by several factors, including bodily functions such as heart rate, blood pressure, and breathing often triggered by seizures.[14,24] Respiratory dysfunction, including cessation of breathing and abnormally slow breathing after a seizure, is commonly observed in SUDEP cases. This suggests that some individuals may experience fatal breathing suppression following seizures.[14,24] Cardiac dysfunction, particularly in the form of irregular heartbeat caused by seizure-induced autonomic instability, also contributes to the risk of SUDEP.[25] Genetic predispositions affecting the heart can make certain individuals more vulnerable.[25] The risk of dying from SUDEP varies from person to person, with some individuals' risk being more than 100 times that of others.[1] Certain known risk factors further increase the likelihood of SUDEP, and some are listed below:

- Men are at a higher risk than women[1,16]
- Those who start having epilepsy before the age of 16 are at a higher risk than those who start after the age of 16. When epilepsy starts in childhood, the risk of SUDEP is minimal whilst they are young but increases significantly in adulthood.[1]
- Those who have had epilepsy for more than 15 years are at a higher risk than those who have had it for a shorter period.[1] It is, however, not to be assumed that only having seizures for a long time poses a risk as some people have died from SUDEP on their second seizure.[26]
- Those who continue to have seizures are at a greater risk of SUDEP than those with controlled seizures. Improved control of seizures reduces the risk of SUDEP notably.[1,12,16]
- A high occurrence of generalized tonic-clonic seizures increases the risk of SUDEP[1,27,28]

- Lack of treatment increases the risk of SUDEP. This also includes poor compliance to AEDs.[1,12,27,28] Non-compliance is the primary risk factor for SUDEP.[1] If compliance is that crucial, it gives PWE some hope because it is a factor we can do something about. It is within our control to a certain extent. The issue of compliance to medication is quite critical in epilepsy management, not just SUDEP.
- Those on polytherapy are at a higher risk compared with those on one AED.[1] It has not been established whether the higher risk is due to the polytherapy or the severity of the seizures that may at times make it necessary to be on polytherapy.[1,28]
- Having night-time seizures increases the risk of SUDEP.[1] When seizures happen at night, there might be no one to monitor what is happening, thereby increasing the risk of SUDEP.
- A family history of epilepsy or sudden cardiac death may also point to an inherited risk of SUDEP, suggesting a role for genetic studies in better understanding predispositions[25]
- Changing AEDs because of poor outcomes also increases the risk of SUDEP[1]
- When epilepsy surgery fails, the risk of SUDEP is elevated.[1,8]
- Having an intellectual disability increases the risk of SUDEP.[27,28]

The risk factors listed above suggest that SUDEP is strongly associated with uncontrolled seizures. Research consistently shows that the most effective intervention to reduce SUDEP risk is achieving seizure control.[29] Without effective seizure management, the risk of SUDEP remains significantly elevated. The issue of the epilepsy treatment gap becomes a big concern with regards to SUDEP.

The epilepsy treatment gap is the difference between the number of people with active epilepsy and the number whose seizures are being appropriately treated in a given population at a given point of time, expressed as a percentage. Includes diagnostic and therapeutic deficits.[30]
Meinardi, H., Scott, R. A., & Reis, R.

Research has established that the epilepsy treatment gap in developing countries can be as high as 90%.[31] A study carried out in

Zimbabwe under the Global Campaign Against Epilepsy (2010) revealed an epilepsy treatment gap in Zimbabwe of 83.6%.[32] The situation in LMICs is really a concern as a lot of PWE are at risk of SUDEP because of continuing seizures due to the epilepsy treatment gap.

Risk assessment tools and monitoring

Risk assessment tools, such as the SUDEP-7 Inventory, provide clinicians with a structured way to estimate SUDEP risk for individual patients based on factors like seizure frequency and nocturnal seizures.[9] Additionally, advances in seizure monitoring technology are enhancing the ability to detect nocturnal seizures and respiratory changes, which could mitigate the risk of SUDEP in high-risk patients.[33] These monitoring devices, particularly wearable devices with alarm systems, aim to alert caregivers to potentially dangerous post-seizure states, thus allowing for rapid intervention. Several epilepsy foundation websites list these monitoring devices. The value of these tools lies not only in providing peace of mind but in potentially reducing the frequency of fatal postictal events. The devices may be useful, but not everyone can afford them, and they may not be available in certain countries. Another way to alert people would be using seizure-alert dogs.[1] Seizure-alert dogs have been found to be useful as they can detect a seizure, sometimes even before it happens, and can help alerting others to offer first aid when there is a need.[1]

Pharmacologic and non-pharmacologic interventions

Poorly controlled seizures, especially GTCS, are among the most significant risk factors for SUDEP. Therefore, adherence to AEDs is critical.[34] This strategy works for people whose seizures respond to AEDs. However, challenges such as DRE highlight the need for alternative therapeutic approaches. Non-pharmacologic interventions, such as vagus nerve stimulation (VNS), have shown promise in reducing seizure frequency and, by extension, lowering the risk of SUDEP.[14] VNS is thought to influence autonomic pathways, potentially mitigating the autonomic dysfunction seen in SUDEP cases.[14] While VNS and other devices are good alternatives to AEDs, the main focus in arresting

SUDEP is on achieving complete seizure control through individualized treatment strategies.

Socioeconomic and cultural factors

Differences in SUDEP incidence can be seen among people from varying socioeconomic backgrounds. SUDEP is more prevalent in poor communities where access to healthcare is limited.[20] In countries with limited access to neurologists or monitoring technology, PWE are at higher risk of SUDEP as seizures remain uncontrolled due to reduced access to and unavailability of AEDs.[20] Cultural beliefs also influence SUDEP awareness and epilepsy management.[23] In some communities, epilepsy is stigmatized or associated with superstitions, which can discourage individuals from seeking necessary medical care or adhering to prescribed treatments.[23] Superstition creates doubt, which in turn impacts adherence. Addressing cultural and socioeconomic barriers is essential to reducing SUDEP incidence globally.

Counseling and communication with patients and families

Transparent communication about SUDEP risk is critical to effective epilepsy care. Studies reveal that discussing SUDEP with patients and families can improve medication adherence and encourage the use of safety measures, such as night-time monitoring devices.[8,35] In a survey of 519 neurologists and neuro-pediatricians, only 2.7% indicated they discussed SUDEP with their clients.[36] The main reason cited for not discussing this topic with clients was more to do with lack of clinical practice guidelines.[36] Despite the importance of SUDEP counseling, many physicians encounter barriers, including time constraints, patient anxiety, and concerns about instilling fear. As such, physician practices regarding SUDEP counseling vary widely.[22] Relatives of SUDEP victims feel the doctors are leaving them in the dark by not giving them information related to SUDEP.[8] They feel they have a right to know about SUDEP, so that they can take precautions rather than only getting to know about SUDEP after their loved one has died.[8]

SUDEP should not be downplayed as doing so will only worsen the situation.[12] The issue of concealment of the problem is a major contributory factor to coming up with SUDEP preventive strategies.

Leading medical experts and patient advocates emphasize that individuals should be fully informed, with guidelines addressing all possible medical situations.[26] For families affected by SUDEP, support and information from epilepsy foundations and healthcare providers are essential. Encouraging standardized counseling guidelines may help address these challenges and improve patient education on SUDEP.

In some LMICs, people are not very keen on postmortems, especially when they consider the deceased a "known ill person." Considering that, it is possible some people are succumbing to SUDEP and because no autopsy is conducted it is never recorded, leading to under-reporting. Most literature on SUDEP is from well-resourced countries. When something is under-reported, it may appear less concerning because the available numbers indicate it is a rare occurrence. The fact that SUDEP is not common was cited as one of the reasons why doctors never discuss it with their clients.[36] They are afraid of causing unnecessary anxiety. The question becomes, is SUDEP rare or is it under-reported?

Future directions

This is neither a scientific book nor a medical textbook, therefore I will not want to venture too much into this subject, save to mention that people should watch out for SUDEP. Even if your doctor never mentioned this to you, be advised that SUDEP is real in epilepsy. Should anyone with epilepsy die from unknown causes, relatives should cooperate with authorities to have an autopsy done so that researchers can work on identifying underlying causes for SUDEP to save more lives in future. Researchers are also encouraging relatives to donate the brain of the deceased to help in determining the actual cause of SUDEP[1] to reduce its incidence. It is still a challenge that most people in LMICs live far from hospitals, so when someone dies, there is no way people will take the body to a hospital for a postmortem when they failed to take them there for treatment. Many cases will remain unreported.

SUDEP usually occurs after a seizure.[16] Studies show there are two mechanisms of SUDEP.[1] The first one being the "dangerous change in heart rhythm" that is likely after a seizure and the second one being that a seizure affects the function of the "respiratory center in the brain" and a person may not recover that function after a seizure. Two things that can be done to reduce cases of SUDEP: compliance to medication to reduce occurrence of seizures and using different devices or seizure-alert dogs to alert people around when one is having a seizure so that they can assist with first aid.[1] Advances in monitoring technology, particularly those for night-time supervision, are anticipated to enhance preventive strategies. These devices are still questionable as to their effectiveness in terms of accuracy, but the affected people need to know about these for them to make decisions about whether to use them.

Taking omega-3 supplements has been proved to be "effective on the brain structure, the biochemistry, the physiology and thus the function of the brain."[37,38] Though omega-3 has not been proven to reduce epilepsy seizures, it has been proved to be safe in PWE,[4] so it may be of benefit for PWE to take.

SUDEP is real and all PWE need to know the risks. Family and relatives need to be educated as well. This is not to scare anyone, but to equip people with knowledge so that they will be on alert for risks that can be avoided. The most basic message contained in this chapter is compliance and adherence to medication so that seizures are eliminated or reduced and the risk of SUDEP can thus be lowered. Safeguarding life should be another goal of epilepsy treatment.[12]

Conclusion

SUDEP represents a complex and multifaceted issue within epilepsy care. With improved awareness, counseling, and seizure management, there is potential to reduce SUDEP incidence. Technological advances in monitoring, combined with ongoing research into the mechanisms underlying SUDEP, may further improve outcomes for those at risk. By fostering open communication and taking proactive steps in clinical practice, healthcare providers, patients, and families can work together to address the challenges posed by SUDEP.

References:

1. Tomson, T., Surges, R., Delamont, R., Haywood, S., & Hesdorffer, D. C. (2016). Who to target in sudden unexpected death in epilepsy prevention and how? Risk factors, biomarkers, and intervention study designs. *Epilepsia, 57*, 4-16. https://doi.org/10.1111/epi.13234
2. Thurman, D.J., Hesdorffer, D.C. & French, J.A. (2014). Sudden unexpected death in epilepsy: Assessing the public health burden. *Epilepsia, 55*:1479–1485. https://doi.org/10.1111/epi.12666
3. Chapman, D., Moss, B., Panelli, R., & Pollard, R. (2011). Sudden unexpected death in epilepsy. https://www.researchgate.net/profile/Rosemary-Panelli/publication/238772752_Sudden_Unexpected_Death_in_Epilepsy_-_a_global_conversation/links/58d3338c92851c319e56f642/Sudden-Unexpected-Death-in-Epilepsy-a-global-conversation.pdf
4. Terra, V. C., Arida, R. M., Rabello, G. M., Cavalheiro, E. A., & Scorza, F. A. (2011). The utility of omega-3 fatty acids in epilepsy: more than just a farmed tilapia! *Arquivos de neuro-psiquiatria, 69*, 118-121. https://doi.org/10.1590/S0004-282X2011000100022
5. Devinsky, O., and Nashef, L. (2015). SUDEP the death of nihilism, *Neurology, 85*(18), 1534-1535. https://doi.org/10.1212/WNL.0000000000001948
6. Buchhalter, J. & Cascino, G.D. (2017). An important cause of premature mortality in epilepsy across the life spectrum, *Neurology, 89*(2), 114-115. https://doi.org/10.1212/WNL.0000000000004099
7. Duncan, J. S., Sander, J. W., Sisodiya, S. M., & Walker, M. C. (2006). Adult epilepsy. *The Lancet, 367*(9516), 1087-1100. https://cumming.ucalgary.ca/sites/default/files/teams/122/education/neurosurgery/5.-epilepsy-review-lancet-april-2006.pdf
8. Stevenson, M.J. & Stanton, T.F. (2014). Knowing the risk of SUDEP - Two family's perspectives and The Danny Did Foundation. Epilepsia, 55(10):1495–1500. https://doi.org/10.1111/epi.12795
9. Novak, J.L., Miller, P.R., Markovic, D., Meymandi, S.K. & DeGiorgio, C.M. (2015). Risk Assessment for Sudden Death in Epilepsy: The SUDEP-7 Inventory. *Frontiers in Neurology.* 6/252: 1-6. https://doi.org/10.3389/fneur.2015.00252
10. Panelli, R. J. (2020). SUDEP: A global perspective. *Epilepsy & Behavior, 103*, https://doi.org/10.1016/j.yebeh.2019.07.018
11. Shankar, R., Donner, E. J., McLean, B., Nashef, L., & Tomson, T. (2017). Sudden unexpected death in epilepsy (SUDEP): What every neurologist should know. *Epileptic Disorders, 19*(1), 1-9. http://dx.doi.org/10.1684/epd.2017.0891
12. Nashef, L., & Sander, J. W. A. S. (1996). Sudden unexpected deaths in epilepsy—where are we now? *Seizure-European Journal of Epilepsy, 5*(3), 235-238. https://www.seizure-journal.com/article/S1059-1311(96)80042-2/pdf
13. Nashef, L. (1997). Sudden unexpected death in epilepsy: Terminology and definitions. *Epilepsia, 38*, S6-S8. https://doi.org/10.1111/j.1528-1157.1997.tb06130.x
14. Ryvlin, P., So, E. L., Gordon, C. M., Hesdorffer, D. C., Sperling, M. R., Devinsky, O., ... & Friedman, D. (2018). Long-term surveillance of SUDEP in drug-resistant epilepsy patients treated with VNS therapy. *Epilepsia, 59*(3), 562-572. https://doi.org/10.1111/epi.14002
15. Devinsky, O., Bundock, E., Hesdorffer, D., Donner, E., Moseley, B., Cihan, E., ... & Friedman, D. (2018). Resolving ambiguities in SUDEP classification. *Epilepsia, 59*(6), 1220-1233. https://doi.org/10.1111/epi.14195

16. Kloster, R. & Engelskjøn, T. (1999). Sudden unexpected death in epilepsy (SUDEP): a clinical perspective and a search for risk factors. *Journal of Neurology, Neurosurgery and Psychiatry. 67:439-444.* https://doi.org/10.1136/jnnp.67.4.439
17. Sveinsson, O., Andersson, T., Carlsson, S., & Tomson, T. (2017). The incidence of SUDEP: A nationwide population-based cohort study. *Neurology, 89*(2), 170-177. https://doi.org/10.1212/WNL.0000000000004094
18. Sveinsson, O., Andersson, T., Mattsson, P., Carlsson, S., & Tomson, T. (2020). Clinical risk factors in SUDEP. *Neurology, 94*: 419-429. http://dx.doi.org/10.1212/WNL.0000000000008741
19. Verducci, C., Hussain, F., Donner, E., Moseley, B. D., Buchhalter, J., Hesdorffer, D., ... & Devinsky, O. (2019). SUDEP in the North American SUDEP Registry: The full spectrum of epilepsies. *Neurology, 93*(3), 227-236. https://doi.org/10.1212/WNL.0000000000007778
20. Cihan, E., Hesdorffer, D. C., Brandsoy, M., Li, L., Fowler, D. R., Graham, J. K., ... & Friedman, D. (2020). Socioeconomic disparities in SUDEP in the US. *Neurology, 94*(24), e2555-e2566. https://doi.org/10.1212/WNL.0000000000009463
21. Saetre, E., & Abdelnoor, M. (2018). Incidence rate of sudden death in epilepsy: a systematic review and meta-analysis. *Epilepsy & Behavior, 86*, 193-199. https://doi.org/10.1016/j.yebeh.2018.06.037
22. Asadi-Pooya, A. A., Trinka, E., Brigo, F., Hingray, C., Karakis, I., Lattanzi, S., ... & Gigineishvili, D. (2022). Counseling about sudden unexpected death in epilepsy (SUDEP): a global survey of neurologists' opinions. *Epilepsy & Behavior, 128.* *https://doi.org/10.1016/j.yebeh.2022.108570*
23. Chin, J. H. (2012). Epilepsy treatment in sub-Saharan Africa: closing the gap. *African health sciences, 12*(2), 186-192. http://dx.doi.org/10.4314/ahs.v12i2.17
24. Barot, N., & Nei, M. (2019). Autonomic aspects of sudden unexpected death in epilepsy (SUDEP). *Clinical Autonomic Research, 29*(2), 151-160. https://doi.org/10.1007/s10286-018-0576-1
25. Whitney, R., Sharma, S., Jones, K. C., & RamachandranNair, R. (2023). Genetics and SUDEP: challenges and future directions. *Seizure: European Journal of Epilepsy.* https://doi.org/10.1016/j.seizure.2023.07.002
26. Morton, B., Richardson, A., and Duncan, S. (2006). Sudden unexpected death in epilepsy (SUDEP): don't ask, don't tell? *Journal of Neurology, Neurosurgery, and Psychiatry, 77*(2), 199–202. http://doi.org/10.1136/jnnp.2005.066852
27. Young, C., Shankar, R., Palmer, J., Craig, J., Hargreaves, C., McLean, B., ... & Hillier, R. (2015). Does intellectual disability increase sudden unexpected death in epilepsy (SUDEP) risk? *Seizure, 25*, 112-116. https://doi.org/10.1016/j.seizure.2014.10.001
28. Hesdorffer, D. C., Tomson, T., Benn, E., Sander, J. W., Nilsson, L., Langan, Y., ... & ILAE Commission on Epidemiology; Subcommission on Mortality. (2011). Combined analysis of risk factors for SUDEP. *Epilepsia, 52*(6), 1150-1159. https://doi.org/10.1111/j.1528-1167.2010.02952.x
29. Terra, V. C., Scorza, F. A., Sakamoto, A. C., Pinto, K. G., Fernandes, R. M., Arida, R. M., ... & Machado, H. R. (2009). Does sudden unexpected death in children with epilepsy occur more frequently in those with high seizure frequency? *Arquivos de neuro-psiquiatria, 67*, 1001-1002. https://doi.org/10.1590/S0004-282X2009000600007
30. Meinardi, H., Scott, R. A., Reis, R., & On Behalf of The Ilae Commission on the Developing World, J. S. (2001). The treatment gap in epilepsy: the current situation and ways forward. *Epilepsia, 42*(1), 136-149. https://doi.org/10.1046/j.1528-1157.2001.32800.x

31. Reynolds, E. H. (2024). The origins and early development of the ILAE/IBE/WHO global campaign against epilepsy: Out of the shadows. *Epilepsia Open, 9*(1), 77-83. https://doi.org/10.1002/epi4.12850
32. Global Campaign Against Epilepsy, (2010). "Demonstration Project on Epilepsy in Zimbabwe" http://www.globalcampaignagainstepilepsy.org/demonstration-project-on-epilepsy-in-zimbabwe/
33. van der Lende, M., Hesdorffer, D. C., Sander, J. W., & Thijs, R. D. (2018). Nocturnal supervision and SUDEP risk at different epilepsy care settings. *Neurology, 91*(16), e1508-e1518. http://dx.doi.org/10.1212/WNL.0000000000006356
34. Sveinsson, O., Andersson, T., Mattsson, P., Carlsson, S., & Tomson, T. (2020). Pharmacologic treatment and SUDEP risk: a nationwide, population-based, case-control study. *Neurology, 95*(18), 2509-2518. https://doi.org/10.1212/WNL.0000000000010874
35. Young, C., Shankar, R., Henley, W., Rose, A., Cheatle, K., & Sander, J. W. (2018). SUDEP and seizure safety communication: Assessing if people hear and act. *Epilepsy & Behavior, 86*, 200-203. https://discovery.ucl.ac.uk/id/eprint/10054847/1/Sander_SUDEP%20and%20seizure%20safety%20communication.%20Assessing%20if%20people%20hear%20and%20act_AAM.pdf
36. Strzelczyk, A., Zschebek, G., Bauer, S., Baumgartner, C., Grond, M., Hermsen, A., ... & Rosenow, F. (2016). Predictors of and attitudes toward counseling about SUDEP and other epilepsy risk factors among Austrian, German, and Swiss neurologists and neuropediatricians. *Epilepsia, 57*(4), 612-620. https://doi.org/10.1111/epi.13337
37. Bourre, J. M. (2005). Dietary omega-3 fatty acids and psychiatry: mood, behaviour, stress, depression, dementia and aging. *The Journal of Nutrition, Health & Aging, 9*(1), 31-38. https://www.researchgate.net/profile/Heba-Elsalahy/post/Do-omega-3-fatty-acids-have-any-protective-role-against-dementia/attachment/5d46eeb63843b0b9825dc943/AS%3A788186519314433%401564929718858/download/Bourre+2005_DIETARY+OMEGA-3+FATTY+ACIDS+AND+PSYCHIATRY_+MOOD%2C+BEHAVIOUR%2C.pdf
38. Bourre, J. M. (2006). Effects of nutrients (in food) on the structure and function of the nervous system: update on dietary requirements for brain. Part 2: macronutrients. *Journal of Nutrition Health and Aging, 10*(5), 386. http://www.bourre.fr/pdf/publications_scientifiques/260.pdf

CHAPTER 9 – STATUS EPILEPTICUS

Status epilepticus is a life-threatening neurological emergency that requires prompt diagnosis and treatment.
Sánchez & Rincon[1]

Introduction

Status epilepticus (SE) is a prolonged or recurrent seizure state that is recognized as one of the most severe manifestations of epilepsy. It has been defined as:
- A single seizure lasting more than 5 minutes or
- Two or more seizures without full recovery in between.[2]

This timeframe is critical because seizures lasting more than 5 minutes are unlikely to stop on their own, and the risk of brain damage is increased. SE is associated with high death rates and severe life-long medical complications.[3] Though SE cases vary between regions, in LMICs, SE is estimated to impact up to 40 cases per 100,000 individuals.[4] The actual numbers are believed to be higher as the true incidence may be underreported due to diagnostic challenges.[4] SE is a medical emergency that needs immediate attention.[1] Long-lasting seizure episodes increase the risk of long-term brain complications and can result in death in severe cases.[1]

Classification of status epilepticus

SE can be divided into several subtypes based on clinical presentation, response to treatment, and underlying causes. The primary categories are:
- **Convulsive SE:** This type is easier to diagnose because it involves physical signs seen in tonic-clonic seizures where there is jerking and muscle stiffness.[5]
- **Non-convulsive SE:** This type is more subtle because there is no jerking or muscle stiffness. However, the individual may show signs of confusion, compromised consciousness, and unusual behavior. It can be identified through EEG only.[6] Further subtypes include:

Refractory SE (RSE): Does not respond to first- and second-line treatments. This type affects up to 30% of SE cases. RSE requires extended stay in the intensive care unit (ICU) and the treatment outcomes are not good.[7]

Super-refractory SE (SRSE): The SE persists for more than 24 hours or recurs 24 hours after starting strong treatments of anesthetic therapy, or seizures return after the withdrawal of anesthetic agents.[5] SRSE requires constant monitoring due to anticipated and severe side effects, including low blood pressure and reduced immunity, leading to increased infection risk.[8] Classifying SE accurately is essential because each subtype may require different management strategies, impacting outcomes and prognosis significantly.[9]

Functional changes in the body (pathophysiology)

SE is associated with loss of balance between brain stimulants and suppressants.[10] Under normal circumstances, stimulating neurotransmitters like glutamate and suppressing neurotransmitters such as GABA work together to regulate brain activity. In SE, the levels of glutamate are higher and GABA is lower than normal, leading to an overactive brain.[10] This shift leads to excitotoxicity, a state that damages neurons, increasing the risk of additional seizures.[11] SE causes the withdrawal of GABA receptors, resulting in reduced suppressant signals and worsening seizure activity.[12] The prolonged seizure activity also causes cellular energy wastage, leading to metabolic dysfunction. The brain's inability to replenish adenosine triphosphate (ATP), the primary energy carrier in living things, leads to ionic imbalance, calcium overload, and ultimately neuronal death. These effects are further compounded by inflammatory processes that worsen brain injury and may contribute to secondary conditions such as cognitive decline.[10] Pathophysiological understanding of SE guides pharmacological interventions. For example, treatments like benzodiazepines target GABA receptors to restore inhibition, while other agents aim to reduce excitatory signals.[13]

Etiology and risk factors

SE has numerous causes, varying by patient demographics and co-morbidities.

Acute causes include traumatic brain injury, stroke, infections, and metabolic imbalances such as low blood sugar or electrolyte disturbances.[14]

Age-related causes: Among the elderly, all conditions that affect blood vessels supplying the brain are the major cause.[15] In younger people, genetics and fever-related seizures are the major causes.[15]

Lifestyle and health factors: Other common risk factors for SE include a history of epilepsy, withdrawal from AEDs, alcohol, and illegal drugs.[16]

Social factors: People in low socioeconomic groups have higher rates of SE and worse outcomes.[17] Delayed or limited access to healthcare and limited resources contributes to this higher incidence.[17] Addressing these economic gaps could help reduce the incidence of SE.

Clinical presentation and diagnosis

The clinical presentation of SE varies significantly between convulsive and non-convulsive forms as already described under types of SE. Convulsive SE can lead to low oxygen supply to vital organs and increased pressure in the brain.[6] Non-convulsive SE is harder to diagnose due to its subtle nature and requires an EEG.[18] Early diagnosis is important to minimize brain injury and improve outcomes.[18] EEG remains the gold standard for SE diagnosis, especially for non-convulsive cases, where visual confirmation of seizure activity is not possible. Innovations such as portable or wireless EEG systems have shown promise in emergency rooms, allowing rapid diagnosis and immediate treatment initiation.[19] MRI and CT scans are used to identify underlying causes of SE.

Management and treatment approaches

The aim of treatment in SE focuses on the rapid cessation of seizures. First-line treatments typically include benzodiazepines such as lorazepam or midazolam, administered through the vein due to their fast-acting nature and strong affinity for GABA receptors.[20] When it is not possible to inject the drug into the vein, some alternative routes include injecting into the muscle or inserting the drug into the rectum.[15]

Clinicians use the second-line treatments like phenytoin, levetiracetam, or valproate if the first line fails.[8] Patient factors, like other conditions the individual may have and previous drug response, determine the second-line treatment choice.[8] The increasing use of levetiracetam, due to its favorable safety profile, reflects an evolving preference for drugs with fewer adverse effects in SE management.[11]

For patients with RSE, third-line treatments may include anesthetic agents like propofol or ketamine. These are administered under intensive care conditions due to their significant side effects, including low breathing and heart instability.[13] Drug-resistant cases may also warrant alternative therapies, such as ketogenic diets or neurostimulation, although these are generally considered last-resort interventions.[21]

Challenges in treatment and refractory status epilepticus

Managing SE becomes more difficult when it progresses to RSE or SRSE because it requires a lengthy stay in the ICU with intensive interventions.[7] Managing RSE requires a careful balance between aggressive seizure control while minimizing adverse effects.[8] Prolonged use of anesthetics can lead to compromised immunity, infections, and nerve damage.[8] Strategies for managing RSE are not standardized and can vary widely across institutions, creating disparities in treatment outcomes.[22] Current research aims to establish protocols for early escalation to anesthetic therapies and optimize dosing regimens to improve efficacy while minimizing complications.

Outcomes and prognosis

Several factors influence SE treatment outcomes, like age, cause, and seizure duration. Studies indicate that prolonged SE can cause permanent intellectual and reduced muscular function, especially in children, in whom the developing brain is more prone to damage.[26] Convulsive SE has higher death rates because of its connection with breathing and heart problems.[23] In the long run, the aftermath of SE could include chronic epilepsy, psychiatric conditions, and cognitive decline.

Preventive strategies, including rapid response systems and community awareness, can help reduce these burdens by promoting early intervention.[24]

Public health implications

The socioeconomic burden of SE is significant, with direct costs including hospital admissions, ICU stays, and long-term rehabilitation.[9] Indirect costs include lost productivity and poor quality of life.[9] Public health initiatives focused on educating at-risk populations and providing resources for prompt diagnosis and treatment are crucial for reducing SE-related deaths and complications.[25] Ensuring access to emergency care and expanding training for early SE recognition can substantially improve outcomes in both developed and resource-limited settings.

Conclusion

SE remains a challenging neurological emergency with significant implications for patient quality of life and healthcare systems. Advances in pharmacotherapy, diagnostic tools, and treatment protocols have improved SE outcomes; however, continued research and public health efforts are necessary to address remaining challenges.[7]

References:

1. Sánchez, S., & Rincon, F. (2016). Status epilepticus: Epidemiology and public health needs. *Journal of Clinical Medicine*, 5(8), 71. https://doi.org/10.3390/jcm5080071
2. Betjemann, J. P., & Lowenstein, D. H. (2015). Status epilepticus in adults. *The Lancet Neurology*, 14(6), 615-624. https://doi.org/10.1016/S1474-4422(15)00042-3
3. Seinfeld, S., Goodkin, H. P., & Shinnar, S. (2016). Status epilepticus. *Cold Spring Harbor Perspectives in Medicine*, 6(3), a022830. https://doi.org/10.1101/cshperspect.a022830
4. Dham, B. S., Hunter, K., & Rincon, F. (2014). The epidemiology of status epilepticus in the United States. *Neurocritical Care*, 20, 476-483. https://doi.org/10.1007/s12028-013-9935-x
5. Trinka, E., Cock, H., Hesdorffer, D., Rossetti, A. O., Scheffer, I. E., Shinnar, S., ... & Lowenstein, D. H. (2015). A definition and classification of status epilepticus–Report of the ILAE Task Force on Classification of Status Epilepticus. *Epilepsia*, 56(10), 1515-1523. https://doi.org/10.1111/epi.13121
6. Bauer, G., & Trinka, E. (2010). Nonconvulsive status epilepticus and coma. *Epilepsia*, 51(2), 177-190. https://doi.org/10.1111/j.1528-1167.2009.02297.x
7. Trinka, E., & Kälviäinen, R. (2017). 25 years of advances in the definition, classification and treatment of status epilepticus. *Seizure*, 44, 65-73. https://doi.org/10.1016/j.seizure.2016.11.001

8. Brophy, G. M., Bell, R., Claassen, J., Alldredge, B., Bleck, T. P., Glauser, T., ... & Neurocritical Care Society Status Epilepticus Guideline Writing Committee. (2012). Guidelines for the evaluation and management of status epilepticus. *Neurocritical care*, *17*, 3-23. https://doi.org/10.1007/s12028-012-9695-z
9. Betjemann, J. P., Josephson, S. A., Lowenstein, D. H., & Burke, J. F. (2015). Trends in status epilepticus—related hospitalizations and mortality: redefined in US practice over time. *JAMA Neurology*, *72*(6), 650-655. https://doi.org/10.1001/jamaneurol.2015.0188
10. Walker, M. C. (2018). Pathophysiology of status epilepticus. *Neuroscience Letters*, *667*, 84-91. https://doi.org/10.1016/j.neulet.2016.12.044
11. Deshpande, L. S., & DeLorenzo, R. J. (2014). Mechanisms of levetiracetam in the control of status epilepticus and epilepsy. *Frontiers in Neurology*, *5*, 11. https://doi.org/10.3389/fneur.2014.00011
12. Fernández, I. S., Goodkin, H. P., & Scott, R. C. (2019). Pathophysiology of convulsive status epilepticus. *Seizure*, *68*, 16-21. https://doi.org/10.1016/j.seizure.2018.08.002
13. Trinka, E., Höfler, J., Leitinger, M., & Brigo, F. (2015). Pharmacotherapy for status epilepticus. *Drugs*, *75*, 1499-1521. https://doi.org/10.1007/s40265-015-0454-2
14. Trinka, E., Höfler, J., & Zerbs, A. (2012). Causes of status epilepticus. *Epilepsia*, *53*, 127-138. https://doi.org/10.1111/j.1528-1167.2012.03622.x
15. Capovilla, G., Beccaria, F., Beghi, E., Minicucci, F., Sartori, S., & Vecchi, M. (2013). Treatment of convulsive status epilepticus in childhood: Recommendations of the Italian League Against Epilepsy. *Epilepsia*, *54*, 23-34. https://doi.org/10.1111/epi.12307
16. Tan, R. Y. L., Neligan, A., & Shorvon, S. D. (2010). The uncommon causes of status epilepticus: A systematic review. *Epilepsy research*, *91*(2-3), 111-122. https://doi.org/10.1016/j.eplepsyres.2010.07.015
17. A., & Rajakulendran, S. (2024). Impact of social factors on the outcome of status epilepticus. *Epilepsy & Behavior*, *161*, 110097. https://doi.org/10.1016/j.yebeh.2024.110097
18. Nair, P. P., Kalita, J., & Misra, U. K. (2011). Status epilepticus: Why, what, and how. *Journal of Postgraduate Medicine*, *57*(3), 242-252. https://doi.org/10.4103/0022-3859.81807
19. Welte, T. M., Janner, F., Lindner, S., Gollwitzer, S., Stritzelberger, J., Lang, J. D., ... & Hamer, H. M. (2024). Evaluation of simplified wireless EEG recordings in the neurological emergency room. *PloS One*, *19*(10), e0310223. https://doi.org/10.1371/journal.pone.0310223
20. Glauser, T., Shinnar, S., Gloss, D., Alldredge, B., Arya, R., Bainbridge, J., ... & Treiman, D. M. (2016). Evidence-based guideline: treatment of convulsive status epilepticus in children and adults: report of the Guideline Committee of the American Epilepsy Society. *Epilepsy currents*, *16*(1), 48-61. https://doi.org/10.5698/1535-7597-16.1.48
21. Zaccara, G., Giannasi, G., Oggioni, R., Rosati, E., Tramacere, L., & Palumbo, P. (2017). Challenges in the treatment of convulsive status epilepticus. *Seizure*, *47*, 17-24. https://doi.org/10.1016/j.seizure.2017.02.015
22. Riviello, J. J., Claassen, J., LaRoche, S. M., Sperling, M. R., Alldredge, B., Bleck, T. P., ... & Neurocritical Care Society Status Epilepticus Guideline Writing Committee. (2013). Treatment of status epilepticus: An international survey of experts. *Neurocritical care*, *18*, 193-200. https://doi.org/10.1007/s12028-012-9790-1
23. Sutter, R., Kaplan, P. W., & Rüegg, S. (2013). Outcome predictors for status epilepticus—what really counts. *Nature Reviews Neurology*, *9*(9), 525-534. https://doi.org/10.1038/nrneurol.2013.154
24. Sculier, C., Gaínza-Lein, M., Sánchez Fernández, I., & Loddenkemper, T. (2018). Long-term outcomes of status epilepticus: a critical assessment. *Epilepsia*, *59*, 155-169. https://doi.org/10.1111/epi.14515

25. Lv, R. J., Wang, Q., Cui, T., Zhu, F., & Shao, X. Q. (2017). Status epilepticus-related etiology, incidence and mortality: a meta-analysis. *Epilepsy Research*, *136*, 12-17. https://doi.org/10.1016/j.eplepsyres.2017.07.006
26. Legriel, S., Azoulay, E., Resche-Rigon, M., Lemiale, V., Mourvillier, B., Kouatchet, A., ... & Bedos, J. P. (2010). Functional outcome after convulsive status epilepticus. *Critical Care Medicine*, *38*(12), 2295-2303. https://doi.org/10.1097/CCM.0b013e3181f859a6

CHAPTER 10 – EPILEPSY MYTHS AND MISCONCEPTIONS

Rarely is epilepsy featured in the entertainment business without a reference to 'flashing lights'. In fact, less than 5% of PWE have photosensitive epilepsy seizures that may be triggered by flashing lights.
Sallie Baxendale[1]

Introduction

Despite being one of the most common neurological disorders, affecting more than 65 million people worldwide, epilepsy is often misunderstood. Prevailing myths and misconceptions reinforce stigma and discrimination against those affected by it. These myths and misconceptions have been passed from generation to generation making them sound authentic. This chapter aims to address some of the most common myths surrounding epilepsy and to provide accurate information, supported by current research and literature. These myths not only perpetuate inaccurate perceptions but also significantly impact the quality of life, mental health, and social standing of PWE.[1,2] Understanding and dispelling these myths is crucial to fostering more supportive and inclusive communities. These beliefs, no matter how one may try to trivialize them, shape the way society relates to people with this condition.

Historical origins of epilepsy myths

Epilepsy has long been shrouded in myth and superstition across various cultures. In ancient Greece and Rome, epilepsy was often attributed to divine forces, with terms like the "sacred disease" used to describe it.[3] Many people believed that seizures were a sign of divine possession or punishment by the gods, an idea that persisted well into the Middle Ages in Europe.[4,5] Similarly, in other regions, epilepsy was sometimes viewed as a curse or as the result of demonic influence.[6,7] These historical associations with supernatural causes were largely due to the dramatic and unpredictable nature of seizures, which lacked a clear explanation in the absence of scientific understanding.[8,9] As medical knowledge expanded, epilepsy began to be recognized as a neurological disorder, yet these early beliefs continue to influence contemporary attitudes in certain cultures.

Common myths and misconceptions about epilepsy

Despite advancements in medical science and public awareness, myths and misconceptions about epilepsy continue to circulate globally, creating obstacles for PWE and reinforcing stigma. These misconceptions vary by region and cultural background but share common threads that misrepresent the nature, causes, and treatment of epilepsy. Here is an exploration of some of the most persistent myths from various sources.

Epilepsy is caused by supernatural forces or demons

In many parts of Africa, Asia, and the Middle East, epilepsy is viewed as a curse or a consequence of demonic possession, stemming from longstanding beliefs in the supernatural.[10,11,12] Some communities believe that seizures are evidence of an evil spirit or ancestor's curse, leading people to consult spiritual healers instead of medical professionals.[10,11,12] This belief is so strong in some regions that PWE are subjected to exorcisms, ritual cleansings, or isolation from the community to prevent "contamination" by the supposed supernatural forces.[10,11] Such treatment not only isolates PWE but often leads them to forego medical care, worsening their health outcomes.

Epilepsy is contagious

In certain regions, especially in parts of Africa and Asia, epilepsy is believed to be contagious, especially if one is in contact with the person's body fluids (breath, saliva, blood, sperm, or genital secretions).[2,5,6,13,14] This myth likely originates from misunderstandings of how epilepsy manifests and a lack of information on its neurological basis. Many people foam at the mouth or drool, and this causes them to be avoided by people who could give them first aid during a seizure, because they are afraid of catching the condition. Some people have confirmed that they have witnessed PWE being burnt without being able to do anything to help them because they were afraid of catching the disease.[14] Writing about his experience with seizures, Walter narrated his ordeal as he was attacked by a dog during an epileptic seizure and onlookers did nothing about it.[38] He was badly hurt by the dog, which only stopped biting him after the convulsions had stopped. He had to be admitted to hospital for several weeks due to the dog bites and not the seizure. Some even go to the extent of disowning their relatives because they are convinced if they continue relating to them as before, the epilepsy can pass down the bloodline and they will be affected as well, especially by those from the father's side.[10] From the time of early writings about 3,000 years ago, PWE have lived in isolation because everyone was afraid of catching the disease.[15] As a result, many people avoid physical contact with PWE, fearing they might "catch" the condition through touch or proximity.[11,16] This misconception not only isolates PWE but can discourage family members from caring for or comforting them during a seizure, increasing the risk of injury during episodes.[11] One professor is said to have written that even speaking to PWE was risky as one could contract the condition.[6] Nothing is further from the truth: epilepsy is not contagious.

Mental illness and cognitively challenged

A prevalent myth across various cultures is that epilepsy is a form of mental illness or psychiatric disorder. This misconception likely arises from the visible nature of seizures, which are often dramatic and unpredictable, sometimes causing confusion, unconsciousness, or unusual behaviors.[4,8] In some parts of Asia and Latin America, epilepsy is equated with mental instability, leading to the belief that PWE cannot function normally in society or are unable to control their actions.[8,17] This myth contributes to social exclusion and discrimination, as people fear that those with epilepsy are "unpredictable" or "dangerous."[8] When real issues are being discussed in families, a PWE will be excluded as they are considered "an ill person" in a negative way and treated as a minor.[14,18] Some organizations whose mandate is to fight for the cause of the PWE will not have PWE taking pivotal positions in those organizations, because according to them, PWE have nothing to contribute at boardroom tables. People without the condition will run the organizations and make decisions about epilepsy for PWE. PWE are regarded as cognitively challenged starting in their families, the community, and even organizations for PWE. One day I asked my sister-in-law, Dorothy, what she thought or knew about epilepsy.[18] Unknown to her that I have the condition, she went to great lengths to explain to me that PWE could not contribute anything fruitful to the family or society. I asked her seeking to understand the first reaction. I eventually told her I had the condition, and she was genuinely surprised because I was taking care of her during her illness. I had driven to her rural home and brought her to the city. I would take her to the doctor every week until she got well. Now she had been healed of her disease, and I was just asking her about epilepsy, without knowing she spoke her "truth" on what she believed. This belief that PWE cannot contribute anything positive to society is common. Nothing can be further from the truth as it is observed that many prominent and influential people in history had the condition.

PWE should not have children

A particularly harmful myth is that PWE should avoid parenthood, either due to fears that epilepsy will be passed down genetically or that they cannot safely care for children. Many people think that PWE cannot have children.[2] This misconception is prevalent in several regions, including parts of the Middle East and South Asia, where epilepsy is misunderstood and associated with hereditary "defects" or instability.[19,20,21] Historically, PWE were not allowed to marry to contain the condition as many believed it to be hereditary. Probably, people would associate this with the LMICs, but in the USA and UK, PWE were not allowed to marry.[6] The law was only repealed as late as 1970 in the UK and the last state to repeal the law in the US did so in 1980.[6] To make sure these people never reproduced, some states in the US allowed them to be sterilised.[3,6]

This myth has scared even some people with the condition to the extent that many women refuse to get married because they are not sure they will be able to bear children. Others are afraid that if they do have children, there is a risk of passing on their condition. Another dimension is that when a woman with epilepsy becomes pregnant, her husband may end the relationship, with no support whatsoever given to his former spouse and child.[10] In reality, while certain forms of epilepsy can have a genetic component, most PWE are fully capable of becoming responsible parents, and the risk of transmitting epilepsy to children is generally low.[19,20] Such myths deprive PWE of the opportunity to experience family life. The myth contributes to a sense of inadequacy and exclusion. This topic will be discussed in greater detail in Chapter 13, which deals with gender issues. What can be said under this section is that low fertility rates in PWE are mainly attributed to the way society perceives them and not from having epilepsy.

PWE can swallow their tongue during a seizure

A common myth in both Western and non-Western societies is that PWE may swallow their tongue during a seizure, leading some people to try to "protect" them by inserting objects into their mouth.[1] This misconception is dangerous, as attempting to place objects in a seizing person's mouth can result in choking and dental injuries. The risk of tongue-swallowing during a seizure is non-existent, as it is physically impossible to swallow one's tongue.[1,14,22] The seizure should be left to run its course and any objects that might cause injury to the person during a seizure removed. Educating the public about seizure first aid is essential to dispel this myth and ensure that PWE receive appropriate assistance during a seizure.

Seizures are always triggered by flashing lights

Another myth, particularly common in Western countries, is that flashing lights always trigger seizures in PWE. This belief stems from depictions of epilepsy in the media, where flashing lights are often portrayed as seizure triggers.[23,24] However, only a small percentage of PWE, estimated at 3–5%, experience photosensitive epilepsy, where flashing lights can indeed induce a seizure.[23,24] Most PWE do not have this sensitivity, and their seizures are typically triggered by factors such as stress, sleep deprivation, or illness.[23,24] Misunderstandings about seizure triggers can limit the activities PWE feel they can safely participate in, contributing to unnecessary restrictions on their lives.[23,24] As discussed in the chapter for seizure triggers, it is important for every person living with the condition to understand what triggers their seizures.

Epilepsy can only be cured by traditional or alternative practices

In regions with limited access to medical treatment, there is a strong belief that epilepsy can only be cured by traditional or alternative practices.[10,11,12] Many families turn to herbal remedies, religious practices, or even harmful methods like burning or branding in an attempt to "cure" epilepsy.[10,11,12] In African and Asian cultures, where traditional healers hold a respected role, PWE often delay or avoid seeking medical treatment, opting instead for these non-medical approaches due to the belief that they address the "spiritual" or "cultural" cause of epilepsy.[10,11] While alternative treatments can be supportive, epilepsy is a chronic condition typically requiring medical management, and such misconceptions prevent PWE from accessing effective care. In LMICs, hospitals may be far away, so people end up seeking help from spiritualists, making it hard to break free and seek medical help based on what the spiritualist will have identified as the cause of the illness.

PWE cannot participate in sports or physical activities

A widespread myth, particularly in Western societies, is that PWE should avoid physical activities or sports to prevent triggering seizures or risking injury.[7,18] Physical activity could be beneficial in managing epilepsy, reducing stress, and improving overall health in PWE. Discouraging PWE from such activities works against their overall health outcomes.[7,18] While certain activities, like swimming alone, may require precautions, many PWE can safely engage in sports, especially with proper supervision or tailored adjustments. This myth restricts PWE from fully participating in recreational or fitness opportunities, impacting their quality of life and social engagement.[7,18]

Epilepsy is a rare condition

In many communities, epilepsy is considered a rare or unusual condition, resulting in a lack of understanding or support for PWE.[3] Epilepsy is one of the most common neurological conditions worldwide, affecting approximately 1% of the global population.[3,5,24] Almost every person knows someone with the condition, and it is not rare. The myth of rarity not only limits awareness and education efforts but also contributes to the isolation of PWE, as they may feel "alone" in their condition or struggle to find others who share their experiences.[3,5,24] Raising awareness about epilepsy's prevalence can foster greater empathy and encourage communities to provide resources and support for PWE.

Epilepsy is solely characterized by convulsive seizures

A misconception common even among healthcare providers is that epilepsy is solely characterized by convulsive seizures.[13,25,26] Epilepsy can manifest in a variety of ways, including non-convulsive seizures, absence seizures, and focal seizures, which may not involve visible convulsions.[13,25,26] Some PWE experience subtle symptoms, such as staring spells, repetitive movements, or sensory disturbances. This narrow understanding of epilepsy limits accurate diagnosis and appropriate management, as people with non-convulsive forms of epilepsy may go undiagnosed or misunderstood.[13,25,26]

Epilepsy limits intellectual ability

The notion that epilepsy negatively affects intelligence is widespread and contributes to educational and employment discrimination.[7] Many people wrongly assume that PWE have cognitive impairments, are slower to learn, or are incapable of handling complex tasks. This misconception has resulted in limited educational opportunities for children with epilepsy, particularly in regions where awareness is low and school policies may restrict PWE from attending class.[27,28] In workplaces, this myth leads to bias in hiring, as employers often question the capabilities of PWE, perceiving them as less capable or less productive.[6,7] Many highly qualified PWE are under-employed, meaning they are working in roles that do not fully utilize their skills, education, or availability for work. Epilepsy does not inherently impair cognitive abilities, and many PWE are just as intellectually capable as anyone without the condition.[27,28]

Despite the myths and stigma, many prominent individuals with epilepsy have made significant contributions to society, challenging stereotypes about the disorder. Notable figures such as Vincent van

Gogh, Julius Caesar, Sir Isaac Newton, Theodore Roosevelt, Pythagoras, Levy Mwanawasa, Napoleon Bonaparte, Agatha Christie, Charles Dickens, Alfred Nobel, Alexander the Great, Michelangelo, Aristotle, Socrates, Chanda Gunn, just to name a few, have achieved remarkable success in their respective fields.[3,29,30] PWE lead normal lives and do challenging jobs like everybody else.[2] Epilepsy is neither a "form of mental illness nor does it cause mental illness."[31] Given the opportunity, PWE can lead normal productive lives. Their stories can help change public perceptions by illustrating that PWE can lead fulfilling, impactful lives. Raising public awareness about these individuals and their accomplishments is a valuable tool in reducing stigma and fostering positive attitudes toward epilepsy.[3]

Epilepsy is a permanent disorder

Epilepsy is not a permanent condition in all people. In Zimbabwe, I have heard people saying epilepsy can be treated if the PWE has not been burnt before. Once someone gets burnt during a seizure, they have epilepsy for life. This is not true as most forms of epilepsy, especially those that start in childhood, are usually outgrown in adolescence. Parents must not isolate or hide their children with epilepsy. If the epilepsy resolves later in life, the child will continue thriving in society as they have always been a part of it. In some communities, a child with epilepsy is kept locked away so that no one will know about them. During one of my interactions speaking with parents of children with epilepsy, a couple disclosed and confirmed they had kept their child locked in a room for 3 years. The father was a pastor at a local church, and he did not want society to know he had a child with epilepsy. A neighbor found out that a child was being kept locked away and alerted social services. The parents only started attending these group sessions of parents after being discovered that way. At that meeting, the father expressed regret, but he was grateful to the neighbor who had reported them because now they could find help for their child. Hiding a child away only makes the situation worse, and their recovery will be almost impossible. There are some types of epilepsy that are permanent, but if managed well, a person can lead a normal life like everybody else. No human being deserves to be kept in isolation because of a non-contagious medical condition.

Sexual intercourse with a woman with epilepsy will make you rich

Another myth that has led to abuse of women is that if one has sexual intercourse with a woman with epilepsy, they will become rich.[10] This myth seems prevalent in some African countries.[10] If wealth can come from having sex with someone with epilepsy, then many are willing to do it, though the myth of being contagious in this case helps scare away some people.[10] A lot of women have suffered sexual abuse, especially when they are unconscious. Some will never know what happened to them because by the time they regain consciousness, the man will have left. Some women have contracted sexually transmitted diseases, including HIV and AIDS, from people they do not know. Others have been impregnated by strangers.

PWE are aggressive

The myth that PWE are predisposed to aggression and religious ecstasy also needs attention.[6] This led to the development of the term "epileptic character."[6] Some scholars argue that this so-called epileptic character could be a result of reactions to society.[6] Society makes it impossible for PWE to function properly as they meet stumbling blocks at every turn.[6] In a way, we can say the epileptic character is a creation of society. Stereotyping is not good in any society. Each person should be assessed on their own merits and not just painted with the same brush.

Every seizure should be taken to emergency room

Some people are in the habit of calling an ambulance every time someone has a seizure. This is unnecessary unless a seizure lasts more than 5 minutes or the person has been injured due to the convulsions. By the time the ambulance arrives, the person will have regained consciousness. The ambulance will drive back or if they insist on carrying the patient, by the time they get to a medical facility, nothing will be done to the patient because the seizure will have run its course, and the person needs no medical attention anyway. The person will still need to pay for the ambulance even if it was not necessary to call it in the first place, and will also need to find their way home.

Epilepsy is non-fatal

Many people regard epilepsy as a "non-fatal and non-disabling condition."[16] This is not true as the mortality rate of PWE is up to three times higher than that of the general population.[4] Most of these deaths are attributable to SUDEP, status epilepticus, suicide, and injuries because of seizures. Epilepsy can be fatal and disabling, so needs to be taken seriously.

Every seizure needs an EEG or a specialist to diagnose epilepsy

Medical professionals want to refer every suspected epilepsy patient to a specialist for an EEG. This may be practical in highly resourced countries, but in countries where there is only one neurologist and one EEG machine, this is not practical. Epilepsy is a clinical condition that can be diagnosed at the primary healthcare level if people are equipped with the necessary skills to diagnose and manage it. An EEG is not the answer to epilepsy diagnosis. It should only be used to confirm a diagnosis and not as the basic test to prove someone has epilepsy. This misconception has contributed to too many people going for months or years without treatment because they are waiting for an appointment with a neurologist. In Africa, many countries do not have neurologists. The "median number of neurologists in sub-Saharan Africa is estimated at 3 per 10 million people" against Europe's median of "484 per 10 million people"[16] and this complicates the situation for someone in need of urgent treatment.

Impact of myths on the daily lives of PWE

Epilepsy myths and misconceptions affect the daily lives of PWE, impacting their social interactions, career opportunities, educational experiences, and mental health. Misunderstandings about the condition create significant challenges, as myths are often internalized by both society and PWE themselves, resulting in reduced quality of life, limited access to opportunities, and heightened feelings of isolation and stigma.

Social isolation and relationships

Myths about epilepsy often lead to social exclusion, as many people mistakenly believe epilepsy is contagious or associated with supernatural influences. In several countries across Africa and Asia, for instance, epilepsy is seen as a sign of demonic possession or spiritual affliction, making PWE targets of fear and ostracism. Consequently, PWE may be excluded from family gatherings, social events, and community spaces, particularly in rural communities where beliefs in the supernatural are strong.[10,11,12,16,20] In some communities, families may even hide relatives with epilepsy to avoid shame or dishonor, leading to a life of seclusion for these individuals.[10,11]

Social isolation can extend to romantic relationships and marriage prospects. In parts of the Middle East and South Asia, epilepsy is often seen as an obstacle to marriage, with families refusing to allow PWE to marry or limiting their interactions with potential partners due to fears that epilepsy makes someone unsuitable for family life.[19,20,21,32] Such stigma leads to reduced marriage prospects, depriving PWE of the opportunity to form family units and participate in cultural and social rites of passage that are critical in many societies.[20,33] This restriction on forming intimate relationships can contribute to feelings of inadequacy and loneliness among PWE.

Barriers to employment and education

In many regions, misconceptions about epilepsy's impact on cognitive abilities and productivity create significant barriers to employment for PWE. Employers may assume that PWE are less reliable, fearing that seizures will disrupt productivity or create safety risks.[6,7] These attitudes contribute to higher unemployment rates among PWE and limited access to career growth and advancement. This employment discrimination is particularly prominent in settings that lack legal protections for people with disabilities, leaving PWE vulnerable to workplace exclusion.[7,34] Even when PWE are employed, they may feel compelled to hide their condition out of fear of discrimination or job loss, which can lead to additional stress and impact job performance.

Education is another area where myths about epilepsy have detrimental effects. In various parts of Asia, Africa, and Latin America, school administrators, teachers, and peers often lack awareness about epilepsy, leading to unfair treatment or exclusion of PWE from classroom settings.[27,28,35] For example, some school systems may restrict PWE from attending school altogether, fearing that they could disrupt class or pose a "threat" to other students.[27,28] This denial of education deprives PWE of the opportunity to develop academic skills and limits their potential career prospects, trapping many in cycles of poverty and dependence. Educational discrimination can also affect students' self-esteem, as they internalize the stigma and begin to view themselves as incapable or "less than" their peers.

Mental health implications

The impact of epilepsy myths extends deeply into the mental health of PWE, contributing to increased rates of depression, anxiety, and low self-esteem.[6,7] In Western societies, PWE often report experiencing covert forms of discrimination, such as subtle social exclusion or lowered expectations from friends and colleagues. These experiences contribute to feelings of alienation and inferiority, as individuals may feel like they are constantly being judged or misunderstood.[6,7] Additionally, fear of having a seizure in public, especially due to widespread misunderstandings, can lead to self-imposed isolation and a reluctance to engage in social activities.[6,7]

In regions where epilepsy is viewed as a curse or spiritual punishment, such as parts of Africa, the Middle East, and Asia, PWE often endure heightened psychological distress. The perception that they are "cursed" or "damaged" can create a profound sense of shame and self-blame, leading many to feel that they are responsible for their condition or inherently unworthy of a "normal" life.[10,16,19,21] This internalized stigma can severely impact self-esteem and may result in mental health disorders that compound the difficulties of living with epilepsy.

Limited access to healthcare and treatment

Myths about epilepsy often lead PWE to pursue alternative or traditional treatments instead of medical care, impacting their health and well-being. In many cultures where epilepsy is believed to be spiritual or supernatural, families may turn to spiritual healers, traditional medicine, or religious rituals rather than consulting neurologists or epilepsy specialists.[10,11,12] In Africa, for example, reliance on traditional healers is common due to beliefs that seizures are caused by ancestral or demonic forces.[10,11,12] This can lead to poorly managed epilepsy, as traditional treatments rarely address the underlying neurological issues. Furthermore, fear of stigma can discourage families from seeking medical help, particularly if they worry about judgment from the community for pursuing "foreign" or "modern" medical solutions.[10,11,12]

Even when PWE seek medical care, myths and stigma can affect the quality of treatment they receive. Medical professionals in some regions may hold misconceptions about epilepsy, leading to inadequate treatment or a lack of empathy in patient interactions. This lack of understanding from healthcare providers can discourage PWE from following treatment plans or returning for follow-up care, thereby worsening health outcomes.[12,34]

Economic consequences

The combined impact of social isolation, employment discrimination, and limited educational access can lead to financial instability for PWE. In areas where epilepsy is highly stigmatized, families may face economic hardship, as PWE are often unable to contribute to household income or require financial support for their care.[11,12] This strain can create a cycle of poverty, as families may need to allocate resources to alternative treatments or deal with the consequences of unemployment or underemployment due to pervasive myths.[7,11,12]

In some cases, these financial consequences extend to the community level, as stigma-related barriers to employment and education prevent PWE from participating fully in the local economy. This exclusion reduces economic productivity and increases the demand on social support systems, particularly in communities where access to government assistance or disability benefits is limited.[11,12]

Self-esteem and identity

The stigma and social exclusion generated by epilepsy myths often lead PWE to internalize negative beliefs about themselves, damaging their self-image and sense of identity. Many PWE report feeling like outsiders or burdens to their families, leading them to withdraw from social engagement and miss out on opportunities to develop a positive self-concept.[6,7,20] This isolation can be particularly damaging for children and young adults, who are still forming their identities and rely heavily on social interactions to build self-esteem.

For many, the persistent belief that they are "different" or "broken" fosters a sense of inadequacy and hopelessness.[6,7] This internalized stigma can be as detrimental as external stigma, as it reinforces feelings of inferiority and reduces motivation to seek personal growth, further education, or professional development.[6,7,20] Without positive social reinforcement or a sense of belonging, PWE may struggle with low self-worth, increasing their susceptibility to mental health disorders like depression and anxiety.[6,7]

The myths and misconceptions surrounding epilepsy create profound challenges for PWE across all areas of life, affecting their social connections, employment, education, mental health, and self-esteem. Addressing these myths requires comprehensive public awareness campaigns, improved medical education, and community-level interventions that foster understanding and empathy for PWE. By dismantling these myths, societies can create a more inclusive environment that enables PWE to lead fulfilling, integrated lives without the added burden of stigma and discrimination.

Regional perspectives on epilepsy myths and misconceptions

Africa

In many African countries, epilepsy is still deeply misunderstood and is often regarded with fear and suspicion. In Nigeria, Ghana, and other parts of sub-Saharan Africa, epilepsy is commonly linked to supernatural beliefs, including associations with witchcraft, spiritual possession, and curses. Many communities believe that epilepsy results from spiritual afflictions or demonic forces, leading to the marginalization and social isolation of PWE.[10,11,12,20] Some families in rural areas may restrict PWE from attending community gatherings, fearing that seizures will bring misfortune or indicate that the family is cursed.[10,12] This stigma can prevent PWE from seeking medical treatment, with many opting for traditional or spiritual healers who may use ritualistic practices that lack any medical basis.[12,16]

Efforts to change these perceptions are underway. Public health campaigns and education programs initiated by non-governmental organizations (NGOs) and government agencies in countries such as Tanzania, Uganda, and Kenya aim to dispel myths through community outreach, providing accurate information on epilepsy and its medical causes. These campaigns emphasize that epilepsy is a neurological disorder rather than a supernatural affliction and encourage families to seek medical treatment from healthcare facilities.[11,12] Programs that incorporate community leaders, religious figures, and educators have been particularly effective, as they leverage trusted sources to communicate accurate information and reduce stigma.[11]

Asia

In Asia, epilepsy myths are varied, with cultural beliefs, religious practices, and social norms playing a significant role in shaping perceptions. In India and Pakistan, epilepsy is sometimes viewed as an impurity or bad omen, and PWE may be ostracized or considered unsuitable for marriage.[20,27,33] Family honor and societal expectations around marriage can influence perceptions, leading to family members concealing the condition of a relative with epilepsy to avoid damaging prospects for marriage and social standing. In Pakistan, for example, epilepsy is often considered a "hidden" illness, with many families opting not to disclose a diagnosis due to fears of stigma and shame.[20]

The stigma surrounding epilepsy also affects treatment-seeking behaviors in Asia, where traditional and alternative medicine are popular options. In some areas, PWE may turn to Ayurvedic or herbal medicine, homeopathy, or religious rituals rather than pursuing conventional medical treatment, partly due to concerns about side effects or doubts about the effectiveness of Western medicine.[20,34] However, increased advocacy for epilepsy awareness and mental health initiatives is gradually shifting perceptions, especially in urban centers where medical resources are more accessible.[27,34] Organizations such as the Indian Epilepsy Association have spearheaded public awareness campaigns and support groups that aim to increase understanding of epilepsy and support the rights of PWE.[34]

Middle East

In Middle Eastern societies, epilepsy remains highly stigmatized, often associated with perceptions of unpredictability and incapacity. In countries such as Saudi Arabia, Jordan, and Lebanon, epilepsy is frequently misunderstood, with many believing that PWE cannot fulfill normal social roles, such as being suitable for marriage or capable of parenting.[19,21,32] This belief significantly impacts the social standing of PWE, with some families discouraged from allowing their children with epilepsy to participate fully in family and community life. In Saudi Arabia, for instance, marriage restrictions are prevalent due to the belief that epilepsy is an insurmountable barrier to fulfilling family roles, and PWE are sometimes seen as unfit for marriage or having children.[19,32]

Beyond social stigma, epilepsy myths in the Middle East also contribute to delays in seeking treatment. Many families believe that traditional healing methods, religious practices, or even exorcisms are effective ways to manage epilepsy, leading to a reliance on these methods over medical intervention.[32] Addressing these misconceptions requires engagement with religious and cultural leaders who can advocate for better understanding and encourage acceptance of medical treatment for epilepsy. Education programs, particularly those endorsed by respected community leaders, have shown some success in reducing stigma and promoting treatment adherence.[32]

Western perspectives

In Western countries, misconceptions about epilepsy have evolved over time, with earlier beliefs rooted in the idea of epilepsy as a "sacred disease" or evidence of madness. While the perception of epilepsy as a divine or demonic phenomenon has largely dissipated, residual myths and stereotypes persist. Some Western societies still view epilepsy as an indicator of mental instability, particularly when psychiatric co-morbidities are present. PWE may encounter subtle forms of discrimination in workplaces, where employers might mistakenly assume that individuals with epilepsy are less reliable or productive.[6,7,34]

The effects of stigma on mental health and self-esteem among PWE in Western societies are significant, even if the form of discrimination is less overt. For instance, PWE often report feelings of isolation, fear of having a seizure in public, and reluctance to disclose their condition to friends, colleagues, or even employers.[6,7] To combat this, many organizations, such as the Epilepsy Foundation in the USA and Epilepsy Action in the UK, actively promote epilepsy awareness through national campaigns and educational programs. These initiatives aim to provide the public with accurate information about epilepsy, challenge stereotypes, and support PWE in social and professional environments.[34]

Latin America

In Latin America, particularly in rural and indigenous communities, epilepsy is often misunderstood, and myths about the condition reflect a mix of indigenous beliefs and colonial-era attitudes.[28,35] In some areas, epilepsy is still viewed as a spiritual affliction, leading families to consult traditional healers or religious figures instead of seeking medical care. Fear of contagion is also common in certain parts of Latin America, where people may believe that seizures can be transmitted through physical contact.[28,35] This fear often results in social isolation, with some PWE excluded from social gatherings and communal activities to avoid perceived "risks" of contagion.[35]

Efforts to increase epilepsy awareness in Latin America face unique challenges, as healthcare infrastructure and resources for neurological care are limited in many regions. Despite these challenges, several countries, including Brazil, Argentina, and Mexico, have implemented programs to train healthcare providers, promote epilepsy education, and work with local communities to dispel myths.[28,35] Collaborations between NGOs, local healthcare providers, and government agencies have been crucial in promoting accurate information and reducing the stigma associated with epilepsy in both rural and urban settings.[35]

Oceania

In Oceania, particularly in indigenous Australian and Polynesian communities, traditional beliefs and cultural practices shape the perception of epilepsy. Indigenous Australian communities, for example, may have cultural interpretations of epilepsy that see it as a spiritual or ancestral issue, rather than a medical condition.[8,9] This perspective may lead individuals to seek guidance from elders or spiritual healers rather than medical treatment. In some Polynesian cultures, epilepsy is sometimes seen as a source of shame, resulting in social marginalization for PWE and their families.[8]

Public health initiatives in Oceania aim to bridge the gap between cultural beliefs and medical understanding. Organizations work with indigenous leaders and community representatives to raise awareness about epilepsy as a neurological disorder and to encourage people to seek appropriate medical treatment. Efforts to incorporate cultural sensitivity into these initiatives have proven effective, as they respect traditional perspectives while promoting modern healthcare options.[8,9]

Conclusion

Across diverse cultural contexts, epilepsy myths and misconceptions manifest in distinct yet impactful ways. These regional beliefs influence treatment-seeking behaviors, social inclusion, and the mental health of PWE. Efforts to address and dispel these myths require culturally tailored education programs, support from community leaders, and partnerships between health organizations and local stakeholders to foster a more informed, accepting approach to epilepsy worldwide.

Education and advocacy play crucial roles in dispelling myths about epilepsy and promoting accurate understanding. Medical organizations, NGOs, and advocacy groups work globally to educate communities about epilepsy, offering resources and information to reduce stigma.[13,24,36] Initiatives in schools and workplaces further reinforce understanding, promoting a culture of empathy and support for PWE.[36,37]

Epilepsy myths and misconceptions not only perpetuate stigma but also significantly impact the lives of PWE in terms of their social, professional, and medical experiences. From beliefs about contagion and possession to misconceptions about parenting and tongue swallowing, these myths create barriers that limit the opportunities and support available to PWE. Through ongoing efforts in education and advocacy, communities can correct these misconceptions and support a more inclusive, empathetic environment for all.

References:

1. Baxendale, S. (2009). Dangerous Myths About Epilepsy. http://news.bbc.co.uk/2/hi/health/8413404.stm
2. VA Epilepsy Center of Excellence. (2023). Facts and myths about epilepsy. http://www.disabled-world.com/health/neurology/epilepsy-information.php#ixzz2AZtXDRlq
3. Schachter, S.C. ed. 2004. "Epilepsy History" in: http://www.epilepsy.com/EPILEPSY/HISTORY.
4. Carpio, A., Bharucha, N. E., Jallon, P., Beghi, E., Campostrini, R., Zorzetto, S., & Mounkoro, P. P. (2005). Mortality of epilepsy in developing countries. *Epilepsia, 46*, 28-32. https://doi.org/10.1111/j.1528-1167.2005.00404.x
5. Carod-Artal, F.J. and V´azquez-Cabrera, C.B. (2007). An anthropological study about epilepsy in native tribes from Central and South America. *Epilepsia, 48*(5):886–893. https://doi.org/10.1111/j.1528-1167.2007.01016.x
6. International League against Epilepsy. (2003). The History and Stigma of Epilepsy. *Epilepsia, 44*(Suppl. 6): 12–14. https://doi.org/10.1046/j.1528-1157.44.s.6.2.x
7. Nasif, M. B., Koubeissi, M., & Azar, N. J. (2021). Epilepsy–from mysticism to science. *Revue Neurologique, 177*(9), 1047-1058. https://doi.org/10.1016/j.neurol.2021.01.021
8. Kaddumukasa, M., Kaddumukasa, M. N., Buwembo, W., Munabi, I. G., Blixen, C., Lhatoo, S., ... & Sajatovic, M. (2018). Epilepsy misconceptions and stigma reduction interventions in sub-Saharan Africa, a systematic review. *Epilepsy & Behavior, 85*, 21-27. https://doi.org/10.1016/j.yebeh.2018.04.014
9. Alhagamhmad, M. H., & Shembesh, N. M. (2018). Investigating the awareness, behavior, and attitude toward epilepsy among university students in Benghazi, Libya. *Epilepsy & Behavior, 83*, 22-27. https://doi.org/10.1016/j.yebeh.2018.03.021
10. Komolafe, M. A., Sunmonu, T. A., Fabusiwa, F., Komolafe, E. O., Afolabi, O., Kett, M., & Groce, N. (2011). Women's perspectives on epilepsy and its sociocultural impact in southwestern Nigeria. *African Journal of Neurological Sciences, 30*(2). https://www.ajol.info/index.php/ajns/article/view/77320
11. Dugbartey, A.T. & Barimah, K.B. (2013). Traditional beliefs and knowledge base about epilepsy among university students in Ghana. *Ethnicity & Disease, 23*(1):1-5. https://www.researchgate.net/publication/236050024_Traditional_beliefs_and_knowledge_base_about_epilepsy_among_university_students_in_Ghana
12. Makasi, C. E., Kilale, A. M., Ngowi, B. J., Lema, Y., Katiti, V., Mahande, M. J., ... & Mmbaga, B. T. (2023). Knowledge and misconceptions about epilepsy among people with epilepsy and their caregivers attending mental health clinics: A qualitative study in Taenia solium endemic pig-keeping communities in Tanzania. *Epilepsia Open, 8*(2), 487-496. https://doi.org/10.1002/epi4.12720
13. Ball, D. E., Mielke, J., Adamolekun, B., Mundanda, T., & McLean, J. (2000). Community leader education to increase epilepsy attendance at clinics in Epworth, Zimbabwe. *Epilepsia, 41*(8), 1044-1045. https://doi.org/10.1111/j.1528-1157.2000.tb00292.x

14. Diop, A.G., de Boer, H.M., Mandlhate, C., Prilipko, L. & Meinardi, H. (2003). The global campaign against epilepsy in Africa. *Acta Tropica. 87*(1): 149-59. https://doi.org/10.1016/s0001-706x(03)00038-x
15. Fater, M. [s.a]. Living Life Unpredictably http://www.scientiareview.org/pdfs/120
16. Chin, J. H. (2012). Epilepsy treatment in sub-Saharan Africa: Closing the gap. *African Health Sciences, 12*(2), 186-192. http://dx.doi.org/10.4314/ahs.v12i2.17
17. Kaddumukasa, M., Smith, P. J., Kaddumukasa, M. N., Kajumba, M., Almojuela, A., Bobholz, S., ... & Koltai, D. C. (2021). Epilepsy beliefs and misconceptions among patient and community samples in Uganda. *Epilepsy & Behavior, 114.* https://doi.org/10.1016/j.yebeh.2020.107300
18. Zifo, D. (2012). Interview with Dorothy Zifo, a 77-year-old woman. Harare, Zimbabwe.
19. Al-Dossari, K. K., Al-Ghamdi, S., Al-Zahrani, J., Abdulmajeed, I., Alotaibi, M., Almutairi, H., ... & Alhatlan, O. (2018). Public knowledge awareness and attitudes toward epilepsy in Al-Kharj Governorate Saudi Arabia. *Journal of Family Medicine and Primary Care, 7*(1), 184-190. https://doi.org/10.4103/jfmpc.jfmpc_281_17
20. Noor, S., Saeed, F., & Aslam, M. A. (2017). Prevalence of Various Myths about Epilepsy among Families of Epileptic Patients in Pakistani Society. *Journal of Fatima Jinnah Medical University, 11*(1). http://jfjmu.com/index.php/ojs/article/download/23/15
21. Al Kayed, Z. S., Al Ali, S. M., & Otoum, A. M. F. (2023). Perceived Causes of Epilepsy from Society Perspective and its Relationship to Some Variables in Jordan. *Journal of Namibian Studies: History Politics Culture, 34,* 6208-6228. https://namibian-studies.com/index.php/JNS/article/download/2558/1739
22. Vageriya, V., & Sharma, A. (2020). Misconceptions and traditional treatment practices regarding childhood epilepsy in Central Gujarat of India: A community perspective. *Indian Journal of Public Health Research & Development, 11*(3). https://openurl.ebsco.com/EPDB%3Agcd%3A8%3A13755064/detailv2?sid=ebsco%3Aplink%3Ascholar&id=ebsco%3Agcd%3A145376295&crl=c
23. Elmazny, A., Alkharisi, M. A. A., Ibrahim, Y. S. J., Albarakati, A. B. A., Almutairi, S. S., Altalhi, L. A., ... & Dahshan, A. (2024). Public misconceptions and attitudes towards persons diagnosed with epilepsy in the Kingdom of Bahrain: A cross-sectional study. *Epilepsy & Behavior, 153.* https://doi.org/10.1016/j.yebeh.2024.109731
24. Musekwa, O. P., Makhado, L., Maphula, A., & Mabunda, J. T. (2020). How much do we know? assessing public knowledge, awareness, impact, and awareness guidelines for epilepsy: A systematic review. *The Open Public Health Journal, 13*(1). http://dx.doi.org/10.2174/1874944502013010794
25. Yeni, K. (2023). Stigma and psychosocial problems in patients with epilepsy. *Exploration of Neuroscience, 2*(6), 251-263. https://doi.org/10.37349/en.2023.00026
26. Eltibi, R., & Shawahna, R. (2022). Knowledge and attitudes of physical educators toward epilepsy and students with epilepsy: A cross-sectional study from Palestine. *Epilepsy & Behavior, 126.* https://doi.org/10.1016/j.yebeh.2021.108460
27. Javed, T., Awan, H. A., Shahzad, N., Ojla, D., Naqvi, H. B., Arshad, H., ... & Abrar, S. (2023). Unraveling the myths around epilepsy: A cross-sectional study of knowledge, attitude, and practices among Pakistani individuals. *Cureus, 15*(5). https://doi.org/10.7759/cureus.39760
28. Rani, A., & Thomas, P. T. (2019). Parental knowledge, attitude, and perception about epilepsy and sociocultural barriers to treatment. *Journal of Epilepsy Research, 9*(1), 65. https://doi.org/10.14581/jer.19007
29. Disabled World. (2023). Famous people who had or have epilepsy, http://www.disabled-world.com/artman/publish/epilepsy-famous.shtml

30. Geloo, Z. [2006]. Zambia Goes To the Polls. http://archive.niza.nl/docs/200609232233446486.pdf?&username=guest@niza.nl&password=9999&groups=NIZA&workgroup=
31. Slowik, G. (2012). What is Epilepsy? http://ehealthmd.com/content/what-epilepsy
32. AlHarbi, F. A., Alomari, M. S., Ghaddaf, A. A., Abdulhamid, A. S., Alsharef, J. F., & Makkawi, S. (2021). Public awareness and attitudes toward epilepsy in Saudi Arabia: a systematic review and meta-analysis. *Epilepsy & Behavior*, *124*. https://doi.org/10.1016/j.yebeh.2021.108314
33. Gosain, K., & Samanta, T. (2022). Understanding the role of stigma and misconceptions in the experience of epilepsy in India: findings from a mixed-methods study. *Frontiers in Sociology*, *7*. https://doi.org/10.3389/fsoc.2022.790145
34. Braga, P., Hosny, H., Kakooza-Mwesige, A., Rider, F., Tripathi, M., & Guekht, A. (2020). How to understand and address the cultural aspects and consequences of diagnosis of epilepsy, including stigma. *Epileptic Disorders*, (5), 531-547. https://doi.org/10.1684/epd.2020.1201
35. Bashir, M. A., & Khalid, A. (2023). Misconceptions in Epilepsy and its Differentiation from Psychogenic Nonepileptic Events in Pakistan: The Dilemma in Underdeveloped Regions. *International Journal of Epilepsy*, *9*(01/02), 033-036. https://doi.org/10.1055/s-0044-1789251
36. Murthy, M. K. S., Rajaram, P., Mudiyanuru, K. S., Marimuthu, P., Govindappa, L., & Dasgupta, M. (2019). Potential for increased epilepsy awareness: Impact of health education program in school on teachers and children. *Journal of Neurosciences in Rural Practice*, *10*(4), 625. https://doi.org/10.1055/s-0039-3399473
37. Dwajani, S., Krithika, S., Meghana, K. S., & Adarsh, E. (2021). Knowledge, attitude and practice among parents towards children with epilepsy. *European Journal of Biomedical*, *8*(9), 429-431. https://www.researchgate.net/profile/Dr-Dwajani-S/publication/357016506_Knowledge_attitude_and_practice_among_parents_towards_children_with_epilepsy/links/63245a930a70852150fb3eb4/Knowledge-attitude-and-practice-among-parents-towards-children-with-epilepsy.pdf
38. International Bureau for Epilepsy. (2012). The dilemma of epilepsy – Personal short stories. https://www.ibe-epilepsy.org/wp-content/uploads/2012/07/IBE-Story-Book-Final.pdf

CHAPTER 11 – EPILEPSY AND RELIGION

Diseases were often seen either as caused by supernatural forces: gods, demons, or spirits and treated through spiritual means, or as natural conditions managed with physical remedies. Epilepsy, displaying both physical and psychological symptoms, was especially significant in this divide, interpreted both as a medical condition and a spiritual affliction.[1]
Owsei Temkin

Introduction

Culture and religion influence the way people perceive illness and how they seek healing.[2] Religion is defined as the practice of serving and worshiping a deity or supernatural forces.[3] The American Psychiatric Association[4] defines culture as the philosophy, perceptions, laws, and customs that are acquired and passed down through generations. Religious views can impact health outcomes in both positive and negative ways. When these views inspire people, provide a support system and assuagement, they should be promoted.[5] They become undesirable when they are associated with self-condemnation and retribution. At times religious beliefs make one feel that some external force is in control, hence the ill person must comply with the requirements of this external force to be well again. The beliefs can lead to delayed treatment in some cases as people try to please this external being.[2]

Historically, religious beliefs, customs, and culture have shaped the understanding of epilepsy. Epilepsy is understood as a reflection of varying cultural attitudes toward health and sickness. As mentioned in earlier chapters, epilepsy being referred to as the "sacred disease" in ancient times was because people could not understand its manifestations and quickly linked it to divine or supernatural forces.[6,7] This perception not only contributed to stigma, but influenced how PWE would be treated for centuries. Various cultures and religions have diverse views on epilepsy, but there is one common area everyone seems to converge on—superstition.

Epilepsy has been closely related with religion, with some people attributing it to possession by gods or evil spirits.[5] Many key prophets have been said to have had epilepsy. The mystical experience mainly associated with key religious figures is a seizure phenomenon.[5] Studies have demonstrated that prayer reduces physical stress, irrespective of which deity or spiritual force is being worshipped.[8] In this chapter, I will examine how epilepsy was viewed in ancient times as well as take into consideration different cultures and a few selected religions. The chapter delves into how different religious perspectives, from ancient traditions to contemporary practices, have viewed and impacted the experience of individuals with epilepsy.

The world view of epilepsy

Throughout history, the interpretation of epilepsy has varied significantly across cultures. PWE were considered either chosen or possessed, influencing their care and social acceptance.[9] In ancient Greece, Hippocrates dismissed the belief that epilepsy was a sacred or divine illness, promoting an understanding to view it as a natural condition.[7,10] With the spread of Christianity, people began seeking healing from saints and relics.[1] A boy reportedly became seizure-free after visiting St. Nicetius' grave. St. Valentine and St. Bibiana became patron saints of epilepsy, and a monastery dedicated to Bibiana served as a healing center. Patients underwent rituals including three Masses, during which they received powdered hulwort in the name of the Holy Trinity, then visit the grave of the saint. Those unable to visit Rome would receive the powder remotely and follow the same rites.[1] Many cultures continued to hold spiritual beliefs regarding epilepsy, with treatment approaches often involving rituals, prayers, and exorcisms.[5,11] Understanding epilepsy as both a medical and spiritual condition still prevails in many communities and continues to influence beliefs and practices.[12,13] If someone believes epilepsy is spiritual, they will handle it differently from one who believes it is a physical medical condition.

Epilepsy is caused by offending the gods

In Zimbabwe's *Shona* culture, when a child develops epilepsy, the ancestral spirits on the mother's side are usually said to be angry with some ritual not being done, or not being done to the ancestors' satisfaction.[14] The mother and child are usually excommunicated to avoid "spoiling" the whole clan. In several African societies, spirits are considered the source or drivers of evil.[15] It is believed that a dead person's spirit can enter another living person's spirit and manifest as epilepsy or mental illness. The dead person will be angry about something, so their spirit returns and torments the living in the form of this condition.[15]

PWE are prophets

The view that PWE are prophets is held by many people from all walks of life. Some scholars argued that most of the biblical and prominent prophets exhibited clear signs of epilepsy.[10,11,16] Signs exhibited by some prophets, like recurrent collapsing and periods of being mute are associated with some types of epileptic seizures. Some prophets are said to have showed signs consistent with temporal lobe epilepsy (TLE), which is associated with being highly religious.[10,11,16] These religious leaders usually transitioned into states of altered consciousness, heard voices, saw visions, and showed various signs associated with TLE.[10,16] Hearing voices and seeing visions allowed the prophets to communicate with God and relay the message to the people.[10,16] Many people believe PWE are prophets especially when they bring a message from God from the seizure episode.[10,16] However, some scholars argue that the idea of biblical prophets having epilepsy remains an area needing further research, as drawing definitive conclusions is challenging with the current information: when the Bible says a prophet fell, it may signify a custom of worshipping and not necessarily epilepsy.[17,18]

PWE are witches

Some people are excommunicated from their families because once they start having epileptic seizures, they are accused of being witches.[19] This is very serious to an extent that paternal relatives usually want to distance themselves from a PWE.[19] Some have been disowned by their fathers. Their siblings are told not to even mention that they are related, because their blood will also be tainted with the epilepsy, hence becoming witches.[19] Most people with the condition end up living in isolation if the maternal relatives are not forthcoming as well.

Buddhism and epilepsy

In Buddhism, the focus on understanding suffering as part of the human experience extends to the way epilepsy is viewed. The concept of *Dukkha* (suffering) is central to Buddhist teachings, which encourage compassion and non-judgmental support for individuals facing health challenges.[20,21] Buddhist teachings are centered on "cause-effect and reincarnation."[20] It is believed that when one does good, it results in positive effects and the opposite is true (karma).[20] The bad deeds that can result in negative consequences may not necessarily have been done by the person who suffers the consequences: they can be generational. The bad karmas often manifest in the form of diseases, epilepsy included.[20] Epilepsy is considered a punishment and an atonement to reduce the weighty effects that could result from the past karmas.[20] Though Buddhism does not prohibit followers from accessing proper medical treatment, PWE are urged to atone for previous wrongdoings, engage in virtuous behavior, and give offerings.[20] Meditation and holistic approaches such as herbal medicine are often integrated into care, reflecting the Buddhist emphasis on balancing mind and body.[21,22]

Since some of the bad karmas are generational, it is not clear how one with epilepsy can confess to a deed done maybe two or three generations before them. How do they know what to confess in such a case? Epilepsy in Buddhist-majority regions has been approached with acceptance, however, emphasizing that suffering could be related to past karma and should be met with mindfulness and kindness.[20,23]

Sikhism and epilepsy

Sikhism, which originated in the Punjab region of India, emphasizes equality and community support. While the Sikh scriptures may not explicitly reference epilepsy, the tenets of Sikhism promote caring for all individuals with compassion and without discrimination.[5,24] The principle of *sewa* (selfless service) underpins the Sikh approach to supporting those with health issues, encouraging collective responsibility and empathy.[24,25] Prayer and collective worship (*ardas*) are often invoked for healing, reinforcing the idea that spiritual and practical support go hand in hand.[5,26]

Hinduism and epilepsy

Hinduism is associated with worshipping many deities. Siva is regarded as the third person of the Hindu Triad and is a destroyer.[27] In the work of destruction, Siva gives beings a new form and is therefore also called the re-creator.[27] He is also called the physician or healer. Siva manifests in different forms and is said to have a thousand names depending on one's circumstances. When people pray for recovery from illness, they pray to him under the name of Panchanana.[27] In the case of epilepsy, however, it is believed that the person will be possessed by Panchanana, hence prayers are conducted to persuade him to depart.[27] Though Panchanana is regarded as the healer of other illnesses, when it comes to epilepsy, he seems to be the cause.

In Hindu mythology, "Apasmara was a dwarf who represented ignorance and epilepsy."[28] Hindu texts, including the *Atharva Veda* and Ayurvedic literature, describe epilepsy as *apasmara*, associating it with a loss of consciousness and divine retribution.[12,27] Apasmara literally means loss of consciousness.[12] The demon Apasmara, often depicted under Siva's foot, symbolizes ignorance and disease, implying that overcoming epilepsy is linked to divine intervention and spiritual growth.[27,29] Killing Apasmara would destroy harmony in the world, so Siva took the form of Sri Nataraja and suppressed Apasmara.[28]

Treatments in traditional Hindu practice include rituals, mantras, and herbal remedies designed to appease deities and correct spiritual imbalances.[8,30] Additionally, the principle of karma suggests that epilepsy may be seen because of actions from past lives, impacting how communities perceive those affected by the condition.[28,29] Epilepsy is attributed to past sins in both Hinduism and Sikhism.[2] In Hinduism, the role of the nine planets in the life of a person is brought to the fore. The nine planets are referred to as *Navagraha* and are revered as gods.[31] It is believed that worshipping them averts any calamities and brings peace and harmony to the worshipper.[31] The planets are believed to influence humanity, even before birth.[31]

Epilepsy was once linked to astrological beliefs, such as Jupiter rising or the moon aligning with Saturn. The moon was thought to influence a child's health and intellect. Those born during its waning phase were considered more prone to epilepsy, while those born without a visible moon were believed to be weak, sickly, or intellectually impaired.[31]

Islam and epilepsy

According to Akhtar and Aziz,[32,33] there is no mention of epilepsy or anything close to it in The Holy Quran, but there is mention of a woman with the condition in the Hadith. The Hadith is a collection of Prophet Mohammed's life, actions, and deeds. The Hadiths and teachings of Prophet Mohammad emphasize seeking treatment for illnesses while maintaining faith in divine will, promoting an integrated approach of prayer, charity, and modern medical care.[34,35]

Though the Quran does not mention anything about epilepsy, Islamic medical literature does have a lot of information on epilepsy. Historical Islamic scholars, including Avicenna (Ibn Sina), contributed to medical understandings of epilepsy, viewing it as a physical condition rather than purely a result of possession or divine punishment.[16,36] Avicenna, a Persian physician, is said to have been the first person to use the term *epilepsy* as meaning being influenced or dominated by an external power.[32]

Islamic literature[34,36] states that there are two types of epilepsy: one caused by evil spirits (jinns) and another that is physical. Allah has given permission to the jinn and the devil to torment humanity, even causing them to have epilepsy.[36,37] Epilepsy's portrayal in Islamic teachings reflects a balance between supernatural and medical interpretations. Despite this, cultural practices in some Islamic communities still link epilepsy to jinn or spiritual interference, leading to the use of *Ruqyah* (recitation of Quranic verses) as a form of spiritual healing.[16,38] According to these documents, doctors can only treat the physical epilepsy and cannot do anything about the other type.[34,36,37] The documents also claim that even Hippocrates acknowledged the presence of this type of epilepsy.[34,36]

Believing in these two types of epilepsy necessitates being able to distinguish one from the other. The epilepsy caused by the jinn or devil is believed to involve the jinn invading the human body, punching and toppling the person, who loses consciousness. The jinn then communicates through the person, possibly stating the reason for the affliction.

Epilepsy that is caused by evil spirits is treated in two parts. The first segment addresses the person with the condition and the second segment addresses the person treating them.[34] The afflicted individual must seek strength and trust in Allah, as must the healer, so the jinn can be cast out in the name of Allah. Reading verses from the Quran has also been said to cure epilepsy.[39] The *Tibb al-Nabi*, a medical document produced by Mohammed's followers after his death, suggests "sniffing of the narcissus flower" as a remedy against epilepsy.[33] The document does not link epilepsy to any demonic influences.[33] Beating a PWE is also recommended in some instances.[34,37] This is based on the understanding that the treating person will be beating the evil spirit and not the physical person. Some of the beating can be very severe, but according to these documents,[34,37] after the beating, the person is set free from epilepsy and does not show any signs of assault.

According to Abbas,[36] diagnosing spiritual epilepsy requires skill, experience, and the willingness of Allah. This is very important in that not just anyone should label every PWE as being possessed by a jinn. Having a symptom of spiritual epilepsy does not in any way imply that the person is suffering from spiritual epilepsy.[36]

Judaism and epilepsy

In ancient Jewish culture, epilepsy was understood through religious texts such as the Talmud, which described symptoms of seizures and possible spiritual interpretations.[17,40] The Talmud teaches that demons are more numerous than humans.[41] For every person, there are 11,000 demons.[41] Epilepsy has always been associated with demons.[42] In ancient times, the Jews referred to PWE as a *nikpeh*, meaning "one who writhes" or "one who is bent or forced over." Later the term *holi nophel*, meaning falling sickness, began to be used.[42]

To avoid epilepsy, several things are recommended. Men are discouraged from marrying someone with a family history of epilepsy even if the woman does not have epilepsy.[42] This is because epilepsy is considered hereditary and contagious. Men are discouraged from having sex with their spouses immediately after leaving the toilet;[41] if they do not observe this, the child that is conceived will have epilepsy.[41] Another cause for epilepsy is standing nude in front of a candle.[41]

While epilepsy was occasionally associated with divine punishment, it was also recognized as a medical condition that required practical intervention.[43] Dietary and herbal treatments were often recommended, showing a balance between religious and practical responses to the condition.[43,44] Modern Judaism generally supports medical treatment for epilepsy, complemented by prayer and religious rituals as sources of comfort.[24,40]

Christianity and epilepsy

Christianity's approach to epilepsy has evolved significantly over time. Early Christian interpretations often linked epilepsy to demonic possession, a view reinforced by biblical accounts in which Jesus exorcised demons from individuals with seizure-like symptoms.[1,4,11] This belief contributed to the stigmatization of PWE, leading to practices aimed at spiritual "cleansing."[45,46] However, with advancements in medical understanding during the Renaissance and beyond, the Christian view shifted to embrace medical explanations alongside spiritual care.[4,47] Modern Christian denominations support medical treatments and encourage compassionate pastoral care, promoting a holistic approach that combines prayer and medical intervention.[13,24,45]

Epilepsy is not mentioned in the Old Testament. The Bible mentions epilepsy in six different verses in the New Testament. Three of them are parallel passages in the three synoptic gospels (Matthew 17:14–20; Mark 9:17–25; Luke 9: 38–42). In summary, these verses narrate the story of a man who brought his son, who was possessed by a violent spirit that caused seizures, to Jesus after the disciples failed to heal him. Jesus expressed frustration over the lack of faith and asked for the boy to be brought to him. Upon seeing Jesus, the spirit triggered another seizure. The boy's father explained the condition had afflicted his son since childhood and begged for help. Jesus told him that all things are possible for those who believe. The father, in tears, declared his belief and asked Jesus to help his doubt. Jesus then commanded the unclean spirit to leave the boy and never return.

Below are some of the views on epilepsy found in the church today. They are not universal to all Christians; most of the issues discussed are based on my personal lived or observed experience.

Epilepsy is a demonic attack

So, to this group, everyone with epilepsy is demon possessed and needs deliverance. I have heard many preachers equating demons to epilepsy like the two words are synonyms.
Clotilda Chinyanya

As described in the story above, some people in the church regard epilepsy as a sign of demonic possession. In the early church, PWE were segregated as the priests feared the communion plate and cup would be defiled.[9] Many people have concluded that since Jesus personally commanded this spirit to leave and it left, it means it was an unclean spirit. So, to this group, everyone with epilepsy is demon-possessed and needs deliverance. I have heard many preachers equating demons to epilepsy like the two words are synonyms.

Epilepsy is due to unconfessed sin

According to Koch,[48] when people confess their sinful practices, especially involvement in the occult, they are assured of healing. When these people refuse to confess their sins, the epilepsy will not recede. Many people who suffer from epilepsy are told to confess their sins if they want healing. If they do not confess, they are blamed for their predicament and people usually isolate them.

Epilepsy is a sign of having no faith

Nowadays, we have preachers on the various television channels expressing the view that if anyone is not healed of their condition, it is because of lack of faith. This is also happening in many churches and puts a heavy burden on the already ill person as they are blamed for their condition. People suffering from chronic illnesses are told not to put their trust in the medicines they take, and to show that they have accepted the message, they are asked to bring all their medicines and throw them at the pulpit for burning. After throwing away the medicines, they are assured of healing if they have faith in God.[49,50]

This is a very scary situation in that abrupt withdrawal of AEDs can cause serious convulsions, which can lead to status epilepticus. There is real danger of SUDEP, but no one ever takes responsibility for asking them to stop taking their medicine if the PWE dies, and just say it was God's timing. When someone refuses to let go of their medicine, they are ostracized. How many pastors or church leaders have led their congregants to death because of this practice?

My question is, "How much faith does one need to be healed or for God to intervene in any situation the person may be in?" Where does the issue of "little faith" when a person is not healed come from? Where do we get this theology that people need to have great faith to be healed by God, or for God to intervene in their situations? The Bible is full of stories of people who had little faith, but when they called on God, He answered them.

We also see that someone else's faith can bring healing to a sick person as detailed in the account in Mark (2:3–11). This is a challenge to those who claim the people they are praying for are not getting healed because they lack faith. They themselves should have faith, and the person they will be praying for will receive healing because of their faith if it is true that every time people pray, God should respond in the positive.

Epilepsy is a sign of unbelief or not being saved

In our day, if anyone suffers from any illness, epilepsy included, and they are prayed for and not healed, this is taken as a sign of unbelief. This puts pressure on the afflicted person as they are not sure how they are to demonstrate their belief. According to some pastors, it is not possible to be born again and have epilepsy at the same time. When a member of the church starts suffering from epilepsy, they are asked to receive Christ as their Lord and personal Savior.

Epilepsy is a sign of a poor prayer life

According to our text in Mark (9:29), Jesus told His disciples that the situation they wanted to deal with but failed required prayer and fasting. This then becomes the next point of argument for those who pray for people who do not heal. The ill person is accused of not praying hard enough. They can even be forced to go on a fast to ensure they get healed. The reason people start blaming those in such situations is that they make people believe they are used mightily of God and can heal any disease. When the person does not get healed, they say it is the fault of the person so that the preacher's reputation is not damaged.

In summary, a person who does not receive healing carries all the blame for their condition. It is unfortunate that epilepsy is one condition one can never pretend not to have because it can just manifest when and where you do not want it to. In the end, many people end up avoiding going to church or other places where they feel they will attract negative attention. This directly leads to isolation of these members of our society. Any discomfort on the part of a Christian is attributed to a poor relationship with God in many Christian circles. Many Christians are being ostracized for not receiving healing, as if it is their fault.[49,50]

EPILEPSY SPIRITUAL BELIEFS FOR SPECIFIC REGIONS

African traditional religions

In many African cultures, epilepsy has traditionally been linked to spiritual and mystical beliefs, often deeply intertwined with cultural beliefs about health, illness, and spirituality. It is often regarded as an expression of witchcraft, ancestral spirits, or possession by supernatural entities.[15,19,51] These beliefs vary across regions and countries and shape the approach to treatment, including consulting traditional healers or spiritualists, rituals, and the use of herbal remedies aimed at addressing the spiritual roots of the condition.[19,52] Despite modernization, these traditional beliefs continue to coexist with contemporary medical approaches in many African communities.[25,52] In some cases, they can interfere with medical care. The stigma associated with epilepsy often leads to social isolation and fear. Ongoing public health efforts are aimed at changing these perceptions through education and community-based interventions.[51,53]

Treatment practices and rituals

Treatment of epilepsy within African traditional religions (ATR) combines spiritual rituals, herbal medicine, and community support. In Nigeria, traditional healers might use a variety of herbs known to counteract evil spirits in combination with rituals designed to remove curses or spirits.[19,52] Ceremonies involving drumming, chanting, and animal sacrifices may also be performed to seek protection from ancestors or gods.[33,51]

In South Africa, particularly among Zulu communities, epilepsy is sometimes treated through rituals conducted by *sangomas* (traditional healers). The *sangoma* will enter a trance-like state, to consult the individual's ancestors to gain insight on how to restore spiritual balance.[15,54] Herbal concoctions with both physical and spiritual healing properties are used as part of the treatment process. It is also believed epilepsy can be transferred to another living thing, such as a chicken or goat, or a non-living object, like rocks, soil, or furniture, as part of the ritual practices.[19,29] Once the spirit of epilepsy is transferred into an animal, the animal is then let go to roam freely in the wild. In Zimbabwe, they call this practice *kurasirira*.

Social implications and stigma

The way people in many African communities associate epilepsy with the supernatural often results in far-reaching social consequences. Individuals with epilepsy may be excluded from social events, marriage prospects, or even basic community interactions rooted in fears of spreading the illness or spiritual uncleanness.[52,55] In Ethiopia, for instance, PWE are sometimes considered possessed by evil spirits, leading to social ostracism and limited opportunities for education and employment.[25,51]

In Benin, the influence of *Vodun* (commonly known as Voodoo) is significant in how epilepsy is perceived and treated. Epilepsy is a result of interactions with spirits. Rituals to appease the spirits involve offerings and spiritual appeals with the help of a *houngan* or *mambo* (Vodun priest or priestess) who conducts cleansing rituals to alleviate the condition.[54,56] These practices highlight the role of spiritual leaders in providing not only treatment but also comfort and social inclusion for affected individuals.

The traditional beliefs in Ghana associate epilepsy with the wrath of river gods. People living along rivers may consult priests to perform appeasement rituals.[53,57] The blending of indigenous beliefs with Christian prayer meetings, especially in Pentecostal churches, is common, and faith-based healing practices coexist with traditional spiritual beliefs.[30,58]

In Mali and Burkina Faso, epilepsy is sometimes perceived as a condition that requires the intervention of village elders or griots, who act as oral historians and spiritual guides. These figures may hold ceremonies to seek divine intervention or blessings, accompanied by community gatherings that reinforce collective support for the affected individual.[23,59]

The role of traditional healers today

Traditional healers continue to play a vital role in the management of epilepsy, serving as both medical practitioners and spiritual guides. In many African countries, these healers are often the first point of contact for those experiencing seizures, especially in regions with limited access to modern healthcare.[52,59] Their role extends beyond treatment; they help maintain cultural practices that reinforce social cohesion and provide an accessible framework for understanding and coping with illness.[23,60]

Asia and the Middle East

Historical beliefs and interpretations

In Asia and the Middle East, epilepsy has long been influenced by spiritual and cultural interpretations that differ widely across communities and countries. Historically, in India, epilepsy was viewed within the framework of Ayurvedic medicine, where it was believed to be caused by imbalances in the body's fundamental energies (*doshas*) and influenced by supernatural elements.[10,51] The condition, known as *Apasmara*, was sometimes attributed to karmic consequences or the displeasure of deities, reflecting the connectedness between physical health and spiritual well-being.[50,52]

In ancient Persia, epilepsy was viewed as either a divine or demonic affliction. People consulted Zoroastrian priests to interpret and treat seizures. Evidence found in the Avesta, the sacred texts of Zoroastrianism, includes references to rituals and prayers meant to protect against such conditions.[32,61] Similarly, traditional Chinese medicine viewed epilepsy as a disruption of the *Qi* (vital energy) and yin–yang balance, often associating it with spirit possession or malevolent forces.[17,62]

Treatment practices and rituals

In India, Ayurvedic treatment of epilepsy involved the use of herbal remedies such as *Bacopa monnieri* and *Centella asiatica*, combined with meditation and rituals to harmonize the body's energies.[19,27] These treatments were often managed by *vaidya* (traditional physicians) and included dietary adjustments and specific prayers to counteract the spiritual side of epilepsy.[2,46]

In the Middle East, Islamic traditions have historically influenced epilepsy treatment. While the Quran acknowledges that all ailments, including epilepsy, are part of divine will, traditional practices have included recitation of verses for healing purposes, known as *ruqyah*.[51,54] Traditional healers incorporate herbal infusions and oils believed to fend off jinn, which are sometimes considered the cause of seizures.[29,39]

Chinese medicine uses herbal formulas such as *Tian Ma* (*Gastrodia elata*) and acupuncture to treat epilepsy. These interventions are meant to restore balance to the body's energy channels. Additionally, rituals involving the use of magical objects that ward off harm and spiritual consultations address the underlying cause of seizures.[22,40]

Social implications and stigma

The perception of epilepsy as a condition with supernatural origins can be linked to social stigma across many Asian and Middle Eastern societies. In rural India, PWE might be considered cursed or unclean, jeopardizing their chances of marriage and leading to social isolation.[3,53] In more traditional communities of Pakistan and Afghanistan, epilepsy could be seen as spirit possession. This perpetuates stigma, making it harder for PWE to access modern medical care.[63,64]

In parts of China, especially rural areas, epilepsy was traditionally seen as an omen or a sign of a tormented spirit. This perception worsened discrimination, affecting educational and employment opportunities for PWE.[28,65] Similarly, in Middle Eastern countries, while Islamic teachings advocate for compassion, false notions about epilepsy often result in the social isolation of those affected.[29,57]

In Japan, Shinto beliefs historically interpreted epilepsy as related to spiritual purity and impurity. Traditional healers conduct purification rites at shrines to cleanse the afflicted person of any perceived spiritual impurity.[45,66] In Iran, epilepsy treatment within the context of traditional Persian medicine involved a mix of spiritual and physical remedies. Practitioners might recite sections of the Quran or prayers while applying specific herbs known for their calming effects, such as valerian root.[56,67] In rural areas of Nepal and parts of Pakistan, traditional healers may use amulets, prayers, and rituals meant to ward off evil spirits believed to cause seizures.[2,67]

Latin America
Historical beliefs and interpretations
In Latin America, traditional interpretations of epilepsy are deeply influenced by the blending of indigenous beliefs and Catholicism. Among indigenous communities, epilepsy is a supernatural phenomenon where PWE are believed to communicate with gods.[20,68] Depending on the culture and context, epilepsy can be seen either as a gift or a curse.[20,68] In Mesoamerican cultures, such as the Maya and Aztec, seizures are considered a sign of a person being touched by gods or possessed by a spirit. These beliefs have persisted to some extent, influencing how epilepsy is understood in modern rural communities.[3,69]

Treatment practices and rituals
Traditional healers, known as *curanderos* or *shamans*, play a key role in treating epilepsy. They often use a combination of herbal remedies, such as *ruda* (rue) and *epazote*, together with praying, chanting, and the use of sacred items like crosses or images of saints.[52,70] The rituals can include cleansing ceremonies performed using smoke from burning herbs and reciting of traditional invocations to ward off evil spirits.[33,60] In Brazil, the Afro-Brazilian religion of Candomblé includes practices where epilepsy is associated with *orixás* (deities), particularly those linked to health and misfortune. Rituals may involve drumming, dancing, and offerings to gain favor and healing from these deities.[57,71]

Social implications and stigma

The social implications of epilepsy in Latin American countries are complex, shaped by religious and cultural attitudes. Individuals with epilepsy may be viewed with suspicion or awe, depending on the perceived cause of their seizures. PWE in rural Mexico are sometimes feared as they are believed to have been touched by evil spirits, leading to social isolation.[2,55] The influence of Catholicism has reframed epilepsy as an affliction to be borne with faith, promoting a sense of empathy.[39,46]

In Peru, epilepsy is associated with mountain spirits or *apus*. The shamans lead rituals that include offerings to these spirits to bring about healing.[4,72] In Haiti, Vodou practices often interpret seizures as a manifestation of spirit possession, with *houngans* or *mambos* performing ceremonies to address these spiritual causes.[44,59]

Europe

Historical beliefs and interpretations

Historically in Europe, religion influenced views on epilepsy. During medieval times, epilepsy was known as the "sacred disease," believed to be a sign of divine intervention or demonic possession, depending on the era and region.[21,73] In ancient Greece, epilepsy was both a blessing and a curse, associated with the god Apollo. This idea influenced later European Christian interpretations.[32,61]

Treatment practices and rituals

In medieval Europe, treatments for epilepsy often involved religious rituals, including prayer, exorcisms, and the use of holy water to repel evil forces. Saints such as Valentine, Bibiana and Dymphna were frequently called upon for their presumed ability to heal epilepsy.[1,34,50] Remedies from folk medicine included the use of herbs like valerian and mistletoe, believed to have protective qualities.[24,43]

Social implications and stigma

In Italy, folk beliefs linked epilepsy to the influence of the *malocchio* (evil eye), with traditional healers performing rituals involving prayers and the use of protective amulets.[33,58] In Ireland, epilepsy was once seen as connected to the *fae* (fairies), and local healers would perform rituals to protect individuals from supernatural harm.[62,74]

North America

Historical beliefs and interpretations

In North America, the diverse cultural fabric, shaped by Indigenous populations and later European settlers, has influenced how epilepsy was traditionally perceived. Some Native American tribes viewed epilepsy as confirmation of their connection to the spirit world. Some tribes considered seizures a sign that a person was chosen by spirits for a special purpose, while others saw it as a spiritual imbalance or affliction needing purification rituals.[20,63]

Treatment practices and rituals

Traditional treatment among Indigenous peoples often involved the use of herbal remedies and spiritual ceremonies. Healers or shamans would use plants such as sage and tobacco in cleansing rituals, and drumming or chanting was performed to call upon spirits for healing.[2,55]

Social implications and stigma

The spiritual interpretations of seizures varied, leading to different social reactions. In Indigenous cultures, PWE might have been given a status of honor. However, in colonial European societies, the condition was a sign of possession or divine punishment, and therefore stigmatizing.[61,75] Sources referencing Indigenous communities in North America mention that some tribes view epilepsy as a spiritual sign or challenge that connects the individual with supernatural forces. Rituals involving medicinal plants, drumming, and the guidance of a shaman are noted as traditional treatment methods.[63] The modern-day understanding has largely moved away from spiritual interpretations, but pockets of these beliefs can still be found in traditional communities.[44]

Australia

Historical beliefs and interpretations

Australian Aboriginal and Torres Strait Islander peoples have rich cultural traditions that frame health and illness within a spiritual context. Epilepsy was viewed as a manifestation of spiritual disharmony or ancestral displeasure. Ceremonial rituals involving music, dance, and the use of sacred objects were used for healing or restoration of balance.[32,60]

Treatment practices and rituals

Traditional practices included the use of medicinal plants and spiritual guidance from elders or healers known as *Ngangkari* in some Aboriginal communities. The healers connected with the spiritual realm to find the cause of the illness and provide spiritual facilitation for recovery.[33,44]

Social implications and stigma

The communal nature of Aboriginal societies meant PWE might be cared for within the community based on the perceived cause. If the perceived cause was not good, the individuals would suffer social stigma. Where it was seen as part of spiritual learning or a connection to ancestors, the reaction was empathetic, while fear of negative spiritual implications could contribute to a different form of exclusion or caution.[37,74]

Sources describe epilepsy in the Australian Aboriginal culture, interpreted within a spiritual framework, where illness is seen as a disruption of harmony or as the result of ancestral displeasure.[32] Healing practices might include consultations with a *Ngangkari* and rituals aimed at restoring balance through spiritual means.[60]

Modern religious perspectives and epilepsy

In recent years, many religious groups have moved toward reconciling traditional beliefs with modern medical knowledge. Studies indicate that strong religious beliefs can enhance adherence to treatment and improve psychological outcomes for PWE.[71,76] However, the interplay between positive religious coping and negative spiritual interpretations must be managed to ensure that individuals receive supportive and informed care.[35,60] Religious organizations are increasingly active in reducing epilepsy-related stigma by fostering awareness programs, workshops, and community discussions that align faith with science.[23,55]

Conclusion

Religious beliefs have historically shaped the understanding and treatment of epilepsy in profound ways. From the divine interpretations in ancient texts to the more balanced approaches seen today, the intersection of faith and epilepsy reveals a spectrum of attitudes and practices. Recognizing these perspectives is essential for healthcare professionals to offer culturally competent care, facilitate supportive religious engagement, and reduce stigma. The integration of modern medicine with respectful spiritual care helps create a comprehensive approach that values both the physical and emotional needs of those living with epilepsy.

After considering all the views, it is apparent that epilepsy is a physical condition, though in some instances, it can be perceived supernatural. Demanding too much from the PWE to get deliverance in the form of confession, *Tauheed, Tawakkul, Taqwa, Tawajjhu*, more faith, repentance, healthy prayer life or fasting is an unnecessary extra burden. The efficacy of AEDs, surgery, a ketogenic diet or vagus nerve stimulation in reducing or eliminating true epileptic seizures should provide proof for those who believe they have a supernatural cause; likewise, a child outgrowing certain forms of epilepsy. It is of utmost importance that whatever belief system a PWE may be involved in they are allowed access to modern, clinically validated medical treatment.

My advice to anyone living with epilepsy is: Do not throw away your AEDs even if someone says you have been healed. Keep them and go to your doctor for proper withdrawal management if necessary. We do not want to lose you to SUDEP, status epilepticus, or any other fatal injuries that can result from sudden withdrawal. Be responsible because we still need you around.

References:

1. Temkin, O. (1971). *The Falling Sickness: A history of epilepsy from the Greeks to the beginnings of modern neurology.* The John Hopkins University Press: Baltimore and London.
2. Ismail, H., Wright, J., Rhodes, P. and Small, N. (2005). Religious beliefs about causes and treatment of epilepsy. *British Journal of General Practice.* 26-31. https://bjgp.org/content/55/510/26.short
3. "Religion" http://www.merriam-webster.com/dictionary/religion
4. American Psychiatric Association. (2013). *Diagnostic and statistical manual of mental disorders (5th ed.).* Arlington, VA: American Psychiatric Publishing.
5. Khwaja, G.A., Singh, G. and Chaudhry, N. (2007). Epilepsy and religion. *Annals of Indian Academy of Neurology.* 10: 165-8. https://doi.org/10.4103/0972-2327.34796
6. Fater, M. [s.a]. Living Life Unpredictably, http://www.scientiareview.org/pdfs/120
7. Schachter, S.C. ed. (2004). Epilepsy history, http://www.epilepsy.com/EPILEPSY/HISTORY

8. Brown, E. (2010). Ayurveda and the "Sacred Disease": Treating epilepsy with ancient Ayurvedic wisdom. www.chopra.com/files/docs/teacherdownloads/.../**Epilepsy**,%20Erin%20**brown**.pdf
9. International League against Epilepsy. (2003). The History and Stigma of Epilepsy. *Epilepsia*, 44(Suppl. 6): 12–14. https://doi.org/10.1046/j.1528-1157.44.s.6.2.x
10. Pickover, C. (2012). Transcendent Experience and Temporal Lobe Epilepsy, http://meta-religion.com/Psychiatry/The_Paranormal/trascendent_experiences.htm
11. Motluk, A. (2001). Old Testament prophet showed epileptic symptoms, http://www.newscientist.com/article/dn1565-old-testament-prophet-showed-epileptic-symptoms.html
12. Manyam, B. V. (1992). Epilepsy in ancient India. *Epilepsia*, *33*(3), 473-475. https://doi.org/10.1111/j.1528-1157.1992.tb01694.x
13. Chirchiglia, D., & Chirchiglia, P. (2020). Epilepsy over the centuries: A disease survived at the time. *Neurological Sciences*, *41*(5), 1309-1313. https://doi.org/10.1007/s10072-019-04214-6
14. Zifo, D. 2012. Interview with Dorothy Zifo, a 77-Year-Old Woman. Harare, Zimbabwe. [6 November 2012].
15. Kasomo, D. (2009). An investigation of sin and evil in African cosmology, *International Journal of Sociology and Anthropology*. 1/8: 145-155. https://academicjournals.org/article/article1379413683_Kasomo%20%20pdf.pdf
16. Margoliouth, D.S. (1905). *Mohammed and the Rise of Islam*. Putnam. 46. https://archive.org/details/mohammedandtheri00marguoft/page/n9/mode/2up
17. Feinsod, M. (2010). "Neurology in the Bible and Talmud" in: *Handbook of Clinical Neurology. Vol.95 (3rd Series):* History of Neurology. Amsterdam: Elsevier. 37-47. https://doi.org/10.1016/s0072-9752(08)02104-0
18. Azad, M. S. Comparative analysis of the controversies among the orientalist about the epilepsy imputed to the Holy Prophet. http://religion.asianindexing.com/images_religion/1/12/Al-Basirah_4_2_13.pdf
19. Komolafe, M. A., Sunmonu, T. A., Fabusiwa, F., Komolafe, E. O., Afolabi, O., Kett, M., & Groce, N. (2011). Women's perspectives on epilepsy and its sociocultural impact in southwestern Nigeria. *African Journal of Neurological Sciences*, *30*(2). https://www.ajol.info/index.php/ajns/article/view/77320
20. Rong-Chi, C. H. E. N. (2004). Buddhist's and Taoist's view on epilepsy. *Neurology Asia*, *9*(1), 61-62. https://citeseerx.ist.psu.edu/document?repid=rep1&type=pdf&doi=30544bbff9bb5aa96a42cc0deaf70f4edf2c065e
21. Rigon, I. B., Calado, G. D. A., Linhares, L. S., Cantu, P. L. M., Moritz, J. L. W., Wolf, P., & Lin, K. (2019). Religiosity and spirituality in patients with epilepsy. *Arquivos de Neuro-Psiquiatria*, *77*, 335-340. https://doi.org/10.1590/0004-282X20190055
22. Aziz, H. (2020). Did Prophet Mohammad (PBUH) have epilepsy? A neurological analysis. *Epilepsy & Behavior*, *103*, 106654. https://doi.org/10.1016/j.yebeh.2019.106654
23. Kiyak, E., Erkal, E., Demir, S., Demirkiran, B. C., Uren, Y., & Erguney, S. (2021). Evaluation of attitudes toward epilepsy and health fatalism in northeastern Turkey. *Epilepsy & Behavior*, *115*, 107495. https://doi.org/10.1016/j.yebeh.2020.107495
24. Mameniškienė, R., Puteikis, K., & Carrizosa-Moog, J. (2022). Saints, demons, and faith–A review of the historical interaction between Christianity and epilepsy. *Epilepsy & Behavior*, *135*, 108870. https://doi.org/10.1016/j.yebeh.2022.108870
25. Gugssa, S. A., & Haidar, J. (2020). Knowledge, attitude, and practice towards epilepsy among religious cleric and traditional healers of Addis Ababa, Ethiopia. *Seizure*, *78*, 57-62. https://doi.org/10.1016/j.seizure.2020.03.006

26. Tirukelem, H., Nigatu, S. G., Angaw, D. A., & Azale, T. (2021). Community attitude towards epilepsy patients and associated factors in South Achefer District, Northwest Ethiopia: A mixed-methods study. *Neuropsychiatric Disease and Treatment*, 365-377. https://doi.org/10.2147/NDT.S292257
27. Wilkins, W.J. (1900). Siva in: *Hindu Mythology, Vedic and Puranic.* 262-284. http://www.sacred-texts.com/hin/hmvp/hmvp33.htm
28. Apasmara. https://en.wikipedia.org/wiki/Apasmara
29. Nasif, M. B., Koubeissi, M., & Azar, N. J. (2021). Epilepsy–from mysticism to science. *Revue Neurologique*, *177*(9), 1047-1058. https://doi.org/10.1016/j.neurol.2021.01.021
30. Thapa, L., Bhandari, T. R., Shrestha, S., & Poudel, R. S. (2017). Knowledge, beliefs, and practices on epilepsy among high school students of Central Nepal. *Epilepsy Research and Treatment*, (1). https://doi.org/10.1155/2017/6705807
31. http://www.findyourfate.com/indianastro/medical-astrology/causesofepilepsy.html
32. Akhtar, S.W. & Aziz, H. (2004). Perception of epilepsy in Muslim history; with current scenario. *Neurology Asia.* 9 (Supplement 1): 59 – 60. https://www.neurology-asia.org/articles/20043_059.pdf
33. Vanzan, A. & Paladin, F. (1992). Epilepsy and Persian Culture: An Overview. *Epilepsia*, 33(6): 1057-1064. https://doi.org/10.1111/j.1528-1157.1992.tb01759.x
34. Prophet's Guidance on treating Epilepsy and possession. http://tibbenabawi.org/index.php?option=com_content&view=article&id=64&Itemid=93
35. Lee, S. A., Choi, E. J., & Ryu, H. U. (2019). Negative, but not positive, religious coping strategies are associated with psychological distress, independent of religiosity, in Korean adults with epilepsy. *Epilepsy & Behavior*, *90*, 57-60. https://doi.org/10.1016/j.yebeh.2018.11.017
36. Abbas, M. (n.d.). Chapter 5 (Spiritual Ailments) Jinn Affliction of Man in: *Quranic Healing – A Clinical Psychological Study.* http://www.quranichealing.net/chp5_p.php?id=41
37. Tibb an Nabawi - The Medicine of the Holy Prophet. (2009). Epilepsy. http://prophetic-medicine.blogspot.com/2009/06/understanding-epilepsy.html
38. Duas And/or Surahs for Seizures. (2014). http://www.shiachat.com/forum/topic/235022789-duas-andor-surahs-for-seizures/
39. Is there a prayer to be read for the disease of epilepsy? http://www.questionsonislam.com/question/there-prayer-be-read-disease-epilepsy
40. Kottek, S. (1988). From the history of medicine: Epilepsy in ancient Jewish sources. *Israel Journal of Psychiatry Related Sci*ence, 25: 3-11. https://pubmed.ncbi.nlm.nih.gov/3075204/
41. The Talmud: Demons & Magick**.** https://watch.pair.com/HR**talmud**.html
42. Hateva, D. (2008). Epilepsy in the Talmud 37-39. www.*download.yutorah.org/2008/1053/724884/epilepsy-in-the-talmud.pdf*
43. Rosner, F. (1975). Neurology in the Bible and Talmud. *Israel journal of medical sciences*, *11*(4), 385-397. https://pubmed.ncbi.nlm.nih.gov/1095529/
44. Diby, T., Khumalo, P. G., Anokyewaa-Amponsah, G., Mustapha, R., & Ampofo, A. G. (2021). Knowledge about epilepsy and factors associated with attitudes toward marrying, employing, and driving people with epilepsy: a cross-sectional survey of Asokore Mampong community dwellers in Ghana. *Epilepsy & Behavior*, *115*, 107646. https://doi.org/10.1016/j.yebeh.2020.107646
45. Summers, M. 1946. *The Malleficarum: (The Witch Hammer) of Heinrich Kramer and James Sprenger Translated with an Introduction, Bibliography and Notes*: Unabridged Online Republication of the 1928 Edition. Introduction to the 1948 Edition is Also Included. Translation, Notes, and Two Introduction by Montague Summers. A Bull of

Innocent VIII. https://library.oapen.org/bitstream/handle/20.500.12657/35002/341393.pdf?sequence=1&isAllowed=y

46. Chinyanya, C.M. (2011). *My Grace is Sufficient for You*. http://www.ibe-epilepsy.org/wp-content/uploads/2012/07/IBE-Story-Book-Final.pdf
47. Tedrus, G. M. A. S., & Pereira, J. B. (2020). Epilepsy characteristics and cognitive, social, and mood functions in relation to intrinsic religiosity. *Epilepsy & Behavior*, *111*, 107326. https://doi.org/10.1016/j.yebeh.2020.107326
48. Koch, K.E. (1970). *Occult Bondage and Deliverance*. Grand Rapids: Kregel Publications.
49. Murombedzi, C. (2013). Healing school or killing school? http://www.herald.co.zw/healing-school-or-killing-school/
50. Murombedzi, C. (2014). The role of faith in healing. http://www.herald.co.zw/the-role-of-faith-in-healing/
51. World Health Organization. (2004). *Epilepsy in the WHO Africa Region: Bridging the Gap: The Global Campaign Against Epilepsy "Out of the Shadows."* Geneva: World Health Organization. https://www.ibe-epilepsy.org/downloads/EPILEPSY%20AFRICAN%20Report.pdf.
52. Bone, I., & Dein, S. (2021). Religion, spirituality, and epilepsy. *Epilepsy & Behavior*, *122*, 108219. https://doi.org/10.1016/j.yebeh.2021.108219
53. Kissani, N., Moro, M., & Arib, S. (2020). Knowledge, attitude and traditional practices towards epilepsy among relatives of PWE (patients with epilepsy) in Marrakesh, Morocco. *Epilepsy & Behavior*, *111*, 107257. https://doi.org/10.1016/j.yebeh.2020.107257
54. Kasimoğlu, N., & Baş, N. G. (2024). The relationship between parental attitude toward childhood epilepsy and spiritual orientation. *Epilepsy & Behavior*, *158*, 109946. https://doi.org/10.1016/j.yebeh.2024.109946
55. Beattie, J. F., Thompson, M. D., Parks, P. H., Jacobs, R. Q., & Goyal, M. (2017). Caregiver-reported religious beliefs and complementary and alternative medicine use among children admitted to an epilepsy monitoring unit. *Epilepsy & Behavior*, *69*, 139-146. https://doi.org/10.1016/j.yebeh.2017.01.026
56. Sostre, S. (2018). The aetiology of epilepsy spiritual or physical? *European Journal of Science and Theology*, *14*(1), 35-46. http://www.ejst.tuiasi.ro/Files/68/4_Sostre.pdf
57. Dhikale, P., Muruganandham, R., & Dongre, A. R. (2017). Perceptions of the community about epilepsy in rural Tamil Nadu, India. *Int J Med Sci Public Health*, *6*, 1.
58. Mahmood, A., Abbasi, H. N., Ghouri, N., Mohammed, R., & Leach, J. P. (2020). Managing epilepsy in Ramadan: guidance for healthcare providers and patients. *Epilepsy & Behavior*, *111*, 107117. https://doi.org/10.1016/j.yebeh.2020.107117
59. Zellmann-Rohrer, M. (2021). Hippocratic Diagnosis, Solomonic Therapy, Roman Amulets: Epilepsy, Exorcism, and the Diffusion of a Jewish Tradition in the Roman World. *Journal for the Study of Judaism*, *53*(1), 69-93. https://doi.org/10.1163/15700631-bja10033
60. Singh, S., Mishra, V. N., Rai, A., Singh, R., & Chaurasia, R. N. (2018). Myths and superstition about epilepsy: A study from North India. *Journal of neurosciences in rural practice*, *9*(3), 359. https://doi.org/10.4103/jnrp.jnrp_63_18
61. da Silva, L. G., de Beltrão, I. C. S. L., de Araujo Delmondes, G., de Alencar, C. D. C., Damasceno, S. S., Silva, N. S., ... & Bandeira, P. F. R. (2021). Beliefs and attitudes towards child epilepsy: A structural equation model. *Seizure*, *84*, 53-59. https://doi.org/10.1016/j.seizure.2020.11.020

62. Lee, S. A., Choi, E. J., Jeon, J. Y., & Paek, J. H. (2017). Attitudes toward epilepsy and perceptions of epilepsy-related stigma in Korean evangelical Christians. *Epilepsy & Behavior, 74*, 99-103. https://doi.org/10.1016/j.yebeh.2017.06.013
63. Tayeb, H. O. (2019). Epilepsy stigma in Saudi Arabia: the roles of mind–body dualism, supernatural beliefs, and religiosity. *Epilepsy & Behavior, 95*, 175-180. https://doi.org/10.1016/j.yebeh.2019.04.022
64. Bhattacharya, S., & Singh, A. (2018). Beliefs of a traditional rural Indian family towards naturalistic and faith healing for treating epilepsy: a case study. *Case Reports, 2018*, bcr-2018. https://doi.org/10.1136/bcr-2018-225405
65. Rani, A., & Thomas, P. T. (2019). Parental knoweldge, attitude, and perception about epilepsy and sociocultural barriers to treatment. *Journal of Epilepsy Research, 9*(1), 65. https://doi.org/10.14581/jer.19007
66. Deegbe, D. A., Aziato, L., & Attiogbe, A. (2020). Experience of epilepsy: Coping strategies and health outcomes among Ghanaians living with epilepsy. *Epilepsy & Behavior, 104*, 106900. https://doi.org/10.1016/j.yebeh.2020.106900
67. Król, A., Majda, A., Pieczyrak-Brhel, U., & Wojcieszek, A. (2024). Spirituality/religiosity in a group of people with epilepsy. *Nursing Problems/Problemy Pielęgniarstwa, 32*(2), 91-96. https://doi.org/10.5114/ppiel.2024.140914
68. Dayapoglu, N., Ayyıldız, N. İ., & Şeker, D. (2021). Determination of health fatalism and the factors affecting health fatalism in patients with epilepsy in the North of Turkey. *Epilepsy & Behavior, 115*, 107641. https://doi.org/10.1016/j.yebeh.2020.107641
69. Millogo, A., Ngowi, A. H., Carabin, H., Ganaba, R., Da, A., & Preux, P. M. (2019). Knowledge, attitudes, and practices related to epilepsy in rural Burkina Faso. *Epilepsy & Behavior, 95*, 70-74. https://doi.org/10.1016/j.yebeh.2019.03.006
70. Tuft, M., Nakken, K. O., & Kverndokk, K. (2017). Traditional folk beliefs on epilepsy in Norway and Sweden. *Epilepsy & Behavior, 71*, 104-107. https://doi.org/10.1016/j.yebeh.2017.03.032
71. Lee, S. A., Ryu, H. U., Choi, E. J., Ko, M. A., Jeon, J. Y., Han, S. H., ... & Jo, K. D. (2017). Associations between religiosity and anxiety, depressive symptoms, and well-being in Korean adults living with epilepsy. *Epilepsy & Behavior, 75*, 246-251. https://doi.org/10.1016/j.yebeh.2017.06.005
72. Toudou-Daouda, M., & Ibrahim-Mamadou, A. K. (2020). Teachers' knowledge about epilepsy and their attitudes toward students with epilepsy: a cross-sectional survey in the city of Tahoua (Niger). *Neuropsychiatric Disease and Treatment*, 2327-2333. https://doi.org/10.2147/NDT.S276691
73. Hodzi, T. 2012. "Introduction to Theology." Harare: Harare Theological College. [Term 3].
74. Valeta, T., & Valeta, T. (2017). *History of Epilepsy* (pp. 1-5). Springer International Publishing. https://doi.org/10.1007/978-3-319-61679-7_1
75. Paladin, A.V. (1995). Epilepsy According to the Christian, Jewish and Islamic religions: An overview, *Epilepsy, 1*, 38-41. www.journalagent.com/epilepsi/pdfs/epilepsi_1_1_38_41.pdf
76. Lin, C. Y., Saffari, M., Koenig, H. G., & Pakpour, A. H. (2018). Effects of religiosity and religious coping on medication adherence and quality of life among people with epilepsy. *Epilepsy & Behavior, 78*, 45-51. https://doi.org/10.1016/j.yebeh.2017.10.008

Chapter 12 – Epilepsy in Children

Some children respond very well to AED therapy to an extent that they can live a seizure-free life, but what price do they pay for being seizure-free in terms of learning?
Clotilda Chinyanya

Introduction

Epilepsy is a leading neurological disorder in the pediatric population, affecting roughly 1 in 150 children globally.[1,2] The effects of epilepsy in children go beyond seizure frequency and impact, to affecting cognitive development, learning, and social skills.[3,4] Pediatric epilepsy comprises various and distinct epilepsy syndromes, demanding a specialized approach to diagnosis and treatment.[2] Early diagnosis is critical to prevent epileptic encephalopathy, where persistent seizures impair brain function and cause developmental delays.[5] Diagnosing epilepsy in children is complicated because seizures are usually age-dependent, with signs like staring spells, jerky movements, and unexplained episodes of confusion that may go unnoticed or misdiagnosed.[6] This complexity emphasizes the need for increased awareness among caregivers and clinicians to provide early intervention and treatment.[5]

Epilepsy in children often requires a collaborative, multidisciplinary approach to treatment, integrating neurological, psychological, and social considerations.[13] Family-centered care is critical because childhood epilepsy extends to family life, influencing parental roles, sibling dynamics, and the need for support systems.[5,7] A tailored treatment strategy that accounts for individual needs, syndrome-specific characteristics, and lifestyle factors is essential to support optimal outcomes and quality of life for children with epilepsy and their families.[2,8,9]

In a family setting, there are many challenges that children with epilepsy face together with their siblings. I will discuss some of the challenges and see how best they can be addressed.[10,12,13] Mental health, behavior, and sociological issues, as well as those related to AED therapy, will be discussed in this chapter.[3,8,14]

Common childhood epilepsy syndromes

An epilepsy syndrome is recognized by a distinct set of clinical and EEG characteristics, often accompanied by specific underlying causes such as structural, genetic, metabolic, immune, or infectious factors.[2,6,15] The specific epilepsy syndrome is useful for guiding treatment and predicting outcomes. These syndromes often present at specific ages and come with unique co-morbidities.[16] Understanding the specific syndrome helps in identifying potential causes and helps avoid worsening of seizures linked to certain medications.[5,7] Classifying epilepsy syndromes can be based on the age when seizures begin or the type of epilepsy. Some syndromes can be outgrown or self-limiting, while others are chronic.[2,17,18] Table 9 summarizes the known childhood epilepsy syndromes according to age of onset. I will discuss only four of the syndromes in depth.

Table 9: Childhood epilepsy syndromes

Age of onset	Syndrome
Neonate/infant *(from birth to 24 months)*	**Self-limited** · Self-limited (familial) neonatal epilepsy (SeLNE) · Self-limited familial neonatal-infantile epilepsy (SeLFNIE) · Self-limited (familial) infantile epilepsy (SeLIE) · Genetic epilepsy with febrile seizures plus (GEFS+) spectrum · Myoclonic epilepsy in infancy (MEI) **With developmental and epileptic encephalopathy (DEE)** · Early infantile developmental and epileptic encephalopathy (EIDEE) · Epilepsy of infancy with migrating focal seizures (EIMFS) · Infantile epileptic spasms syndrome (IESS) · Dravet syndrome (DS)

Childhood *(2 years to puberty)*	**Self-limited focal epilepsy syndromes (SeLFEs)**
	Remission expected in all cases by adolescence
	  o Self-limited epilepsy with centrotemporal spikes (SeLECTS)
	  o Self-limited epilepsy with autonomic seizures (SeLEAS)
	Remission expected in most cases by adolescence
	  o Childhood occipital visual epilepsy (COVE)
	  o Photosensitive occipital lobe epilepsy (POLE)
	Genetic generalized epilepsy syndromes
	· Epilepsy with eyelid myoclonia (EEM)
	· Epilepsy with myoclonic absence (EMA)
	Idiopathic generalized epilepsy syndrome
	· Childhood absence epilepsy (CAE)
	With developmental and/or epileptic encephalopathy (DE, EE, or DEE)
	· Epilepsy with myoclonic atonic seizures (EMAtS)
	· Lennox–Gastaut syndrome (LGS)
	· Developmental and/or epileptic encephalopathy with spike-wave activation in sleep (DEE-SWAS, EE-SWAS)
	· Febrile infection-related epilepsy syndrome (FIRES)
	· Hemiconvulsion-hemiplegia-epilepsy syndrome (HHE)

Adapted from International League Against Epilepsy (2024). Diagnostic Manual. www.epilepsydiagnosis.org/index.html[19]

Absence epilepsy

Childhood absence epilepsy (CAE) typically begins between the ages of 4 and 10, peaking around age 6.[19] Absence seizures are brief (lasting 10–20 seconds). The child may stare blankly, and, in some cases, display mild automatisms such as lip smacking or eye fluttering.[19] While these seizures are usually less dramatic and stop with age, they can occur many times throughout the day and disrupt daily activities, including learning and concentration. Teachers may report the child daydreams in class, yet those will be seizure episodes. CAE is often genetically determined, and it has a generally favorable prognosis, with most children responding well to first-line AEDs like ethosuximide or valproate.[15,20]

Lennox–Gastaut syndrome

Lennox–Gastaut syndrome (LGS) is a severe form of epilepsy that typically begins between the ages of 3 and 5. It involves several seizure types, including tonic, atonic, and atypical absence seizures.[19] Children with LGS often have intellectual disability and other neurodevelopmental issues. Management of LGS is challenging because the syndrome is resistant to AEDs. Management involves multiple therapies, including AEDs, dietary therapy, and sometimes surgical interventions.[15] The treatment outcomes for LGS are uncertain because it is drug-resistant and has potential for lasting cognitive impairment and seizures for life.[15]

Dravet syndrome

Dravet syndrome is a rare but severe epilepsy syndrome beginning in the first year of life, often triggered by fever or warm temperatures.[19] The seizures are typically prolonged and initially focal or generalized clonic in nature. The seizure types change with age, and may include myoclonic, focal, and generalized tonic-clonic seizures.[19] The syndrome is frequently caused by mutations in the *SCN1A* gene, which encodes a sodium channel protein. Most AEDs are ineffective or may even worsen seizures in Dravet syndrome, making it very difficult to manage. Treatments often include a combination of AEDs, dietary therapies, and, in some cases, cannabidiol.[15,20]

Benign Rolandic epilepsy

Also known as benign epilepsy with centrotemporal spikes, benign rolandic epilepsy (BRE) is one of the most common pediatric epilepsy syndromes, typically occurring between ages 5 and 10.[19] It is characterized by focal seizures that often involve the face and may include tingling sensations and/or a momentary inability to speak.[19] Seizures usually occur at night, and the treatment outlook for BRE is favorable, with many children outgrowing the condition by adolescence.[19] AEDs are generally only needed if seizures are frequent or disruptive, as the syndrome is often self-limiting.[15,20]

Table 10: Clinical characteristics of childhood epilepsy syndromes

	Childhood absence epilepsy	**Lennox–Gastaut syndrome**	**Dravet syndrome**
Seizure types and patterns	Brief seizures with no recovery period. Blank stares and automatisms (lip smacking, eye fluttering).	Long and disruptive tonic, atonic, and atypical absence seizures	Prolonged seizures that change with age, including myoclonic, focal, and generalized tonic-clonic seizures
Age of onset and developmental progression	Begins between the ages of 4 and 10	Begins between the ages of 3 to 5 years	Begins by age of 1 year
Cognitive and behavioral effects	Normal cognitive development, but learning and attention can be disrupted	Cognitive impairments, developmental delays, and behavioral issues such as hyperactivity, aggression, and social difficulties	Cognitive impairments, developmental delays, and behavioral issues such as hyperactivity, aggression, and social difficulties
Genetic influences	Mutations in the *GABRG2* or *SLC2A1* genes		Mutations in the *SCN1A* gene
Environmental triggers		Secondary brain injury, structural abnormalities	Fever or warm temperatures
Interactions between genetic and environmental factors	Environmental factors may trigger or worsen the syndrome	Environmental factors may trigger or worsen the syndrome	Environmental factors may trigger or worsen the syndrome

Adapted from International League Against Epilepsy (2024). Diagnostic Manual. www.epilepsydiagnosis.org/index.html[19]

Clinical characteristics

Seizure types and patterns

Each epilepsy syndrome in children has distinctive seizure types and patterns, which help in diagnosis. For example, the absence seizures in CAE are brief, with no recovery period, while the tonic and atonic seizures seen in LGS are often longer and more disruptive, sometimes leading to sudden falls and injuries.[19] In Dravet syndrome, seizures tend to be prolonged and febrile, and children often present with several seizure types over time.[19] Recognizing these patterns is crucial for clinicians to establish the correct syndrome diagnosis, which in turn guides treatment options and possible treatment outcomes.

Age of onset and developmental progression

The age of onset can also be a key diagnostic marker. For instance, LGS typically appears between the ages of 3 and 5, while Dravet syndrome presents within the first year of life.[19] The developmental trajectory also varies: in some syndromes, such as BRE, children usually develop normally, while in others, such as LGS and Dravet syndrome, there is a high risk of developmental regression and intellectual disability over time.[19]

Cognitive and behavioral profiles

Children with syndromes like CAE often have normal cognitive development, though frequent absence seizures can disrupt attention and learning. Conversely, LGS and Dravet syndrome are commonly associated with significant cognitive impairments, developmental delays, and behavioral issues, such as hyperactivity, aggression, and social difficulties. Monitoring cognitive and behavioral development is therefore essential for managing these syndromes and providing appropriate support and interventions.[15]

Genetic influences

Advances in genetic research have illuminated the role of genetic mutations in several childhood epilepsy syndromes, providing valuable insights into their underlying causes and treatment potential. For instance, *SCN1A* gene mutations are implicated in Dravet syndrome, while mutations in the *GABRG2* or *SLC2A1* genes have been linked to certain cases of CAE. These discoveries have paved the way for personalized treatment approaches, such as targeting specific ion channels affected by the mutations. Genetic testing is increasingly recommended in cases of severe, early-onset epilepsy syndromes or when there is a family history of epilepsy, as it can help in diagnosing and selecting optimal treatments.[15,19,20]

Environmental triggers
Environmental factors may also play a role in the onset and progression of epilepsy syndromes in children. For instance, fever is a common trigger for seizures in Dravet syndrome, especially early in the disease course. Certain syndromes, such as LGS, may develop secondary to brain injury or structural abnormalities from conditions such as tuberous sclerosis complex or perinatal hypoxic-ischemic injury. Identifying and managing environmental triggers, such as avoiding exposure to extreme heat or rapidly treating fevers, can be a critical component of epilepsy management in specific syndromes.

Interactions between genetic and environmental factors
There is growing recognition of the complex interplay between genetic predispositions and environmental influences in the development of epilepsy syndromes. In genetically susceptible children, environmental factors like infections, head trauma, or perinatal complications may trigger the onset of epilepsy or worsen its course. For example, while a mutation in the *SCN1A* gene is a key driver of Dravet syndrome, external factors such as fever often precipitate seizures. Understanding these interactions can help clinicians develop more nuanced treatment and management plans, especially in identifying preventive measures for high-risk children.[15,20]

Treatment options for pediatric epilepsy
Management of childhood epilepsy involves multiple approaches including AEDs, dietary therapy, CBD therapy, or, in some cases, surgical intervention. The treatment plan will always need regular

adjustments to address seizure control, side effects, and developmental considerations as the child grows.

It has been argued that all major AEDs have adverse cognitive effects, including reduced attentiveness, impoverished memory, and mental slowing, and those patients with more cognitive impairment also have more psychosocial problems
Gus A. Baker

Anti-epileptic drugs

Some children respond very well to AED therapy to an extent they can live a seizure-free life. However, these AEDs can cause certain side effects that may impact the child's development, cognitive functions, and social interactions. AEDs remain the primary treatment for most forms of epilepsy. The selection of AEDs for children requires careful consideration of the specific epilepsy syndrome, the seizure type, age, and the child's overall health profile.[3,5,14] Drug interactions, pharmacokinetics, and side effects are key considerations in childhood epilepsy treatment. For instance, liver enzyme inducers like carbamazepine can reduce the efficacy of other medications, necessitating careful selection and monitoring of AED combinations.

Some commonly used AEDs in pediatric epilepsy include valproate, levetiracetam, lamotrigine, topiramate, and ethosuximide. Valproate, for instance, is frequently used for generalized epilepsy syndromes like absence epilepsy. However, valproate is associated with certain side effects, including weight gain, gastrointestinal issues, and, in some cases, cognitive slowing.[5] Levetiracetam is often preferred for focal and generalized seizures because most of the side effects are less severe. However, levetiracetam can cause behavioral changes such as aggression or irritability in some children.[3,5,14,21] Lamotrigine is very effective in managing focal and generalized seizures and is associated with fewer cognitive side effects, making it the ideal option for children with cognitive challenges.[14]

Some AEDs affect memory. The drug mainly used in sub-Saharan Africa and some LMICs is phenobarbitone. Though this drug addresses the challenge of seizures and is the most cost-effective drug for epilepsy around, it should be avoided in children because of adverse cognitive effects. Phenobarbitone affects memory and causes drowsiness among its many side effects, so a child taking this drug is likely to perform below their capacity in school.[3] Phenobarbitone affects IQ and though these effects can be reversed when the drug is withdrawn, it is clear that this child may never catch up what their peers learned while they were struggling with compromised IQ because of the AED.[3] Long-term studies indicate that the academic performance of many children who have been treated with phenobarbitone does not fully recover even after they stop taking it.[3] PWE already face stigma, therefore, adding poor academic performances because of AED treatment makes the situation harder.

Countries should come up with treatment protocols that restrict phenobarbitone use to only those cases where it is the only AED that can control seizures in that epilepsy syndrome. In LMICs, it is evident the widespread use of phenobarbitone is for economic reasons, and its risks for children are ignored. Policies should focus on providing safer medications to all children, regardless of where they live or how much money their family has. One wonders why resources are provided for most ailments except epilepsy. Why is it that resources only become limited when dealing with epilepsy, but seem to be abundant for other conditions? Have people lost hope that anything of value can come out of PWE? Safe drugs must be made available to all children.

Research continues to evolve around AEDs, with new drugs being developed to offer improved effectiveness and reduced side effects. Newer drugs such as brivaracetam and perampanel provide alternative options with new modes of action. Perampanel, an AMPA receptor antagonist, has shown promise in treating focal seizures and may be effective for patients who have not responded well to other treatments. Although these new drugs are not yet widely used in childhood epilepsy, ongoing studies are assessing their safety and efficacy in younger populations, potentially expanding treatment options for difficult-to-treat cases in the future.[22,23]

Mechanism of action of AEDs

AEDs control seizures through various mechanisms that involve either suppressing excitatory neurotransmission or boosting inhibitory neurotransmission in the brain.[14] For instance, sodium channel blockers like phenytoin and carbamazepine reduce neuronal excitability by slowing the recovery of sodium channels, which are critical in the propagation of action potentials. GABAergic drugs, such as benzodiazepines, increase the inhibitory effects of GABA, thus reducing the likelihood of seizure activity.[14] Other AEDs, like ethosuximide, target calcium channels specifically, which makes them effective in absence seizures.[14]

Age-specific considerations

The pharmacokinetics of AEDs can vary significantly between children and adults due to differences in metabolism and body composition. Children metabolize drugs faster than adults, and need regular adjustments in dosing frequency and amounts. Young children are also more vulnerable to adverse effects, and some AEDs can impact growth and development, especially if used over extended periods.[3,5] For example, phenobarbitone, although effective, is less commonly prescribed in well-resourced countries due to concerns over its impact on cognitive development and potential for sedation and behavioral side effects.

Efficacy and tolerability

AEDs vary in their effectiveness across different epilepsy syndromes. For instance, ethosuximide is particularly effective in controlling absence seizures, while valproate is useful for generalized epilepsy and certain mixed syndromes. The choice of AED often balances efficacy with tolerability, as some drugs may cause side effects such as sedation, weight gain, behavioral changes, and cognitive impairment. Levetiracetam, which is known for a favorable side-effect profile, is often preferred in pediatric epilepsy as it has less impact on cognition; however, it can occasionally lead to behavioral issues like irritability and aggression, particularly in young children.[5,14]

Cognitive and behavioral impacts

Most AEDs impact cognitive function and behavior in children in a significant way. Cognitive effects can include difficulties with memory, attention, and learning, which may affect academic performance and daily functioning. For instance, topiramate and zonisamide are known for their potential to impair language and cognitive processing. Behavioral effects could include irritability, hyperactivity, and mood changes. These effects can be challenging in a school or social environment. Caregivers and clinicians will need to monitor cognitive function and behavior to ensure treatment does not hinder the child's development or quality of life.[3,24]

Drug interactions and polytherapy

When monotherapy fails to control seizures, polytherapy may be considered. However, combining AEDs increases the risk of drug interactions, which can impact drug efficacy and raise the likelihood of adverse effects (see Chapter 6). Drug interaction considerations in children are very important because children respond differently to adults due to their metabolic rates and developing nervous systems.[3,5]

Monitoring and side effect management

During AED treatment it is critical to monitor blood levels, liver function, and kidney function to ensure drug levels remain within therapeutic ranges and to identify potential toxicities early. Common side effects of AEDs include drowsiness, dizziness, nausea, and gastrointestinal issues.[5,14] Less common, but more severe side effects could lead to liver toxicity, blood-related problems like low platelet count, and serious skin reactions that can be fatal. Balancing the risk of long-term cognitive effects and the benefits of seizure control is particularly important in children.[5,14]

Considerations for withdrawal

Depending on the epilepsy syndrome and risk factors, the general guideline is to consider withdrawing AED therapy if the child has been seizure-free for at least 2 years.[14] Stopping AEDs suddenly can have serious consequences like rebound seizures or status epilepticus. Therefore, the withdrawal process must be done slowly under close medical supervision.[3,14] Factors that influence the decision to discontinue AEDs include seizure type, age of seizure onset, and the presence of any neurological deficits. Patients with generalized epilepsy, for instance, may have a higher risk of seizure recurrence than those with focal epilepsy, and thus may require a more cautious approach to withdrawal.[3,14]

Dietary therapies

The ketogenic diet is an established treatment for DRE, inducing ketosis, a metabolic state believed to have anticonvulsant effects. A typical ketogenic regimen includes high-fat and low-carbohydrate components, which require precise meal planning and monitoring to prevent adverse effects such as kidney stones and nutritional deficiencies.[8] A modified Atkins diet offers a less restrictive, high-fat diet alternative that has shown similar efficacy in some cases. Although dietary therapies are demanding, they provide an option for patients who do not respond to conventional treatments and may also benefit overall neurological health. The ketogenic diet is covered in more detail in Chapter 6.

Cannabidiol therapy

CBD has gained recognition for its role in reducing seizures, especially in DRE, such as Dravet syndrome. Evidence suggests that CBD interacts with neuroreceptors that modulate seizure activity, providing a possible solution to individuals not responding to AEDs.[25] CBD therapy, however, requires careful dosing and monitoring due to possible interactions with other drugs and side effects like diarrhea, sleep disturbances, and fatigue.

Surgical interventions

Surgical interventions, such as lobectomy or corpus callosotomy, are reserved for children with focal epilepsy unresponsive to other treatments. Surgery aims to reduce or eliminate seizures by removing or disconnecting the affected brain area. Although surgery carries risks, successful outcomes can lead to a substantial reduction in seizure frequency or complete seizure freedom, significantly enhancing the child's quality of life.[26] Post-operative support, including rehabilitation and cognitive therapy, is often necessary to maximize benefits and address any cognitive or motor impairments. Epilepsy surgery is covered in more detail in Chapter 6.

Sudden unexpected death in epilepsy in children

Although SUDEP is less common in children than adults, it poses a significant concern, particularly for children with frequent GTCS. SUDEP prevention strategies focus on achieving optimal seizure control and educating families about monitoring practices, especially during sleep, as most SUDEP cases occur at night.[27] Enhanced seizure detection devices and supervised sleep environments are emerging as additional preventive measures that may reduce SUDEP risk in high-risk pediatric populations. SUDEP is covered in more detail in Chapter 8.

Challenges and special considerations in pediatric epilepsy management

Drug-resistant epilepsy

DRE, also known as refractory epilepsy, is when seizures persist despite the use of adequate doses of two or more appropriate AEDs. Around 20–30% of childhood epilepsy cases are classified as drug-resistant, significantly impacting quality of life and often requiring alternative treatment approaches. DRE is particularly challenging in syndromes such as LGS and Dravet syndrome.[28]

Drug resistance in pediatric epilepsy can result from various factors, including the epilepsy syndrome type, the presence of structural brain abnormalities, or underlying genetic mutations. Children who have epilepsy early in life and those with frequent seizures at the time of diagnosis are at greater risk of DRE.[28] When DRE is diagnosed, clinicians may explore treatment options beyond traditional AEDs. Options include ketogenic and modified Atkins diets, CBD therapy, and surgical interventions. For some children with focal epilepsy, surgical resection of the epileptogenic zone can lead to seizure freedom or significant reduction. Moreover, recent advances such as vagus nerve stimulation and responsive neurostimulation have shown promise for children who are not surgical candidates. These neuromodulation approaches can help reduce seizure frequency, improve quality of life, and provide options for managing refractory epilepsy.[8,26]

Impact of epilepsy on children's minds and behavior

Cognitive impact of epilepsy and AEDs

The cognitive impact of epilepsy itself, coupled with the side effects of AEDs, presents unique challenges in pediatric epilepsy. Seizures interfere with normal brain activity and may affect cognitive functions, including memory, attention, language, and executive function. AEDs, especially those with sedative properties, can exacerbate these cognitive issues, impacting school performance and daily functioning. For instance, AEDs like phenobarbitone, topiramate, and zonisamide have been linked to slower mental function, especially in children on long-term treatment. Monitoring cognitive development is thus an essential component of childhood epilepsy management.[3,24]

Behavioral and emotional issues

Many children with epilepsy experience challenges with emotions and behavior. These behavioral changes include hyperactivity, aggression, mood swings, and irritability. These issues come from both the epilepsy itself and the use of AEDs like levetiracetam.[3,24] Emotional struggles with anxiety and depression are common. These emotional effects can impact the child's social interactions and quality of life. Addressing these issues may require collaboration with mental health professionals, behavior therapists, and school counselors to develop tailored interventions and support systems.[3,24]

Learning difficulties and educational challenges

Learning difficulties are a frequent concern in children with epilepsy. Both seizures and side effects of AEDs affect cognitive domains, making it hard for the child to pay attention, concentrate, remember things, and process information quickly.[29,30] These cognitive challenges may lead to academic difficulties and necessitate individualized education plans in school settings.[29,30] Schools and educators must be informed about the child's specific needs, as timely educational support can play a crucial role in mitigating academic challenges. Collaborative efforts between healthcare providers, educational psychologists, and teachers are essential for implementing effective support strategies, including adjustments to classroom instruction and testing accommodations.[29,30] In some locations, these facilities may not be available. In such situations, parents must advocate for their child to get the best education depending on circumstances. Search all possibilities for your child to help them reach their full potential.

Co-occurring disorders in epilepsy (co-morbidities)
Neurodevelopmental co-morbidities

Children with epilepsy are at a higher risk for neurodevelopmental disorders such as attention-deficit hyperactivity disorder (ADHD) and autism spectrum disorder (ASD). ADHD is particularly common and affects up to 30% of children with epilepsy, often leading to difficulties with attention, impulse control, and hyperactivity. The overlap between epilepsy and neurodevelopmental disorders necessitates careful consideration when selecting AEDs, as some medications may worsen hyperactivity or attention issues. Children should be screened for these co-morbidities so that early interventions to address them can be started without losing time.[16,31]

Psychiatric co-morbidities

Psychiatric conditions, such as depression, anxiety, and psychosis, are observed in some children with epilepsy. These conditions could be related to the epilepsy itself or the burden of living with a chronic illness. The presence of psychiatric co-morbidities requires a comprehensive, multidisciplinary approach, often involving neurologists, psychiatrists, and counselors to create integrated treatment plans that address both seizure control and mental health. Regular screening for mood and anxiety disorders, along with early interventions, is essential to support emotional and psychological well-being in children with epilepsy.[16,31]

Impact on family and social life

The chronic nature of epilepsy, coupled with the demands of managing seizures and medication regimens, can place a substantial emotional and financial strain on families.[5,7,13] Caregivers may experience stress, anxiety, and burnout, particularly when dealing with drug-resistant or severe forms of epilepsy.[13,28,32] Siblings of children with epilepsy may also feel neglected or bear additional responsibilities. Family support networks, epilepsy support organizations, and counseling services can help relieve caregiver burden by offering practical assistance, emotional support, and access to respite care.[7,13,29]

Children with epilepsy often face social stigma, which can lead to isolation, discrimination, and low self-esteem. Misconceptions about epilepsy, as covered in Chapter 10, could result in children being excluded or bullied.[4,13,29] The child's family is also at a greater risk of being excluded from social interactions, adding an emotional burden to caregivers. Educational initiatives in schools and communities play a key role in reducing stigma and promoting inclusivity by educating peers and teachers about epilepsy, seizure first aid, and the normalcy of the child's condition outside of seizures.[13,29]

In some communities, giving birth to a child with epilepsy can entail dissolution of the marriage between the parents as people in those communities believe any disability in a child comes from the mother's side.[10,11,12] Either she has unconfessed sin or some avenging spirits from her side want compensation of some sort, and the husband does not want his lineage spoiled. To decisively deal with the situation, the husband sends his wife and disabled child packing so that he can guarantee some purity within his family.[10,11] If the mother is unemployed, the child's upbringing can be very difficult. At times, mothers tell other people how and why they got divorced in the presence of their children, thinking that because they are children, they do not understand what is being discussed. Unfortunately, many children understand these stories and they may start feeling guilty for causing their parents to divorce. My message to mothers is that no matter how devastating it might be, never discuss these issues in the presence of children because the long-term effects can be irreversible.

In Zimbabwe, children are generally viewed as an investment for the future.[11] This can be true of many communities in LMICs. Parents are motivated to take care of their children with the hope that when those children grow up, they will in turn take care of them. This is the reason why some parents neglect taking care of their children with epilepsy to the extent of not giving them the opportunity to go to school because they do not see any hope for the future.[10,11,12] This child, according to the parents, is likely to be dependent on the parents for the rest of their life.

Children with epilepsy are generally isolated from the rest of the world in some communities, especially in LMICs.[10,11,12] In these communities, giving birth to a child with any disability is a disgrace.[29] It brings shame to the whole family, so in some cases, the children are hidden away from the public.[11] That child will not even be mentioned when the members of that family are discussed. If they are the firstborn, the second born will be regarded as the first because the one with epilepsy is considered a person who cannot do anything of value in life.[12] In a family with three children, with one of them living with epilepsy, it is not surprising to hear parents talking as if they only have two children.

When a child with epilepsy is lucky enough to be sent to school, there is a high chance of them being bullied, especially if they have seizures at school. This will be worsened if the child had not been exposed to other children whilst at home because the parents were keeping them indoors. The child can even suggest to the parents that they remove them from school.[13,29] This is undesirable but can be avoided if parents do not over-protect their children. This will help children get exposure to the outside world and prepare them to cope with these pressures. At school, children should participate in all activities (academic, sporting, recreational, and social) because under normal circumstances, all activities are done in the presence of teachers, so these children will be supervised like any other child. Excluding them from some activities will make them feel isolated and that is not desirable. No child should be made to feel different.

Girls with disabilities, especially epilepsy, sometimes have hysterectomies (operation to remove uterus) so that they will not have their monthly menstrual cycles.[10] This is done without the child's consent as no one believes she can make any decision regarding her body. The motivation of those who will be subjecting these girls to these procedures is mainly so that the girl does not reproduce, and in case they are not able to properly take care of themselves hygienically, the issue of menstruation will be eliminated for good.

Some AEDs, when given to children, have negative social side effects. Loring,[3] lists the following social effects of AEDs when given to children:

- Gabapentin: *Hyperactivity, irritability, agitation, and aggression, even in the presence of improved seizure control.*
- Topiramate: *Emotional lability, fatigue, difficulty with attention and concentration and forgetfulness and impaired memory.*
- Vigabatrin: *Antisocial behavior, irritability and excitability.*
- Zonisamide: *Risk of psychiatric side effects, including psychotic episodes.*[3] These effects of zonisamide can happen years after commencement of treatment.[3]

Additional information on some undesirable effects of AEDs is covered at the beginning of this chapter and in Chapter 6. Already we can see that these drugs will contribute to the theories people have that PWE are psychotic, yet these are side effects of the drugs that are supposed to be managing the epilepsy. If a drug is affecting a child this way, it needs to be discontinued. The aim of treatment should be to eliminate seizures with minimal side effects.[14,33] These are major side effects, and a safer drug should be given in that situation.

These behavioral problems can also be triggered by other factors, like the way people relate to the PWE, especially after a seizure. This must be managed at home so that when it happens at school, church or any other gathering, the child will not lose their self-esteem. The home plays a critical role in building the child's self-esteem. Once a child has high self-esteem, negative comments coming from people usually do not affect the child negatively, if at all, and it may even be a motivation to greater determination to prove they can live like anybody else and achieve good grades, if not the best.

Medically, children present a different challenge when it comes to treatment. Children need to have their dosages adjusted as they grow older.[7,8,14] If a child is commenced on a drug at the age of 3 months, by the time they reach 16 years of age, many adjustments will have been made to the dosage and/or the AED. This presents a challenge as these changes can lead to seizures as the body will be adjusting to the variations in drug plasma levels, which will be very difficult to maintain. If the parents are not properly counseled, this is the time they may resort to CAM because they claim their child no longer responds to conventional medicine. Others will just adjust the dose at home because they assume the doctor made an error and this can be very dangerous.

Before any adjustment is made, parents or guardians need to be counseled so that they know what may happen after the adjustment and what they may need to do. Healthcare workers also need to be equipped from the primary care level with how to deal with such issues. When parents come to a healthcare worker seeking clarification on anything, they must get accurate information.

On a positive note, most seizures that start in childhood are usually outgrown except a few that persist for life.[2,17,18] Parents need to do all they can to ensure their child is not isolated. They must ensure the child gets the best education and help the child build good self-esteem. A child who outgrows epilepsy can go on to live independently, unlike those kept in isolation, who remain socially disconnected and dependent on family even after seizures stop.

Educational adjustments and accommodations
School support and individualized education plans

Most children with epilepsy are of normal intelligence and can attend mainstream classes where they compete at the same level as those without disabilities, and many do extremely well. This boosts their confidence levels as they can compete with other children without being confined to "special" classes, which should only be used as a last resort if the child cannot cope in mainstream classes. Special classes should be just that, special classes that cater for the needs of special children. Whatever program is put in place, it must be solely for the benefit of the child. Anything that can cause stigma should be avoided if possible.

Given the cognitive, behavioral, and emotional challenges associated with epilepsy, many children benefit from an individualized education plan. These plans outline specific accommodations, such as extended testing time, seating arrangements, access to note-takers, and allowances for medication administration or breaks when needed. Educators, parents, and healthcare providers collaborate to design these plans, which address the child's academic and medical needs while minimizing disruptions to their education. Schools may also offer specialized resources, such as occupational or speech therapy, to address any developmental delays or cognitive difficulties linked to epilepsy.[29] Such facilities may not be universally available. It may be necessary to collaborate with the local ministry of education to ensure they are provided in all schools. If these facilities are lacking, parents should work with school authorities to develop a suitable plan for their child.

Addressing learning difficulties

Children with epilepsy may experience significant challenges in academic performance due to seizures, AED side effects, or associated cognitive impairments. Learning difficulties may manifest in delayed processing speeds, impaired memory, or difficulty concentrating.[3,24] Classroom accommodations such as tutoring, smaller class sizes, and targeted cognitive therapies can improve learning outcomes. Moreover, fostering a supportive classroom environment that minimizes distractions and promotes a sense of inclusivity can greatly enhance the child's educational experience.[29] Children suffering from absence seizures will have difficulty in concentration and attention.[29] At school, teachers may mistake this as "laziness and a lack of interest."[29] Seizures must be controlled so that learning will not be compromised. This is possible because the brain has the capacity to repair itself, given enough time, but when seizures occur frequently, all the connections lost will never be recovered. This capacity of the brain is called plasticity but diminishes with age.

Children with epilepsy are also prone to mental retardation at an incidence of around 25%. Research has also revealed that 50% of children with epilepsy have some sort of learning difficulty.[29] These learning difficulties directly impact academic achievements, and include those affecting speech and language, attention, memory, and executive functioning.

After a seizure, a child feels extreme fatigue and it takes an average of 5 days for all things to return to normal. The child might be coming to school and participating very well, but there are things that go on behind the scenes that a child may not be able to describe, which affect learning. After a seizure, a child can lose a week of learning even though they are still going to school. A child can have several absence seizures per day. During the time of the seizure, those around the child may not know they are having a seizure due to the nature of absence seizures. If the teacher introduces a new concept during those few seconds, the child misses it. If the teacher asks even a simple question related to what has been taught, the child will not be able to give an answer because they never heard the teacher speak. It is therefore critical that seizures be brought under control to reduce the incidence of learning difficulties in children.

Social integration is another important aspect of educational support, as children with epilepsy may struggle with peer relationships due to stigma, self-consciousness, or behavioral challenges. Educators and counselors can facilitate peer support programs that foster understanding and inclusivity, helping to reduce stigma and promote empathy among classmates. These initiatives can help children with epilepsy feel more accepted and included, which can have positive effects on both their social life and academic engagement. By addressing both academic and social needs, educational systems can play a vital role in enhancing the quality of life for children with epilepsy, enabling them to reach their full potential despite the challenges posed by the condition.

Future directions in pediatric epilepsy care

With advancing knowledge in genetics and pharmacology, researchers are exploring new therapies that may offer better outcomes with fewer side effects. New AEDs with innovative mechanisms, along with gene therapies targeting specific genetic mutations, hold promise for more effective, personalized treatment approaches. Precision medicine approaches aim to identify biomarkers that could guide treatment selection, thus avoiding a trial-and-error approach. Early-stage trials for gene therapies in syndromes like Dravet have shown promising results, suggesting a shift toward more individualized and potentially curative treatment options in the future.[22,23]

For many children, access to specialized epilepsy care remains limited. Initiatives to expand access to diagnostic services, AEDs, and epilepsy specialists are critical to improving outcomes in underserved regions. Efforts to train local healthcare providers, establish telemedicine services, and implement community-based support programs are underway in many areas. Improved access to care can lead to earlier diagnoses, better seizure control, and reduced social stigma associated with epilepsy.[11,12]

Conclusion

Pediatric epilepsy requires a comprehensive, individualized approach to care that incorporates medical, psychological, and social considerations. Advances in diagnosis, treatment options, and support resources continue to improve outcomes, offering hope for children with epilepsy and their families. By addressing both medical and psychosocial needs, clinicians and caregivers can work collaboratively to foster optimal health, development, and quality of life for children living with epilepsy.

References:

1. Beghi, E. (2020). The epidemiology of epilepsy. *Neuroepidemiology*, *54*(2), 185-191. https://doi.org/10.1159/000503831
2. Guerrini, R. (2006). Epilepsy in children. *The Lancet*, *367*(9509), 499-524. https://doi.org/10.1016/S0140-6736(06)68182-8
3. Loring, D. W. (2005). Cognitive side effects of antiepileptic drugs in children. *Psychiatric Times*, *22*(10), 1-6. https://citeseerx.ist.psu.edu/document?repid=rep1&type=pdf&doi=1927c5ce0859b73849f9807193ed4de7929fad5e
4. Nazarov, A. I. (2022). Consequences of seizures and epilepsy in children. https://philpapers.org/rec/NAZCOS
5. Minardi, C., Minacapelli, R., Valastro, P., Vasile, F., Pitino, S., Pavone, P., ... & Murabito, P. (2019). Epilepsy in children: from diagnosis to treatment with focus on emergency. *Journal of Clinical Medicine*, *8*(1), 39. https://doi.org/10.3390/jcm8010039
6. Fisher, R. S., Cross, J. H., D'souza, C., French, J. A., Haut, S. R., Higurashi, N., ... & Zuberi, S. M. (2017). Instruction manual for the ILAE 2017 operational classification of seizure types. *Epilepsia*, *58*(4), 531-542. https://doi.org/10.1111/epi.13671
7. Perucca, P., Scheffer, I. E., & Kiley, M. (2018). The management of epilepsy in children and adults. *Medical Journal of Australia*, *208*(5), 226-233. https://doi.org/10.5694/mja17.00951
8. Rosati, A., De Masi, S., & Guerrini, R. (2015). Antiepileptic drug treatment in children with epilepsy. *CNS drugs*, *29*, 847-863. https://doi.org/10.1007/s40263-015-0281-8
9. Guerrini, R., Zaccara, G., la Marca, G., & Rosati, A. (2012). Safety and tolerability of antiepileptic drug treatment in children with epilepsy. *Drug Safety*, *35*, 519-533. https://doi.org/10.2165/11630700-000000000-00000
10. Marongwe, N., & Mate, R. (2007). Children and disability, their households' livelihoods experiences in accessing key services. *Rome: FAO*. https://www.google.com/url?sa=t&source=web&rct=j&opi=89978449&url=https://rdsjournal.org/index.php/journal/article/download/1121/2585/8549&ved=2ahukewixymlfh8cjaxwedeqihsr-kswqfnoecbsqaq&usg=aovvaw0f2thluqnijf59izy-x8ia
11. Lang, R. et al 2007. DFID Scoping Study: Disability Issues in Zimbabwe. Final Report. https://www.google.com/url?sa=t&source=web&rct=j&opi=89978449&url=https://scholar.google.com/scholar%3Fq%3DLang,%2BR.%2Bet%2Bal%2B2007.%2B%25E2%2580%259CDFID%2BScoping%2BStudy:%2BDisability%2BIssues%2Bin%2BZimbabwe.

%2BFinal%2BReport%26hl%3Den%26as_sdt%3D0%26as_vis%3D1%26oi%3Dscholart&ved=2ahUKEwiM3O2cicCJAxX8LUQIHb1jCc0QgQN6BAgGEAI&usg=AOvVaw1RNp_Q_o_hKtrDFiJ-SiXU

12. Choruma, T. 2006. *The Forgotten Tribe: People With Disabilities in Zimbabwe*. London: Progressio. https://www.progressio.org.uk/sites/default/files/Forgotten-tribe.pdf
13. Baker, G.A. (2002). The Psychosocial Burden of Epilepsy, *Epilepsia, 43* (Suppl. 6):26–30. https://doi.org/10.1046/j.1528-1157.43.s.6.12.x
14. Moosa, A. N. (2019). Antiepileptic drug treatment of epilepsy in children. *CONTINUUM: Lifelong Learning in Neurology, 25*(2), 381-407. https://doi.org/10.1212/CON.0000000000000712
15. Sokka, A., Olsen, P., Kirjavainen, J., Harju, M., Keski-Nisula, L., Räisänen, S., ... & Kälviäinen, R. (2017). Etiology, syndrome diagnosis, and cognition in childhood-onset epilepsy: A population-based study. *Epilepsia Open, 2*(1), 76-83. https://doi.org/10.1002/epi4.12036
16. Record, E. J., Bumbut, A., Shih, S., Merwin, S., Kroner, B., & Gaillard, W. D. (2021). Risk factors, etiologies, and comorbidities in urban pediatric epilepsy. *Epilepsy & Behavior, 115*, 107716. https://doi.org/10.1016/j.yebeh.2020.107716
17. Berg, A.T. & Rychlik, K. (2015). The course of childhood-onset epilepsy over the first two decades: a prospective longitudinal study. *Epilepsia, 56*(1): 40-48. https://doi.org/10.1111/epi.12862
18. Geerts, A., Arts, W. F., Stroink, H., Peeters, E., Brouwer, O., Peters, B., ... & Van Donselaar, C. (2010). Course and outcome of childhood epilepsy: a 15-year follow-up of the Dutch Study of Epilepsy in Childhood. *Epilepsia, 51*(7), 1189-1197. https://doi.org/10.1111/j.1528-1167.2010.02546.x
19. International League Against Epilepsy. (2024). Diagnostic Manual. https://www.epilepsydiagnosis.org/index.html
20. Berg, A. T., Berkovic, S. F., Brodie, M. J., Buchhalter, J., Cross, J. H., van Emde Boas, W., ... & Scheffer, I. E. (2010). Revised terminology and concepts for organization of seizures and epilepsies: report of the ILAE Commission on Classification and Terminology, 2005–2009. *Epilepsia, 51*, 676–685. https://doi.org/10.1111/j.1528-1167.2010.02522.x
21. Jebastine, M. I., & Somasundaram, I. (2024). Safety And Efficacy of Lacosamide and Levetiracetam in Children–A Cohort Study. *African Journal of Biomedical Research, 27*(3S), 639-646. https://www.africanjournalofbiomedicalresearch.com/index.php/AJBR/article/download/2077/1817
22. Yu, X., Che, F., Zhang, X., Yang, L., Zhu, L., Xu, N., ... & Li, Y. (2024). Clinical and genetic analysis of 23 Chinese children with epilepsy associated with KCNQ2 gene mutations. *Epilepsia Open*. https://doi.org/10.1002/epi4.13028
23. Samanta, D. (2024). Evolving treatment strategies for early-life seizures in Tuberous Sclerosis Complex: A review and treatment algorithm. *Epilepsy & Behavior, 161*, 110123. https://doi.org/10.1016/j.yebeh.2024.110123
24. Verche, E., San Luis, C., & Hernández, S. (2018). Neuropsychology of frontal lobe epilepsy in children and adults: Systematic review and meta-analysis. *Epilepsy & Behavior, 88*, 15-20. https://doi.org/10.1016/j.yebeh.2018.08.008
25. Hausman-Kedem, M., Menascu, S., & Kramer, U. (2018). Efficacy of CBD-enriched medical cannabis for treatment of refractory epilepsy in children and adolescents–An observational, longitudinal study. *Brain and Development, 40*(7), 544-551. https://doi.org/10.1016/j.braindev.2018.03.013

26. Dwivedi, R., Ramanujam, B., Chandra, P. S., Sapra, S., Gulati, S., Kalaivani, M., ... & Tripathi, M. (2017). Surgery for drug-resistant epilepsy in children. *New England Journal of Medicine*, *377*(17), 1639-1647. https://doi.org/10.1056/NEJMoa1615335
27. Keller, A. E., Whitney, R., Li, S. A., Pollanen, M. S., & Donner, E. J. (2018). Incidence of sudden unexpected death in epilepsy in children is similar to adults. *Neurology*, *91*(2), e107-e111. https://doi.org/10.1212/WNL.0000000000005762
28. Karaoğlu, P., Yiş, U., Polat, A. İ., Ayanoğlu, M., & Hiz, A. S. (2021). Clinical predictors of drug-resistant epilepsy in children. *Turkish Journal of Medical Sciences*, *51*(3), 1249-1252. https://doi.org/10.3906/sag-2010-27
29. World Health Organization. (2004). *Epilepsy in the WHO Africa Region: Bridging the Gap: The Global Campaign Against Epilepsy "Out of the Shadows."* Geneva: World Health Organization. https://www.ibe-epilepsy.org/downloads/EPILEPSY%20AFRICAN%20Report.pdf
30. Yilmaz, B. S., Okuyaz, C., & Komur, M. (2013). Predictors of intractable childhood epilepsy. *Pediatric Neurology*, *48*(1), 52-55. https://doi.org/10.1016/j.pediatrneurol.2012.09.008
31. Eriksson, K., Erilä, T., Kivimäki, T., & Koivikko, M. (1997). Evolution of epilepsy in children with mental retardation: Five-year experience in 78 cases. *American Journal on Mental Retardation*, *102*(5), 464-472. https://doi.org/10.1352/0895-8017(1998)102%3C0464:EOEICW%3E2.0.CO;2
32. Oskoui, M., Webster, R.I., Zhang, X. & Shevell, M.I. (2005). Factors predictive of outcome in childhood epilepsy. *Journal of Child Neurology*, *20*(11): 898-904. https://doi.org/10.1177/08830738050200110701
33. Ebiai, U. P. (2024). Pharmacological treatment of epilepsy in childhood. https://hdl.handle.net/2437/379302

CHAPTER 13 – EPILEPSY IN WOMEN AND GIRLS

There are many possible causes to a reduced fertility in epilepsy. Social isolation and stigmatisation may contribute, and marriage rates are reported to be lower.
Dr. Torbjörn Tomson[1]

Introduction

Epilepsy presents unique challenges for women, influenced by various physiological changes throughout life, from puberty to menopause. Managing epilepsy in women requires an understanding of gender-specific issues, including hormonal fluctuations, reproductive health, pregnancy, breastfeeding, and bone health, along with the psychosocial aspects of living with epilepsy. A significant concern, particularly in LMICs, is the limited expertise among clinicians in managing epilepsy in women. This gap leads many women to use AEDs that may be harmful during certain periods, risking their own and their unborn children's health. This chapter delves into these aspects in detail, underscoring the importance of personalized treatment and care.

Catamenial epilepsy

For some women, their seizures can be linked to a specific time during their menstrual cycle. They can have seizures throughout the cycle, but the seizures intensify during a specific period in their cycle. This is what is referred to as catamenial epilepsy. This condition affects about one-third of women with epilepsy and presents as increased seizure frequency at specific points in the menstrual cycle.[2] The menstrual cycle is continuous and is repeated every 28 days on average. Research identifies three primary patterns:
- C1: seizures near menstruation
- C2: seizures around ovulation
- C3: increased seizure activity in the luteal phase (after ovulation and before menstruation).[3]

These patterns align with fluctuating estrogen and progesterone levels, with estrogen generally promoting and progesterone suppressing seizure activity.[4] Estrogen is believed to lower seizure thresholds, implying it makes a person prone to seizures, whereas progesterone is believed to work in the opposite direction. Depending on the levels of these hormones in the body during the menstrual cycle, a woman with catamenial epilepsy is likely to have seizures when estrogen levels are high, and progesterone levels are low. It is good to keep a diary of when the seizures happen in relation to the menstrual cycle. When these are properly kept, a trend can be established, and this information can be useful in making sure the woman is at a safe place when seizures are likely to happen.

Effective management of catamenial epilepsy can involve hormonal interventions. Progesterone, for instance, has shown potential in reducing seizure frequency by stabilizing neural excitability. Progesterone therapy, however, has mixed results; for some women, it may reduce seizures, while others experience no significant change.[3] Progesterone-based treatments often use a regimen tailored to individual patterns, such as supplementing progesterone in the luteal phase for those with C1 patterns. However, synthetic hormones used for such treatments can have side effects, including mood changes and weight gain, which complicate long-term use.[5]

Non-hormonal approaches to managing catamenial epilepsy include adjustments to AED regimens during high-risk periods. Physicians may temporarily increase dosages or add supplemental AEDs during the pre-menstrual and peri-ovulatory phases. This approach necessitates close monitoring due to the potential for increased side effects. Emerging research is also exploring the role of lifestyle factors in mitigating catamenial epilepsy. Regular sleep, a balanced diet, and stress management have shown promise in helping some women reduce seizure frequency associated with their menstrual cycles.[6]

Fertility and reproductive health

It is generally accepted from scientific studies that PWE have lower fertility levels compared with the general population. Besides lower fertility levels, chances of live births are also lower than in the general population.[1] These issues stem from various factors, including the potential reproductive toxicity of some AEDs, changes in hormone levels due to epilepsy, and psychosocial factors such as stigma.[7] The reason someone may fail to conceive can be directly related to the AED they are taking. Enzyme-inducing AEDs, such as phenytoin and carbamazepine, can lead to hormonal imbalances, potentially reducing fertility by causing no periods (amenorrhea) or irregular periods. Some AEDs like valproate are associated with polycystic ovarian syndrome (PCOS), which can hinder fertility.[8] PCOS is a type of ovulatory dysfunction, and this obviously leads to reduced fertility.[1]

> *PCOS is increased in women with temporal lobe epilepsy and in women who are taking sodium valproate. This is usually characterized by infrequent menstruation, infrequent ovulation and multiple ovarian cysts. Women with this condition take longer to conceive as they do not release their ova (eggs) regularly. The treatment is usually to lose weight (if they are overweight—BMI >26) and ovulation induction.*[9]
> - *Gerald Madziyire*

Medical options to improve fertility include switching to non-enzyme-inducing AEDs, which may have a less pronounced effect on hormone levels and menstrual regularity. For women with PCOS, lifestyle interventions like weight management and exercise can also help restore fertility. Additionally, hormonal therapies, such as ovulation-inducing agents, are available for women with ovulatory disorders, though these treatments must be carefully monitored in women with epilepsy due to potential seizure triggers.[7] Changing the AED can lead to positive outcomes.

Marriage rates are lower in PWE than in the general population.[10] Besides the issues already mentioned, some parents of girls or young women living with epilepsy do not want to let them go and live independent lives. Parents can be over-protective, making their girl-child a lifelong dependent. They are concerned that their child will not be able to cope with the pressure of a married life, so they will do everything in their power to stop their child from getting married. It does not matter whether the seizures are controlled: they prefer monitoring their girl-child every day rather than leaving that responsibility to the prospective husband. Women with epilepsy may also face societal and cultural obstacles that impact their reproductive choices. In some countries, misconceptions about epilepsy lead to discrimination in marital and reproductive contexts. In Zimbabwe, for example, marriage prospects for women with epilepsy are limited, as epilepsy is often misperceived as a sign of weakness, inadequacy or hereditary illness that could potentially taint the upcoming generations.[10] Addressing these barriers requires a multidisciplinary approach that includes counseling, educational interventions for communities, and improved access to reproductive health services.

Another critical factor is social isolation and stigmatization.[1] It makes sense that one cannot reproduce if they are socially isolated. PWE face stigma every day. This reduces their chances of getting married. For a young woman with epilepsy, her chances of getting married are very slim because of various reasons.[11]

Some women with epilepsy are afraid of getting pregnant for two basic reasons. The first is that their seizures are likely to get worse during pregnancy. This fear is authentic because pregnancy affects the levels of the drug in the body for most AEDs.[12] At times the changes are immaterial, yet with some AEDs and depending on individual patient profiles, the effects can be disabling. The second reason is that they are afraid of the effects of the AEDs on the fetus or infant, which is a particular risk with valproate. Most of the generally used AEDs "cross the placenta in potentially clinically" substantial quantities[12] or are excreted in breast milk. When the AEDs cross the placenta, there is a great risk of major congenital malformations (structural abnormalities with surgical, medical, or cosmetic importance)[13] and no woman would want to take chances of exposing their unborn child to AEDs, yet epilepsy without treatment is also associated with doubling the risk of congenital malformations. It is a tricky situation, so if there is not too much pressure coming from the spouse or the in-laws, an informed woman is likely to choose to remain childless. A PWE can also have other forms of disability, and this significantly reduces their fertility rate.

Contraception and epilepsy

Any woman should be able to actively participate in planning for her family. A woman should be able to determine the number of children she wants to have and at what intervals. The challenge faced by many women with epilepsy is that they end up pregnant without planning for it. At the end of the day, some people will regard them as disorganized because they fail to do simple things like use contraception. Is it true that women with epilepsy forget to take their contraceptives? Is it true that most of them are not using any contraception method at all? Nothing could be further from the truth. The question many will ask is why they seem to fall pregnant without planning for it. This is the purpose of this section.

Contraceptive choice is a critical issue for women with epilepsy, because AED interactions can reduce the efficacy of hormonal contraceptives. Most of the common AEDs, including phenobarbitone, primidone, phenytoin, carbamazepine, and oxcarbazepine, reduce the effectiveness of hormonal oral contraceptives by accelerating the metabolism of estrogen and progesterone, diminishing the effectiveness of combined oral contraceptives (COCs).[1,14,15] Women on these medications are advised to use alternative contraceptive methods, such as non-hormonal intrauterine devices (IUDs) or progestin-only options, which are less affected by AEDs.[7,15,16]

For women preferring hormonal contraception, higher doses of estrogen may counteract the effects of enzyme-inducing AEDs, though this increases the risk of side effects like blood clots and may still be less reliable than non-hormonal methods.[17,18] Long-acting reversible contraceptives (LARCs), such as copper or hormonal IUDs and implants, are highly effective alternatives that do not rely on daily compliance, making them a preferred option for many women with epilepsy.[7,16]

Some oral contraceptives (COCs, combined contraceptive patch, progesterone-only pill, progesterone implant) also reduce the effectiveness of some AEDs,[1,7,16] but most if not all oral contraceptives you are likely to find at the primary healthcare level and government hospitals will interact with enzyme-inducing AEDs (EIAEDs). This puts the woman in a very difficult position because her contraceptive choices are limited. It is known that for women not taking AEDs, many struggle to settle on one type of contraception method, yet they have a wider choice. It must be extremely difficult for someone with epilepsy who only has a limited range of products to choose from. The contraception methods that work in women taking AEDs include injectables like medroxyprogesterone acetate depot injection (Depo-Provera) and hormone-releasing intrauterine systems, all copper-containing IUD, the rhythm method, where sex is avoided during the fertility window and barrier methods like condoms.[1,7,15] For those who have completed their families, tubal ligation (TL) would be most ideal, but if husbands of these women are also willing, they can have a vasectomy so that the wife who is already struggling with epilepsy is spared going to the operating theatre for TL.[7,9,19]

Looking at the limited choices of contraception a woman with epilepsy has, the most logical thing would be to change the AED. However, in most places the newer AEDs are not readily available to the public as most of them are either not yet registered or are too expensive. These EIAEDs are the common ones that are dispensed at the primary care levels in many LMICs.

During patient counseling, these challenges are never mentioned, so the woman just finds herself pregnant and confused. Contraceptive counseling for women with epilepsy must also address potential pregnancy risks associated with specific AEDs. Most clinicians are not sure about which contraceptive method to recommend to women with epilepsy and hence there is a need for a standardized protocol drafted by experts to be circulated to all clinicians and the affected women. Once these standards are in place, the clinicians can easily counsel the women with epilepsy appropriately, which is not the case now. People on AEDs need accurate information for them to manage their lives better.

Pregnancy and epilepsy

If a woman conceives while taking sodium valproate, it can be substituted early in the first trimester; otherwise, she will have to have a close follow-up checking on the possibility that she is carrying a malformed baby. All pregnant women need an anomaly screening (an examination by ultrasound to rule out MCMs) between the eighteenth and twenty second week of pregnancy. A termination of pregnancy is offered if a malformation which is deemed not to be compatible with reasonable quality of life is discovered. The risk of congenital malformations is increased in women taking multiple drugs and it is not clear whether it is due to the severity of their epilepsy or just the drugs. The overall risk of congenital malformation is less than 10% (risk in normal women is 3%), meaning that most women with epilepsy will have normal babies.[9]

-Gerald Madziyire

Pregnancy brings with it several challenges when it comes to managing epilepsy. Pregnancy management for women with epilepsy is complex, as AED use during pregnancy poses potential risks to both the mother and fetus. Pregnant women with epilepsy have an increased risk of complications, including pre-eclampsia, bleeding, and premature labor. The fetal risks associated with AEDs are well documented, with certain medications, such as valproate, showing teratogenic effects, particularly in the first trimester.[13] The teratogenicity of AEDs, especially valproate, underscores the importance of pre-pregnancy counseling for women with epilepsy. Consequently, women with epilepsy who plan to conceive are often advised to transition to safer AEDs before conception, which necessitates a well-coordinated plan involving neurologists and obstetricians.[20] The standard practice is to avoid valproate and to consider alternatives, such as lamotrigine and levetiracetam, which have a lower teratogenic risk.[21]

I want to highlight that should anyone taking AEDs decide to get pregnant she must consult her doctor before she does so. Some AEDs can cause serious side effects, especially affecting the fetus, if taken during the first trimester.[8,22] Most women present to their doctor when they are already pregnant, and this can be avoided if there is awareness. As previously mentioned in the fertility section, some AEDs are associated with major congenital malformations (MCMs). Chances of

MCMs are also doubled when a PWE is not on medication.[13,23] The patient must act as a responsible mother, and the same need for responsibility applies to the doctor. It is recommended that should a woman intend to get pregnant, the following should be done. If she has been seizure-free for at least 2 years, depending on the type of epilepsy, the doctor should consider withdrawing the patient from medication.[7,12,18] If withdrawal is successful, she can become pregnant. If she is on more than one drug, the doctor must try to manage her on one drug only by slowly withdrawing her from one of the drugs. This is because when a person is taking more than one AED, the risk of MCMs is increased.[7,13,18] In case withdrawal fails, if she is on an unsafe AED, she must be managed to migrate to a safer one that also controls her seizures.[18,24] If she is on a high dosage of an AED, the doctor must reduce the dosage to a safe level that ensures she remains seizure-free while reducing the risks of MCMs.[7,18,22] The process of withdrawal takes time, so the woman must not just present at the doctor intending to get pregnant the following month.[25] If the withdrawal process is not done properly, the effects can be negative. There must be adequate time to try different alternatives before the woman can fall pregnant. Ladies, you owe it to your children to act responsibly.

Seizures must be well managed throughout the pregnancy, so proper groundwork must be done prior to falling pregnant. Additionally, during pregnancy, AED blood levels may fluctuate due to physiological changes, affecting seizure control. Regular monitoring of blood drug levels is crucial to adjusting dosages, minimizing seizure activity, and preventing adverse effects on fetal development.[12,18] The risks associated with seizures are many. Besides physical injuries, "women with epilepsy have been shown to be over-represented among maternal deaths in the UK."[1] Continuous GTCS are harmful to the fetus and can even lead to fetal death.[1,7,12] There is a need to balance between being cautious about the side effects of AEDs on the mother or fetus and the risks associated with uncontrolled seizures. This balance is not easy to strike, but effort must be made to ensure the mother is seizure-free as well as taking a safe AED (both to her and the fetus). This requires cooperation on the part of the mother as well as dedication on the part of the doctor. To strike a balance takes time, so all parties involved must be patient and determined to make it work.

Research has shown that sodium valproate is the AED with the greatest risk of MCMs, especially when taken during the first trimester.[8,12] Sodium valproate should be avoided in girls and women of childbearing age, unless there is no other AED that controls their seizures.[8,21,24] Trying to change an AED when a woman is already pregnant could produce negative results, especially on seizure control. As previously mentioned, to change from one AED to another takes time, so to be safe, it is suggested that women with epilepsy observe all the things mentioned above so that they plan their pregnancies well. Once there is an MCM, there is no benefit in changing the AED. If a woman presents to the doctor when she is already in the second trimester (week 13 or later), there is no need to change the AED.

MCMs and other possible effects on children born to women taking AEDs during pregnancy are shown in Table 11.

Table 11: Possible teratogenic effects of AEDs

AED	Specific MCM
Phenytoin	Cleft palate Poor cognitive outcomes Increased risk of small for gestational age (SGA) Increased risk of 1-minute Apgar scores of <7
Carbamazepine	Posterior cleft palate Increased risk of SGA Increased risk of 1-minute Apgar scores of <7
Sodium valproate	Neural tube defects Facial clefts Hypospadias Poor cognitive outcomes Increased risk of SGA Increased risk of 1-minute Apgar scores of <7
Phenobarbitone	Cardiac malformations Reduced cognitive abilities Increased risk of SGA Increased risk of 1-minute Apgar scores of <7

This is a summary from information extracted from the chapter entitled "Anti-epileptics."[14]

Table 11 shows possible MCMs associated with four AEDs. As a rule, sodium valproate must be avoided in women who intend to get pregnant later in life, unless there is no other option.[8] This does not denote that the newer AEDs are safe. They still need the test of time for concluding their safety to the mother and unborn baby. Research is ongoing.

About 50% of pregnant women with epilepsy will experience a change in their seizure threshold, either positively or negatively. These changes are caused by several factors like discontinuation of AEDs during pregnancy, excessive vomiting, stress, lack of sleep, and sub-therapeutic levels of AEDs due to reasons mentioned below. Pregnancy causes noteworthy changes in the way the woman processes the AEDs that she takes. It has been proved that blood concentrations for most AEDs are reduced during pregnancy. This is due to "impaired gastrointestinal absorption, increased volume of distribution, decreased protein binding, increased renal glomerular filtration rate, and changes in metabolizing capacity."[1] It is therefore a requirement that plasma concentrations be monitored throughout pregnancy otherwise there is a great risk of seizures due to low levels of the drug in the body. Plasma concentrations of lamotrigine can go as low as 33%, levetiracetam as low as 50%, and phenobarbitone as low as 60%.[1] Oxcarbazepine and topiramate levels are also reduced significantly.

Women with epilepsy who get pregnant need folic acid supplementation. They should be counseled that most women with epilepsy "will have uneventful pregnancies and give birth to perfectly normal children."[1] This information is not to be used to scare anyone from having children, but everyone must be informed of all the possibilities that are likely because of their epilepsy treatment.

After delivery of the baby, the mother's doses may need re-adjustment if she is taking an AED whose plasma concentrations are affected by pregnancy. The mother will also need to consider if the baby will be breastfed, as this brings its own challenges as shown in the next section. A woman might need to change the AED she will be taking if it affects the baby through breast milk.

Breastfeeding and epilepsy

Breastfeeding is generally encouraged for women with epilepsy, as breast milk offers significant health benefits for the newborn. However, the excretion of AEDs into breast milk is a consideration for many women. Levetiracetam, lamotrigine and oxcarbazepine penetrate breast milk, but are relatively safe during breastfeeding, as their concentrations in breast milk are low and unlikely to cause harm to the infant.[12] However, medications such as phenobarbitone and primidone have higher concentrations in breast milk and may cause sedation in the infant.[7]

Healthcare providers typically recommend breastfeeding mothers on AEDs to monitor their infants for signs of sedation, irritability, or feeding difficulties, particularly during the initial weeks.[7] Additionally, breastfeeding can influence AED metabolism in mothers, as the energy demands of lactation may affect drug clearance, potentially requiring dosage adjustments. Counseling on safe breastfeeding practices and infant monitoring is essential for minimizing risks while promoting the health benefits of breastfeeding. Table 12 is a summary of AED behavior in breast milk[14]: it is clear most of the AEDs in use affect babies somehow. Some of the effects may be of a serious nature, while others may be less severe.

Table 12: AEDs excreted in breast milk and their effects on breastfed babies

AED	Possible effects on breast-fed infant
Carbamazepine	Transient cholestatic hepatitis (rare)
Clobazam, clonazepam, diazepam	Neonatal sedation (avoid breastfeeding)
Ethosuximide	Hyperexcitability and poor suckling (avoid if possible)
Gabapentin, levetiracetam, topiramate	Transferred into breast milk in significant amounts
Lamotrigine	Possible drug accumulation in breast-fed baby
Phenobarbitone, primidone	Sedation and methemoglobinemia (use with caution)
Phenytoin	Rarely methemoglobinemia
Valproate	Rarely thrombocytopenic purpura and anemia
Vigabatrin	Avoid breastfeeding
Zonisamide	To be used only if benefit outweighs risk

This is a summary from information extracted from the chapter entitled "Anti-epileptics."[14]

Some mothers in poor communities may not be able to afford supplementary feeding and rely solely on breastfeeding to nourish their babies. Table 12 could provide information on potential effects on breast-fed babies, but some mothers may not have options. Clinicians should work with mothers to evaluate alternatives so that the infant is not impacted in a significant way.

Menopause and hormonal changes

Menopause is the period where menstruation ceases. It is marked by a change in the balance of sex hormones in the body. This can lead to hot flushes, palpitations, dryness of vaginal canal, and emotional disturbances. Hormonal changes during menopause can significantly affect seizure patterns in women with epilepsy. Estrogen, a hormone with pro-convulsant properties, declines alongside progesterone, which has an anticonvulsant effect. The net impact of these hormonal changes varies among individuals; for some, seizure frequency decreases, while others experience an increase due to hormonal instability.[16,26] This variability requires individualized management.

Seizure risk is increased in the "peri-menopausal" phase and reduced at menopause in women with catamenial epilepsy.[2,9] Another term for perimenopause is "climacteric period."[9] During this phase ovarian function starts declining. Features during this period are: "irregular periods, hot flushes, decreased libido, urine leakage, urinary urgency, worsening of premenstrual syndrome, fatigue, breast tenderness, vaginal dryness, difficulty sleeping and mood swings due to hormonal fluctuations."[9] Perimenopause starts well before menopause—in some cases, up to 10 years earlier.[9]

In women with catamenial epilepsy, these hormonal fluctuations can lower the seizure threshold.[2,5] At menopause, estrogen levels are low, resulting in a lowered risk of seizures.[4,26] As a way of coping with the effects of menopause, many women resort to hormone replacement therapy (HRT). HRT is sometimes prescribed to manage menopausal symptoms, though it can exacerbate seizure frequency in women with epilepsy.[27] Estrogen-based HRT can increase seizure risk in women with catamenial epilepsy due to estrogen's excitatory effects on the brain.[4,9] Menopause causes a change in seizure control if we are to go by the conclusion drawn in the catamenial section where we said estrogen lowers the seizure threshold and progesterone increases it. Alternative treatments, including selective serotonin reuptake inhibitors (SSRIs) and non-hormonal therapies, may offer symptom relief without adversely affecting seizure control.[27]

There is not much literature on epilepsy and menopause, but deducting from other studies, it can be concluded that there is a change in how a woman feels after they have gone into menopause and this general trend can be applied to women with epilepsy as well. Management strategies for women with epilepsy undergoing menopause often involve closely monitoring seizure activity and tailoring AED regimens to mitigate changes in seizure frequency. Lifestyle interventions, such as stress reduction and regular physical activity, may also support seizure stability, offering a holistic approach to menopause management in epilepsy care.[16]

Bone health in women with epilepsy

Women with epilepsy have an increased risk of osteoporosis and fractures, partly due to AED side effects and lifestyle factors.[1] AEDs like phenytoin and phenobarbitone reduce bone density by interfering with the metabolism of vitamin D, which is crucial for calcium absorption.[14] Studies indicate that women with epilepsy, especially those taking enzyme-inducing AEDs, have a higher prevalence of low bone density and fractures, especially post menopause when bone loss accelerates naturally.[28]

Preventive strategies for bone health include regular bone density assessments, calcium and vitamin D supplementation, and engaging in weight-bearing exercise. Some women may also benefit from bisphosphonate therapy, though this should be discussed with healthcare providers due to potential side effects.[29] Awareness of AED-related bone health risks is essential, especially for postmenopausal women, who face a compounded risk of osteoporosis-related complications.[1,28]

Psychosocial aspects and stigma

The psychosocial impact of epilepsy can be especially pronounced for women, affecting their mental health, social relationships, and economic opportunities. In many societies, epilepsy-related stigma leads to social exclusion and limited marital and career prospects for women. In Nigeria, for instance, epilepsy is widely misunderstood, often perceived as contagious or as a sign of mental instability, which diminishes the social standing of affected women.[11]

Living with epilepsy may lead to heightened rates of anxiety and depression, with the stigma amplifying these effects. Educational interventions aimed at demystifying epilepsy for families and communities have proven effective in reducing stigma. Studies indicate that providing accurate information about epilepsy's causes and treatment can help dispel myths and foster greater social acceptance.[9] Psychoeducational support for women with epilepsy can significantly enhance their quality of life, helping to mitigate stigma's adverse effects on mental health.

Conclusion

Women with epilepsy encounter unique medical and social challenges, from hormonal influences on seizure patterns to reproductive health, pregnancy, and bone health concerns. Tailored medical management, including personalized AED selection and lifestyle interventions, is essential to address these complexities. Additionally, addressing stigma through community education can improve social integration and quality of life. By considering the specific needs of women at different life stages, healthcare providers can better support women with epilepsy in achieving improved health outcomes and well-being.

References:

1. Tomson, T. (2012). VIREPA Course on Clinical Pharmacology and Pharmacotherapy: Gender Issues in Antiepileptic Drug (AED) Use. Stockholm: International League Against Epilepsy.
2. Frank, S., & Tyson, N. A. (2020). A clinical approach to catamenial epilepsy: a review. *The Permanente Journal, 24.* https://doi.org/10.7812/TPP/19.145
3. Joshi, S., Sun, H., Rajasekaran, K., Williamson, J., Perez-Reyes, E., & Kapur, J. (2018). A novel therapeutic approach for treatment of catamenial epilepsy. *Neurobiology of Disease, 111,* 127-137. https://doi.org/10.1016/j.nbd.2017.12.009
4. Alshakhouri, M., Sharpe, C., Bergin, P., & Sumner, R. L. (2024). Female sex steroids and epilepsy: Part 2. A practical and human focus on catamenial epilepsy. *Epilepsia, 65*(3), 569-582. https://doi.org/10.1111/epi.17820
5. Voinescu, P. E., Kelly, M., French, J. A., Harden, C., Davis, A., Lau, C., ... & Pennell, P. B. (2023). Catamenial epilepsy occurrence and patterns in a mixed population of women with epilepsy. *Epilepsia, 64*(9), e194-e199. https://doi.org/10.1111/epi.17718
6. Voinescu, P. E. (2019). Catamenial epilepsy. *Neurology and Psychiatry of Women: A Guide to Gender-based Issues in Evaluation, Diagnosis, and Treatment,* 85-94. https://doi.org/10.1007/978-3-030-04245-5_9
7. Stephen, L. J., Harden, C., Tomson, T., & Brodie, M. J. (2019). Management of epilepsy in women. *The Lancet Neurology, 18*(5), 481-491. https://doi.org/10.1055/s-0039-3399473
8. Tomson, T., Marson, A., Boon, P., Canevini, M. P., Covanis, A., Gaily, E., ... & Trinka, E. (2015). Valproate in the treatment of epilepsy in girls and women of childbearing potential. *Epilepsia, 56*(7), 1006-1019. https://doi.org/10.1111/epi.13021
9. Madziyire, M.G. (2013). Interview with Dr. M.G. Madziyire, a Gynaecologist and Obstetrician. Harare, Zimbabwe. [31 July 2013].

10. Mugumbate, J. & Mushonga, J. (2013). Myths, perceptions, and incorrect knowledge surrounding epilepsy in rural Zimbabwe: A study of the villagers in Buhera District, *Epilepsy & Behavior, 27*: 144–147.
11. Komolafe, M. A., Sunmonu, T. A., Fabusiwa, F., Komolafe, E. O., Afolabi, O., Kett, M., & Groce, N. (2011). Women's perspectives on epilepsy and its sociocultural impact in southwestern Nigeria. *African Journal of Neurological Sciences, 30*(2). https://www.ajol.info/index.php/ajns/article/view/77320
12. Harden, C. L., Pennell, P. B., Koppel, B. S., Hovinga, C. A., Gidal, B., Meador, K. J., ... & Le Guen, C. L. (2009). Management issues for women with epilepsy—Focus on pregnancy (an evidence-based review): III. Vitamin K, folic acid, blood levels, and breast-feeding: Report of the Quality Standards Subcommittee and Therapeutics and Technology Assessment Subcommittee of the American Academy of Neurology and the American Epilepsy Society. *Epilepsia, 50*(5), 1247-1255. https://doi.org/ 10.1111/j.1528-1167.2009.02130.x
13. Holmes, L. B., Harvey, E. A., Coull, B. A., Huntington, K. B., Khoshbin, S., Hayes, A. M., & Ryan, L. M. (2001). The teratogenicity of anticonvulsant drugs. *New England Journal of Medicine, 344*(15), 1132-1138. https://www.nejm.org/doi/pdf/10.1056/NEJM200104123441504
14. Sweetman, S.C. et al eds. 2009. "Antiepileptics" in: *Martindale: The Complete Drug Reference. 36th ed.* London: Pharmaceutical Press. 465-516.
15. Gooneratne, I. K., Wimalaratna, M., Ranaweera, A. P., & Wimalaratna, S. (2017). Contraception advice for women with epilepsy. *BMJ, 357*. https://doi.org/10.1136/bmj.j2010
16. Kennedy, J. D., & Chen, M. J. (2019). Women and epilepsy. *Practical Neurology, 63*. https://www.researchgate.net/profile/Jeffrey-Kennedy/publication/336813878_Women_Epilepsy_Biology_unique_to_female_individuals_with_epilepsy_affects_disease_management_significantly/links/5db3825c4585155e270117de/Women-Epilepsy-Biology-unique-to-female-individuals-with-epilepsy-affects-disease-management-significantly.pdf
17. Bosak, M., Słowik, A., & Turaj, W. (2019). Why do some women with epilepsy use valproic acid despite current guidelines? A single-center cohort study. *Epilepsy & Behavior, 98*, 1-5. https://doi.org/10.1016/j.yebeh.2019.06.031
18. Lee, S. K. (2023). Issues of women with epilepsy and suitable antiseizure drugs. *Journal of Epilepsy Research, 13*(2), 23. https://doi.org/10.14581/jer.23005
19. Shawahna, R., & Zaid, L. (2022). Caring for women with epilepsy in Palestine: A qualitative study of the current status. *Epilepsy & Behavior, 130*, 108689. https://doi.org/10.1016/j.yebeh.2022.108689
20. Karlsson Lind, L., Komen, J., Wettermark, B., von Euler, M., & Tomson, T. (2018). Valproic acid utilization among girls and women in Stockholm: impact of regulatory restrictions. *Epilepsia Open, 3*(3), 357-363. https://doi.org/10.1002/epi4.12228
21. Toledo, M., Mostacci, B., Bosak, M., Jedrzejzak, J., Thomas, R. H., Salas-Puig, J., ... & Schmitz, B. (2021). Expert opinion: use of valproate in girls and women of childbearing potential with epilepsy: recommendations and alternatives based on a review of the literature and clinical experience—a European perspective. *Journal of Neurology, 268*, 2735-2748. https://doi.org/10.1007/s00415-020-09809-0
22. Craig, J., & Kinney, M. (2024). Teratogenic risk and aspects of epilepsy relating to women's health. *Comorbidities and Social Complications of Epilepsy and Seizures: The Cognitive, Psychological and Psychosocial Impact of Epilepsy*, 215. https://books.google.com/books?hl=en&lr=&id=l8sVEQAAQBAJ&oi=fnd&pg=PA215

&dq=menopause,+pregnancy,+breastfeeding,+fertility,+contraception,+bone+health+in+epilepsy&ots=MahqZx0Brr&sig=6CPdnHSDPEWSGe0hX2nZM65qnAg

23. Ding, D., Sha, L., Chen, Y., Sha, L., Ding, D., Chen, Y., & Ding, D. (2024). Disease burden of women with epilepsy. In *Women with Epilepsy in Child-bearing Age: Diagnosis and Treatment* (pp. 1-23). Singapore: Springer Nature Singapore. https://doi.org/10.1007/978-981-97-3921-9_1

24. Mostacci, B., Ranzato, F., Giuliano, L., La Neve, A., Aguglia, U., Bilo, L., ... & Galimberti, C. A. (2021). Alternatives to valproate in girls and women of childbearing potential with Idiopathic Generalized Epilepsies: State of the art and guidance for the clinician proposed by the Epilepsy and Gender Commission of the Italian League Against Epilepsy (LICE). *Seizure, 85*, 26-38. https://doi.org/10.1016/j.seizure.2020.12.005

25. Dierking, C., Porschen, T., Walter, U., & Rösche, J. (2018). Pregnancy-related knowledge of women with epilepsy—an internet-based survey in German-speaking countries. *Epilepsy & Behavior, 79*, 17-22. https://doi.org/10.1016/j.yebeh.2017.11.013

26. Hophing, L., Kyriakopoulos, P., & Bui, E. (2022). Sex and gender differences in epilepsy. In *International Review of Neurobiology* (Vol. 164, pp. 235-276). Academic Press. https://doi.org/10.1016/bs.irn.2022.06.012

27. Li, Q., Zhang, Z., & Fang, J. (2024). Hormonal Changes in Women with Epilepsy. *Neuropsychiatric Disease and Treatment*, 373-388. https://doi.org/10.2147/NDT.S453532

28. Tatum, W. O. (2018). Women with Epilepsy. *Common Pitfalls in Epilepsy: Case-Based Learning*, 189. https://books.google.com/books?hl=en&lr=&id=Lq52DwAAQBAJ&oi=fnd&pg=PA220&dq=menopause,+pregnancy,+breastfeeding,+fertility,+contraception,+bone+health+in+epilepsy&ots=s4UyYyjQxT&sig=Tz8OiiSEhzZKC6WF6g9PZ6BIMAc

29. Sazgar, M., Young, M. G., Sazgar, M., & Young, M. G. (2019). Women with epilepsy. *Absolute Epilepsy and EEG Rotation Review: Essentials for Trainees*, 101-113. https://doi.org/10.1007/978-3-030-03511-2_4

Chapter 14 – Stigma in Epilepsy

4,000 years of ignorance, superstition and stigma followed by 100 years of knowledge, superstition and stigma.[1]
R. Kale

"Please remember that though we are talking about epilepsy, we are also talking about people. The disorder is certainly part of the person, but it does not define the person. A person is not epileptic, a person suffers from epilepsy."
M. Giles

Stigma' traces its roots back to the Greek and means a 'mark.' Stigma, a mark with a pejorative taint, silences the communication '........... Stigma is therefore antithetical to the very spirit of psychology.[2]
S. Behnke

Introduction

Epilepsy, a neurological disorder affecting millions worldwide, continues to be misunderstood and stigmatized due to a combination of historical beliefs and persistent myths.[2,3] Social and cultural biases, compounded by limited public awareness, often lead to discrimination, affecting both the social and psychological well-being of those with epilepsy.[4] The repercussions of epilepsy stigma are vast, affecting relationships, employment, and mental health, which underscores the need for comprehensive approaches to dismantling these outdated perspectives.[5,6] Why would I dedicate a whole chapter to the issue of stigma? I will begin with this quote extracted from a paper in the journal *Epilepsia*:

A person with epilepsy faces deep social exclusion and systemic barriers that isolate them from opportunities to work, relationships, and personal fulfillment. Their condition leads to rejection, loss of dreams, and emotional despair, amounting to a spiritual death.[7] ILAE

Stigma is disabling. It diminishes a person's quality of life; it gives the person a low status in society and contributes to prejudice and discrimination. Epilepsy is disabling enough, but to add stigma to that just makes it unbearable. Everyone wants to live their life to their full potential. In my observations, I have noticed that most of the stigma emanates from the myths discussed in Chapter 10. "My people are destroyed for lack of knowledge" (Hosea 4:6). This verse is very applicable to the issue of stigma. We can do something about it. We can obtain knowledge if we try as Proverbs (4:7b) says, "with all your acquiring, get understanding." Once people are equipped with knowledge, the issue of stigma will be a thing of the past.

Definition

What then is stigma? I will go with Weiss and Ramakrishna's definition: "stigma is a social process or related personal experience characterized by exclusion, rejection, blame, or devaluation that results from experience or reasonable anticipation of an adverse social judgment about a person or group identified with a particular health problem."[8]

Origins and history of epilepsy-related stigma

Early civilizations such as those of Mesopotamia and ancient Egypt, associated epilepsy with spiritual possession, causing both social exclusion and stigma for PWE.[9] Similarly, Greeks and Romans saw epilepsy as divine punishment, perpetuating beliefs of epilepsy being caused by the supernatural which shaped public attitudes for centuries.[10] Throughout the Middle Ages, epilepsy was stigmatized in Europe, where it was often linked to sin or moral failings. Under the Pope's instruction, the *Malleus Maleficarum* led to the persecution of people believed to be witches resulting in up to 9 million deaths, including PWE who were also grouped among the witches.[59] Meanwhile, other regions, including parts of Asia and Africa, viewed epilepsy as a sign of spiritual imbalance or curse, leading to the ostracism of affected individuals.[11,12] These views persisted well into the 19th century and have left a lasting imprint on societal beliefs regarding epilepsy.[13] With advancements in neurology in the 19th and 20th centuries, the medical community began to understand epilepsy as a neurological disorder rather than a mystical affliction. Deeply ingrained cultural beliefs have proven difficult to overcome entirely, however.[14,15] That is why stigma is still an issue several millennia after epilepsy's first mention in early medical writings.

Types of stigmata

Epilepsy-related stigma is particularly severe in sub-Saharan Africa, where epilepsy rates are much higher than in developed countries.[10] This heightened stigma is largely fueled by widespread beliefs in supernatural causes and the idea that the condition is contagious.[16] Kale reflects on the historical roots of this stigma, noting "4,000 years of ignorance, superstition, and stigma followed by 100 years of knowledge, superstition, and stigma."[1] Despite increased awareness of epilepsy, Kale notes that superstition and stigma persist. Stigma can be "enacted" or "felt."[10] Enacted stigma is the discrimination that a stigmatized person faces from others.[17] Felt stigma occurs when a stigmatized individual willingly restricts their own actions to avoid facing discrimination from others.[17] Both types pose a significant challenge for PWE.[10]

Public stigma

Public stigma comes from societal misconceptions about epilepsy, already covered in Chapter 10. These myths and misconceptions can make people believe PWE are unreliable or potentially dangerous among many things. Such stereotypes contribute to social exclusion and discrimination in settings like the workplace, where PWE may be denied opportunities due to perceived risks.[18,19]

Courtesy stigma

Courtesy stigma, which may manifest as either enacted or felt stigma, impacts individuals connected to those with epilepsy, including family members, friends, colleagues, worshippers, teachers, and even healthcare providers. In some African communities, this stigma can extend to an entire clan, potentially leading people to disown relatives with epilepsy. This phenomenon also plays a role in cases where women are divorced for having children with epilepsy, as discussed in Chapter 12.

Internalized or self-stigma

Many individuals with epilepsy internalize societal attitudes, leading to feelings of shame and low self-esteem. This self-stigma often discourages people from seeking treatment, participating in social activities, or openly discussing their condition.[20,21] Internalized stigma can also exacerbate mental health challenges, creating a cycle that is difficult to break.[22] In my own lived experience, I found that self-stigma was significantly reduced when I started interacting with others living with epilepsy at the Epilepsy Support Foundation (ESF) in Harare, Zimbabwe. Belonging to this support group and seeing ways I could add value helped me come out of my shell.

Institutional stigma

Structural stigma is reinforced through discriminatory policies, such as restrictions on driving or limitations to insurance access. These institutional barriers perpetuate social exclusion and contribute to reduced opportunities for PWE.[23,24]

Stigma in different countries and regions

High-income countries

Although awareness is generally higher in wealthier nations, individuals with epilepsy still experience discrimination due to lingering stereotypes. In countries like the USA and UK, studies indicate that PWE face social and occupational exclusion, often based on unfounded concerns about safety or reliability.[25] When PWE are employed, they are usually under-employed.

Low- and middle-income countries

In many lower-income regions, stigma is fueled by deep-rooted traditional beliefs about epilepsy.[8,26] For instance, in parts of Africa and South Asia, epilepsy is sometimes attributed to supernatural causes, such as witchcraft or demonic possession, resulting in severe social and family exclusion.[8,26]

Cultural comparisons

The level and intensity of stigma experienced by PWE varies according to local cultural interpretations of epilepsy. Individuals will have differing experiences of stigma based on where they live and the context. In some cultures, epilepsy is considered spiritually significant, whereas in others, it is viewed with negativity or fear. These cultural perceptions influence how PWE are treated and the level of social support they receive.[27,28]

Relationship between knowledge, attitudes, and stigma

Research shows that public knowledge about epilepsy directly impacts societal attitudes. When people are more aware of epilepsy, attitudes towards PWE improves and stigma is reduced.[7,29] Targeting young people and community engagement have been shown to help dismiss myths and misconceptions.[30,31]

When a person starts having epilepsy in adulthood, they need time to process what is happening to them. Acceptance is rarely instant, but given enough time and proper support, a person can start to accept their condition. It requires effort from all angles, starting with healthcare workers. Proper counseling will help the person accept the condition. Clinicians also need to be properly skilled in diagnosing and treating epilepsy. If seizures are controlled, many people will never know that a person has epilepsy. This will help protect the affected person during the time they will be trying to adjust to their new condition. They must be allowed enough time to process it in their own way. It is like grieving. Someone has lost their abilities to do certain things, and you cannot expect that person to take it and move on as if nothing has happened. Some people will no longer be able to drive safely. In some cases, depending on the type of job, PWE lose their jobs for safety reasons. In my own lived experience, the best scenario would be that the affected person gets to a point of sharing information with other people about their condition without feeling ashamed about it. When one gets to this level, the issue of felt stigma has been overcome, but before we get there, a lot of work needs to be done.

Family stigma and interpersonal relationships

Family members of individuals with epilepsy may experience courtesy stigma, whereby they face judgment or exclusion based on their association with someone who has epilepsy. This phenomenon can strain family relationships, particularly in cultures where epilepsy is heavily stigmatized.[32]

Overprotective family behaviors often arise from societal expectations or fear of judgment. If no one knows their family member has epilepsy, they will not suffer courtesy stigma. However, this practice limits the independence of the PWE. While well-intentioned, such behaviors can reinforce feelings of dependency and social isolation for the PWE.[33,34] Consequently, epilepsy stigma impacts family dynamics, support systems, and interpersonal relationships, with family members experiencing secondary social consequences.[35,36]

The family needs to support the person and give them assurance that they are still the same person they were before epilepsy. This process can take years in some people and can be a challenging time especially in cultural settings where some traditional roles and chores are expected. For instance, in many rural African communities, a woman may be stigmatized if she is unable to perform duties like cooking over an open flame due to epilepsy-related limitations. The inability to do those chores can be a source of stigmatization. Some cultures associate burn marks acquired during seizures as a sign of "permanent epilepsy," an affliction they believe cannot be cured. It is like a seal which cannot be removed. Their interpretation is since the scar will never go away, neither will the epilepsy. It is sealed for life and no medication (herbal or conventional) can reverse that.

Cultural expectations put a heavy burden on PWE. For instance, in some LMICs, drinking water is accessed from deep wells, which may not be suitable for those with certain epilepsy syndromes that are triggered by heights. In some Zimbabwe cultures, when there is a funeral in the family, the daughter-in-law is expected to do all chores and ensure all people coming to mourn have a warm bath in the morning, eat hot meals at stipulated times, and sing and dance with everybody else. On such occasions, the extended family, friends, the community at large and neighbors come. If they see that the daughter-in-law is not doing all these chores, they start whispering amongst themselves, why this is so? Someone will tell them in a low voice that "she is ill *ane pfari*" (*pfari* is epilepsy in Shona). After that, if you are observant, you will see people pointing fingers towards the daughter-in-law. They do it in a subtle way and speak with their faces down. These cultural expectations around funerals, where women are expected to manage household responsibilities, can increase stigmatization if they cannot fulfill these roles. This often leads communities to question the woman's ability to perform traditional duties, sometimes even prompting suggestions that the husband should marry a second wife. If the affected woman lives in an urban area, but is not working, her next destination will be her rural home, or if she is not divorced, she will be sent to her husband's rural home, while the new wife stays with him in the city. All this is done in an effort not to bring disgrace to the husband's family. It is also a way of ensuring she does not continue to bear any more children as these will taint the lineage.

The misconception that PWE suffer from mental illness contributes to stigmatization, which leads to isolation and loneliness.[7,10,17] Others consider every PWE as cognitively challenged.[10,17,18] Those who associate with PWE may do so out of pity, rather than respect, which can be demeaning and patronizing. As a person with this condition, I would not want people to associate with me because they feel sorry for me, and I do not think anyone, whether with this condition or not, would want people to associate with them because they feel sorry for them. Any association should be based on love and mutual respect and not out of pity. Others start to distance themselves once they know you have epilepsy. Many people end up not disclosing their condition if possible, so that they can be treated with dignity and respect; this should not be confused with patronizing.[10,34,35]

It should be pointed out here that PWE are not charity cases. Given equal opportunities, they can live quality lives like any other person.[1,37] Stigma starts affecting a neonate because the parents do not want the world to know they have a child with epilepsy. In my interactions with parents of children with epilepsy at CRU and Tose in Harare, some parents disclosed they had hidden their children from the world until someone tipped off social services. The child will never go to school. Some of them are never taken to the clinic to get AEDs. Many seek the help of witchdoctors and "prophets." The child's health usually deteriorates due to uncontrolled seizures.[15,16,17] This child will always be treated like a minor by the parents.[30] If they have other children after this one, the younger children will go to school and get married eventually, yet this one will always be infantilized. At our support group at the ESF, many women identified this as a challenge. Their younger siblings were getting married, but their parents would not even allow them to get into a relationship. In East Timor, a child with epilepsy is not sent to school, and this is common in most developing countries.[15,17,20] What do people expect from a person who is kept from the rest of the world? Their world is their house. They have no friends. They are always under constant supervision. In this case, we see stigma coming from those who are supposed to protect and care for you. How does someone feel when they know they bring shame to their parents?

Some parents send their children with epilepsy to school, but the issue of stigma cannot be trivialized. Teachers and fellow pupils may not know how to handle someone with seizures.[7,10,35] The lack of support often results in children being asked to leave school because their seizures were scaring the rest of the students, limiting their prospects.[15,16,35] The parents are also not empowered to do anything, and they remove their child from school. What is the future of this child with no education? As already discussed, some types of epilepsy syndromes are outgrown by the time the child reaches adolescence. What happens when the epilepsy has gone? Can this child who is now 16 be taken back to grade two? This is quite sad, but this is what is happening around us. When this child reaches adulthood, they will only be able to do menial jobs because of not being educated. This perpetuates the idea PWE cannot perform at the same level as everyone else.[15,16,37] The child was set up for failure from the beginning and achieving anything meaningful in life will require more effort.

Research has shown that men with epilepsy are less likely to get married than their female counterparts.[17,21,35] The reason could be that in many cultures it is the man who approaches a woman to propose marriage. We are talking of a man who has been socially isolated his whole life. How does he even know where to begin? Some have siblings who will take it upon themselves to propose on behalf of their brother, and this has resulted in a few marriages.[14,30] In my view, their main motivation for getting their brother a wife is that the wife will act as a nurse to the man. Since this man cannot live on his own because he has been taught to be dependent on other people his whole life, the siblings do not want to have to look after him, especially if the parents are deceased. For most of the men who eventually get married, stigma associated with bedwetting largely affects them.[14,38] Their wives might leave them because they cannot afford to be seen washing blankets on a regular basis (courtesy stigma) or they are just tired of washing blankets. When the wife leaves, it becomes very complicated socially. To reduce the possibility of a divorce, the siblings will try to get a wife for their brother who has a disability as well, better still, one with epilepsy who will understand and not have many options herself.[14,30,39]

Effects of stigma on quality of life

Social limitations: Individuals with epilepsy often restrict their social interactions to avoid public seizures and subsequent stigmatization. This social withdrawal has a direct negative impact on their overall quality of life, leading to feelings of isolation and alienation.[40,41]

Educational and occupational impact: Stigma also limits educational and employment opportunities. Many employers hold misconceptions about epilepsy, fearing liability or safety risks associated with seizures. This bias creates a considerable barrier to employment and economic stability for PWE.[37,38]

Overall life satisfaction: The combined effects of social, occupational, and educational limitations contribute to decreased life satisfaction. PWE report lower quality of life metrics than the general population, with stigma being a critical factor influencing these experiences.[1,42]

Challenges in cultural contexts

The success of educational initiatives depends on the regional and cultural context. For example, awareness programs in schools and workplaces have successfully shifted attitudes in Western countries, but similar efforts often face resistance in regions where traditional beliefs about epilepsy prevail.[43,44] Tailoring educational materials to address specific cultural misconceptions can enhance the efficacy of these initiatives.[45]

Another significant source of stigma comes from traditional healers or witch doctors. In many African regions, particularly in rural areas, a large portion of the population lives far from healthcare centers, making traditional healers a more accessible option. However, this issue is not limited to rural areas; many urban residents also seek out traditional healers. In these settings, epilepsy is often linked to beliefs in witchcraft, demons, avenging spirits, broken taboos, goblins, or even divine punishment.[17] It is commonly thought that a PWE suffers on behalf of their family or because of a relative's wrongdoing, marking them as deserving of the condition in a manner like a punishment.

Historically, as summarized in one review, the primary driver of discrimination against individuals with disabilities is fear, not the disability itself.[7] Reducing this stigma is crucial, as it stands as one of the greatest obstacles for PWE. Much work is needed to educate communities, individuals with epilepsy, and their families to improve understanding and dismantle harmful misconceptions. This effort requires coordinated action from epilepsy associations, ministries of health and education, and donor organizations to promote awareness and dispel myths.

Pharmaceutical companies also have a role to play in funding sustainable epilepsy awareness campaigns. By bringing epilepsy into the public eye and ensuring accurate information is widely available, we can help reduce the stigma that continues to burden people with this condition. Epilepsy needs to come out of the shadows.

Mental health impact

The stigma associated with epilepsy contributes to elevated rates of mental health disorders among those with the condition. Individuals with epilepsy are significantly more likely to experience anxiety and depression, often due to social rejection and self-imposed isolation.[17,46] Self-stigma and societal discrimination reinforce these mental health challenges, leading to poorer quality of life outcomes.[47]

Additionally, self-esteem is frequently affected by epilepsy-related stigma. Studies reveal that PWE may develop feelings of inadequacy, particularly when facing societal pressure to conceal their condition or avoid public spaces due to fear of a seizure.[39,48]

Stigma and mental health create a harmful vicious cycle. Anxiety and depression exaggerate stigma perception, leading to increased social isolation and lower quality of life, creating a negative feedback loop.[49,50] Stigma and mental health feed off each other.

Strategies for addressing and reducing stigma

Clinicians' role: Medical professionals play an essential role in countering epilepsy stigma. By educating patients, families, and communities about epilepsy, healthcare providers can help dismantle myths and reduce internalized stigma.[16,51]

Public education campaigns: Awareness campaigns aimed at addressing common misconceptions about epilepsy have been shown to be effective, particularly among younger audiences. Success is more likely when these campaigns are culturally sensitive and involve community leaders to address region-specific beliefs.[52,53]

Policy recommendations and advocacy: Legal protections, such as anti-discrimination policies, are essential for addressing institutional stigma. Advocacy organizations work to promote these policies and increase public awareness, improving opportunities and protections for those with epilepsy.[54,55]

Support groups and community engagement: Peer support groups provide safe spaces for PWE to share experiences and mitigate feelings of isolation. Community-based programs that educate the public about epilepsy are also effective in reducing stigma at the local level.[56,57]

Conclusion

Epilepsy-related stigma is a diverse and far-reaching social issue, shaping the experiences of individuals, their families, and the community on multiple levels. No single institution or profession can tackle the issue of stigma in isolation. Addressing it requires a comprehensive approach involving education, policy reform, and social support initiatives that empower individuals with epilepsy to live openly and without fear of discrimination.[4,58]

Although progress has been made, ongoing efforts are essential to challenge outdated perceptions, foster inclusivity, and ensure that PWE can lead lives free from discrimination and social limitations. By prioritizing these goals, society can work toward dismantling epilepsy stigma and enhancing the quality of life for affected individuals.[10,26]

The persistence of stigma continues to shape treatment access. For example, despite the availability of affordable AEDs in East Timor, a study by Amoroso found that 95% of individuals with epilepsy were untreated, largely due to stigma and limited healthcare training.[20] Similar figures, with 65–95% untreated, are seen across sub-Saharan Africa.[17]

References:

1. Kale, R. (1997). Bringing Epilepsy out of the Shadows: Wide Treatment Gap need to be Reduced, *BMJ*. 1997/315: 2-3.
https://pmc.ncbi.nlm.nih.gov/articles/PMC2127052/pdf/9233309.pdf
2. Behnke, S. (2009). Disability as an ethical issue - A law school symposium offers an opportunity for psychologists to reflect on the role of stigma within our own field. 40/6: 62. http://www.apa.org/monitor/2009/06/ethics.aspx
3. Kaufman, K.R. (2016). Epilepsy and secondary perceived stigma in a social setting: A night at the theater, *Epilepsy & Behavior*, 61: 138-140.
https://doi.org/10.1016/j.yebeh.2016.05.003
4. De Boer, H. M., Mula, M., & Sander, J. W. (2008). The global burden and stigma of epilepsy. *Epilepsy & Behavior*, *12*(4), 540-546. https://doi.org/10.1016/j.yebeh.2007.12.019
5. Lee, H. J., Choi, E. K., Park, H. B., & Yang, S. H. (2020). Risk and protective factors related to stigma among people with epilepsy: an integrative review. *Epilepsy & Behavior, 104*. https://doi.org/10.1016/j.yebeh.2020.106908
6. Lee, S.A., Kim, S.J., Kim, H.J., Lee, J.Y., Kim, M.K., Heo, K., Kim, W.J., Cho, Y.J., Ji, K.W., Park, K., Kim, K.K., Lee, E.M. (2020). Family cohesion is differently associated with felt stigma depending on enacted stigma in adults with epilepsy, *Epilepsy & Behavior*, 112, https://doi.org/10.1016/j.yebeh.2020.107446
7. International League against Epilepsy. (2003). The history and stigma of epilepsy. *Epilepsia,* 44(Suppl. 6): 12–14. https://doi.org/10.1046/j.1528-1157.44.s.6.2.x
8. Weiss, M & Ramakrishna, J. (2006). Stigma interventions and research for international health, *Lancet. 367*: 536-538. https://www.thelancet.com/journals/lancet/article/PIIS0140-6736(06)68189-0/abstract
9. Baybaş, S., Yıldırım, Z., Ertem, D.H., Dirican, A., Dirican, A. (2017). Development and validation of the stigma scale for epilepsy in Turkey, *Epilepsy & Behavior, 67*: 84-90. https://doi.org/10.1016/j.yebeh.2016.12.023
10. Bandstra, N.F, Camfield C.S & Camfield P.R. (2008). Stigma of epilepsy, *The Canadian Journal of Neurological Sciences*. 35/4: 436-440.
https://doi.org/10.1017/S0317167100009082
11. Tedrus, G. M. A. S., Sterca, G. S., & Pereira, R. B. (2017). Physical activity, stigma, and quality of life in patients with epilepsy. *Epilepsy & Behavior, 77*, 96-98. https://doi.org/10.1016/j.yebeh.2017.07.039
12. Kuramochi, I., Iwayama, T., & Shimotsu, S. (2023). Perspective Chapter: How can we provide lifelong support for people with epilepsy to reduce their self-stigma? In *Epilepsy During the Lifespan-Beyond the Diagnosis and New Perspectives*. IntechOpen.
https://doi.org/10.5772/intechopen.112136
13. Doganavsargil-Baysal, O., Cinemre, B., Senol, Y., Barcin, E. & Gokmen, Z. (2017). Epilepsy and stigmatization in Turkey,
Epilepsy & Behavior, 73, https://doi.org/10.1016/j.yebeh.2017.05.015

14. Mao, L., Wang, K., Zhang, Q., Wang, J., Zhao, Y., Peng, W., & Ding, J. (2022). Felt stigma and its underlying contributors in epilepsy patients. *Frontiers in Public health, 10.* https://doi.org/10.3389/fpubh.2022.879895
15. Newton, C. R., & Garcia, H. H. (2012). Epilepsy in poor regions of the world. *The Lancet, 380*(9848), 1193-1201. https://www.thelancet.com/journals/lancet/article/PIIS0140-6736(12)61381-6/abstract
16. Mugumbate, J. & Nyanguru, A. (2013). Measuring the challenges of people with epilepsy in Harare, Zimbabwe, *Neurology Asia, 18*/1: 29-33. https://ro.uow.edu.au/cgi/viewcontent.cgi?article=4271&context=sspapers
17. Baskind, R. & Birbeck, G. L. (2005). Epilepsy-associated stigma in sub-Saharan Africa: The social landscape of a disease, *Epilepsy & Behaviour, 7*: 68-73. https://doi.org/10.1016/j.yebeh.2005.04.009
18. Viteva, E. & Semerdjieva, M. (2015). Enacted stigma among patients with epilepsy and intellectual impairment, *Epilepsy & Behavior, 42*: 66-70. https://doi.org/10.1016/j.yebeh.2014.11.020
19. Fernandes, P. T., Salgado, P. C., Noronha, A. L. A., Barbosa, F. D., Souza, E. A., & Li, L. M. (2004). Stigma scale of epilepsy: conceptual issues. *Journal of Epilepsy Clinical Neurophysiology, 10*(4), 213-8. https://www.researchgate.net/profile/Li-Min-40/publication/228838908_Stigma_Scale_of_Epilepsy_conceptual_issues/links/56b8903708ae5ad3605f3eca/Stigma-Scale-of-Epilepsy-conceptual-issues.pdf
20. Amoroso, C., Zwi, A., Somerville, E., & Grove, N. (2006). Epilepsy and Stigma, *Lancet, 367*:1143-1144. https://www.thelancet.com/pdfs/journals/lancet/PIIS0140-6736(06)68503-6.pdf
21. Henning, O., Buer, C., Nakken, K. O., & Lossius, M. I. (2021). People with epilepsy still feel stigmatized. *Acta Neurologica Scandinavica, 144*(3), 312-316. https://doi.org/10.1111/ane.13449
22. Sang-Ahm Lee, S.A. (2021). Felt stigma in seizure-free persons with epilepsy: Associated factors and its impact on health-related quality of life, *Epilepsy & Behavior, 122.* https://doi.org/10.1016/j.yebeh.2021.108186
23. Mayor, R., Gunn, S., Reuber, M., & Simpson, J. (2022). Experiences of stigma in people with epilepsy: A meta-synthesis of qualitative evidence. *Seizure, 94*, 142-160. https://doi.org/10.1016/j.seizure.2021.11.021
24. Fernandes, P. T., Salgado, P. C., Noronha, A. L., de Boer, H. M., Prilipko, L., Sander, J. W., & Li, L. M. (2007). Epilepsy stigma perception in an urban area of a limited-resource country. *Epilepsy & Behavior, 11*(1), 25-32. https://doi.org/10.1016/j.yebeh.2007.02.020
25. Shi, Y., Liu, S., Wang, J., Li, C., & Zhang, J. (2021). Stigma experienced by patients with epilepsy: A systematic review and meta-synthesis of qualitative studies. *Epilepsy & Behavior, 118.* *https://doi.org/10.1016/j.yebeh.2021.107926*
26. Rice, D. R., Cisse, F. A., Hamani, A. B. D., Tassiou, N. R., Sakadi, F., Bah, A. K., ... & Mateen, F. J. (2021). Epilepsy stigma in the Republic of Guinea and its socioeconomic and clinical associations: A cross-sectional analysis. *Epilepsy Research, 177.* https://doi.org/10.1016/j.eplepsyres.2021.106770
27. Austin, J. K., Birbeck, G., Parko, K., Kwon, C. S., Fernandes, P. T., Braga, P., ... & Jette, N. (2022). Epilepsy-related stigma and attitudes: Systematic review of screening instruments and interventions-Report by the International League Against Epilepsy Task Force on Stigma in Epilepsy. *Epilepsia, 63*(3). https://discovery.ucl.ac.uk/id/eprint/10145061/7/Cross_ILAE%20Tools%20and%20Interventions.pdf
28. Herrmann, L. K., Welter, E., Berg, A. T., Perzynski, A. T., Van Doren, J. R., & Sajatovic, M. (2016). Epilepsy misconceptions and stigma reduction: Current status in Western

countries. *Epilepsy & Behavior, 60,* 165-173. https://doi.org/10.1016/j.yebeh.2016.04.003
29. Baker, D., Eccles, F. J., & Caswell, H. L. (2018). Correlates of stigma in adults with epilepsy: A systematic review of quantitative studies. *Epilepsy & Behavior, 83,* 67-80. https://doi.org/10.1016/j.yebeh.2018.02.016
30. Amjad, R. N., Nasrabadi, A. N., & Navab, E. (2017). Family stigma associated with epilepsy: A qualitative study. *Journal of Caring Sciences, 6*(1), 59.
31. Lee, S.A., Han, S.H., Cho, Y.J., Kim, K.T. Kim, J.E., ……. Yeon, G.M. (2020). Factors associated with stigma and depressive symptoms in family members of patients with epilepsy, *Epilepsy & Behavior, 110.* https://doi.org/10.1016/j.yebeh.2020.107129
32. Jacoby, A., Snape, D., & Baker, G. A. (2005). Epilepsy and social identity: the stigma of a chronic neurological disorder. *The Lancet Neurology, 4*(3), 171-178. https://www.thelancet.com/journals/lancet/article/PIIS1474-4422(05)01014-8/abstract
33. Choi, M. (2018). *Korean National and Korean American Social Behavior and Stigma Towards Epilepsy.* California State University, Los Angeles. https://www.proquest.com/openview/ac4eb94be205fd9ae38d3a29ae0ff579/1?pq-origsite=gscholar&cbl=18750&diss=y
34. Benson, A., O'Toole, S., Lambert, V., Gallagher, P., Shahwan, A. & Austin, J.K. (2015). To tell or not to tell: A systematic review of the disclosure practices of children living with epilepsy and their parents, *Epilepsy & Behavior,* 51: 73-95. https://doi.org/10.1016/j.yebeh.2015.07.013
35. Kwon, C. S., Jacoby, A., Ali, A., Austin, J., Birbeck, G. L., Braga, P., ... & Jette, N. (2022). Systematic review of frequency of felt and enacted stigma in epilepsy and determining factors and attitudes toward persons living with epilepsy—Report from the International League Against Epilepsy Task Force on Stigma in Epilepsy. *Epilepsia, 63*(3). https://discovery.ucl.ac.uk/id/eprint/10145060/15/Cross_ILAE%20Stigma%20Attitudes%20and%20Frequency%20.pdf
36. Tombini, M., Assenza, G., Quintiliani, L., Ricci, L., Lanzone, J., De Mojà, R., ... & Di Lazzaro, V. (2019). Epilepsy-associated stigma from the perspective of people with epilepsy and the community in Italy. *Epilepsy & Behavior, 98,* 66-72. https://doi.org/10.1016/j.yebeh.2019.06.026
37. Boling, W., Means, M., & Fletcher, A. (2018). Quality of life and stigma in epilepsy, perspectives from selected regions of Asia and Sub-Saharan Africa. *Brain sciences, 8*(4), 59. https://doi.org/10.3390/brainsci8040059
38. Malik, N. I., Fatima, R., Ullah, I., Atta, M., Awan, A., Nashwan, A. J., & Ahmed, S. (2022). Perceived stigma, discrimination and psychological problems among patients with epilepsy. *Frontiers in psychiatry, 13.* https://doi.org/10.3389/fpsyt.2022.1000870
39. Tedrus, G. M. A. S., Pereira, R. B., & Zoppi, M. (2018). Epilepsy, stigma, and family. *Epilepsy & Behavior, 78,* 265-268. https://doi.org/10.1016/j.yebeh.2017.08.007
40. Chakraborty, P., Sanchez, N. A., Kaddumukasa, M., Kajumba, M., Kakooza-Mwesige, A., Van Noord, M., ... & Koltai, D. C. (2021). Stigma reduction interventions for epilepsy: a systematized literature review. *Epilepsy & Behavior, 114. https://doi.org/10.1016/j.yebeh.2020.107381*
41. Luna, J., Nizard, M., Becker, D., Gerard, D., Cruz, A., Ratsimbazafy, V., ... & Preux, P. M. (2017). Epilepsy-associated levels of perceived stigma, their associations with treatment, and related factors: a cross-sectional study in urban and rural areas in Ecuador. *Epilepsy & Behavior, 68,* 71-77. https://doi.org/10.1016/j.yebeh.2016.12.026
42. Er, D. & Aktaş, B. (2023). An investigation of stigma and self-management in individuals diagnosed with epilepsy, *Epilepsy & Behavior, 149.* https://doi.org/10.1016/j.yebeh.2023.109494

43. Ak, P.D., Atakli, D., Yuksel, B., Guveli, B.T., Sari, H. (2015). Stigmatization and social impacts of epilepsy in Turkey, *Epilepsy & Behavior,* 50: 50-54. https://doi.org/10.1016/j.yebeh.2015.05.014
44. Gosain, K., & Samanta, T. (2022). Understanding the role of stigma and misconceptions in the experience of epilepsy in India: Findings from a mixed-methods study. *Frontiers in Sociology, 7.* https://doi.org/10.3389/fsoc.2022.790145
45. Shi, Y., Wang, S., Ying, J., Zhang, M., Liu, P., Zhang, H., & Sun, J. (2017). Correlates of perceived stigma for people living with epilepsy: A meta-analysis. *Epilepsy & Behavior, 70,* 198-203. https://doi.org/10.1016/j.yebeh.2017.02.022
46. Blixen, C., Ogede, D., Briggs, F., Aebi, M. E., Burant, C., Wilson, B., ... & Sajatovic, M. (2020). Correlates of stigma in people with epilepsy. *Journal of Clinical Neurology (Seoul, Korea), 16*(3), 423. https://doi.org/10.3988/jcn.2020.16.3.423
47. Yeni, K., Tulek, Z., Bebek, N., Dede, O., Gurses, C., Baykan, B., & Gokyigit, A. (2016). Attitudes towards epilepsy among a sample of Turkish patients with epilepsy, *Epilepsy & Behavior, 62*: 66-71. https://doi.org/10.1016/j.yebeh.2016.06.022
48. Lalatović, S., Milovanović, M., & Krstić, N. (2022). Stigma and its association with health-related quality of life in adults with epilepsy. *Epilepsy & Behavior, 135.* https://doi.org/10.1016/j.yebeh.2022.108874
49. Baulac, M., De Boer, H., Elger, C., Glynn, M., Kälviäinen, R., Little, A., ... & Ryvlin, P. (2015). Epilepsy priorities in Europe: A report of the ILAE-IBE epilepsy advocacy Europe task force. *Epilepsia, 56*(11), 1687-1695. https://doi.org/10.1111/epi.13201
50. Fernandes, P. T., Noronha, A. L. A., Sander, J. W., & Li, L. M. (2008). Stigma scale of epilepsy: the perception of epilepsy stigma in different cities in Brazil. *Arquivos de Neuro-Psiquiatria, 66,* 471-476. https://doi.org/10.1590/S0004-282X2008000400006
51. Sleeth, C., Drake, K., Labiner, D.M. & Chong, J. (2016). Felt and enacted stigma in elderly persons with epilepsy: A qualitative approach, *Epilepsy & Behavior, 55,* https://doi.org/10.1016/j.yebeh.2015.12.026
52. Baker, G. A., Brooks, J., Buck, D., & Jacoby, A. (2000). The stigma of epilepsy: A European perspective. *Epilepsia, 41*(1), 98-104. https://doi/pdf/10.1111/j.1528-1157.2000.tb01512.x
53. Deleo, F., Quintas, R., Pastori, C., Pappalardo, I., Didato, G., Giacomo, R.D., de Curtis, M. & Villani, F. (2020). Quality of life, psychiatric symptoms, and stigma perception in three groups of persons with epilepsy, *Epilepsy & Behavior, 110,* https://doi.org/10.1016/j.yebeh.2020.107170
54. Yildirim, Z., Ertem, D.H., Dirican, A.C., Baybas, S. (2019). Who is the bigger stigmatizor?: The loved one or the society, *Epilepsy & Behavior, 96*: 13-22. https://doi.org/10.1016/j.yebeh.2019.04.013
55. Yıldırım, Z., Ertem, D. H., Dirican, A. C., & Baybaş, S. (2018). Stigma accounts for depression in patients with epilepsy. *Epilepsy & Behavior, 78,* 1-6. https://doi.org/10.1016/j.yebeh.2017.10.030
56. Lim, K. S., & Tan, C. T. (2014). Epilepsy stigma in Asia: the meaning and impact of stigma. *Neurology Asia, 19*(1). http://www.neurology-asia.org/articles/neuroasia-2014-19(1)-001.pdf
57. Karakaş, N., Sarıtaş, S.C., Aktura, S.C., Karabulutlu, E.Y. & Oruç, F.G. (2022). Investigation of factors associated with stigma and social support in patients with epilepsy in Turkey: A cross-sectional study, *Epilepsy & Behavior, 128,* https://doi.org/10.1016/j.yebeh.2022.108572
58. Benson, A., O'Toole, S., Lambert, V., Gallagher, P., Shahwan, A. & Austin, J.K. (2016). The stigma experiences and perceptions of families living with epilepsy: Implications for

epilepsy-related communication within and external to the family unit, *Patient Education and Counseling, 99*(9), 1473-1481. https://doi.org/10.1016/j.pec.2016.06.009

59. Summers, M. 1946. *The Malleus Maleficarum: (The Witch Hammer) of Heinrich Kramer and James Sprenger Translated with an Introduction, Bibliography and Notes*: Unabridged Online Republication of the 1928 Edition. Introduction to the 1948 Edition is Also Included. Translation, Notes, and Two Introduction by Montague Summers. A Bull of Innocent VIII.
https://library.oapen.org/bitstream/handle/20.500.12657/35002/341393.pdf?sequence=1&isAllowed=y

CHAPTER 15 – ACCOMMODATIONS FOR PWE

Research shows that job candidates with disabilities are viewed more favorably when their condition is physical, not mental or neurological, and perceived as blameless and less visible.
Ann Jacoby, Joanne Gorry, Gus A. Baker[1]

Introduction

Epilepsy can make everyday tasks harder for PWE. Accommodations play a vital role in ensuring that individuals with epilepsy can navigate academic, workplace, and social environments with ease. Epilepsy, characterized by recurrent and unprovoked seizures, can impose significant physical, emotional, and social challenges. These accommodations are given by making certain adjustments to allow individuals to fully participate in daily activities. The implementation of accommodations is essential not only for practical reasons, such as managing seizure risks, but also to combat the stigma and discrimination associated with epilepsy. By tailoring environments to meet their unique needs, individuals with epilepsy can achieve greater independence, productivity, and quality of life.[2,3,4]

This chapter provides a comprehensive overview of the current state of accommodations for PWE and highlights actionable steps to drive meaningful change. I will explore the various accommodations available to individuals with epilepsy, focusing on academic, workplace, social, and family settings. I also discuss barriers to effective accommodations, perspectives on accommodation needs, successful case studies, and recommendations for improvement.

Legislative framework and rights

Legal protections play a critical role in securing the rights of individuals with epilepsy. In the United States, the Americans with Disabilities Act (ADA) ensures that PWE are protected from discrimination in education, employment, and public services.[3] Under the ADA, epilepsy is recognized as a disability, and employers, educators, and other stakeholders are required to provide reasonable accommodations.[3,5] Examples of these accommodations include flexible scheduling, access to rest areas, and seizure-response training for colleagues.

Additionally, the Equal Employment Opportunity Commission (EEOC) provides guidelines on epilepsy in the workplace, emphasizing that individuals with epilepsy should not face unfair treatment due to their condition.[6] Globally, efforts to protect the rights of individuals with epilepsy vary. While some countries with strong disability rights frameworks offer comprehensive protections, others lack sufficient policies, leaving individuals vulnerable to discrimination.[7,8]

Academic accommodations

Due to epilepsy's impact on classroom performance, teachers should understand both the condition and how to effectively manage its potential effects.
Juliet E Hart Barnett & Catherine Gay[9]

Students with epilepsy face unique challenges in educational settings due to the unpredictable nature of seizures, the cognitive impact of both seizures and medications, and the potential for stigma among peers and staff. Academic accommodations are vital for leveling the playing field and supporting students' educational and social success. These accommodations not only address physical safety concerns but also promote an inclusive environment that encourages participation and minimizes the risk of academic setbacks. Not every student will require the same accommodations because the seizures are different for everyone. Just as in the tailored treatment approach per individual, the same applies to accommodations. The key accommodation strategies are discussed as follows:

Flexible scheduling

Seizures and their aftereffects, such as fatigue, confusion, and difficulty concentrating, can interfere with a student's ability to maintain a standard class schedule. Flexible scheduling provides students with the opportunity to adjust their academic routines in response to their condition.[7,9] Under this type of accommodation, schools can allow students to arrive late, leave early, or attend classes part-time depending on their seizure patterns and recovery needs. For instance, a student who experiences seizures in the early morning might benefit from starting their school day later to accommodate recovery time. Similarly, schools may permit students to take breaks during long class sessions to manage fatigue or other side effects of their condition or medications.[7,9]

This accommodation allows students with epilepsy to focus on education without feeling overwhelmed by inflexible schedules. It also reduces stress, which is a known seizure trigger, allowing students to prioritize their health while still meeting academic goals.[10] Schools may need to adapt attendance policies or collaborate with parents to ensure flexible scheduling aligns with educational requirements. While administrators might initially view flexibility as disruptive, training and awareness programs can help staff understand its critical role in supporting students with epilepsy.

Modified testing environments

Examinations and assessments increase the risk of seizures due to the elevated stress levels associated with these activities. Modified testing environments help reduce stress by providing students with a more customizable examination experience without undue pressure. Common modifications include providing extended time for tests, offering quiet and distraction-free environments, and permitting breaks during exams. Other options can be explored depending on the individual student's circumstances. For instance, a student might be allowed to pause during a seizure episode and resume their test once they have recovered. Schools may also allow alternative assessment formats, such as oral presentations or projects, for students who find written exams particularly challenging due to the cognitive side effects of their medications.[9,11]

Such accommodations empower students with epilepsy to perform at their best without being penalized for factors beyond their control. This approach acknowledges that traditional timed exams may not accurately reflect a student's abilities and promotes equity in academic evaluations.[7,10] Educators might need additional resources or training to implement testing accommodations effectively. In schools with large student populations, finding suitable testing spaces or scheduling extended exam times can require extra planning. However, the benefits for the student often outweigh these logistical concerns.

Seizure action plans

A seizure action plan is a document that outlines steps for school staff to take in the event a student experiences a seizure. This accommodation focuses on safety and ensures a quick, informed response, reducing the likelihood of complications during an episode. Seizure action plans are typically developed in collaboration with the clinician, parents, and school staff. These plans include specific information such as:
- A description of the student's seizure type(s)
- Steps for responding to a seizure, including first aid procedures
- Emergency contact information and when to call for medical help
- Medication details, including administration instructions if the student requires rescue medication at school.

For example, a school nurse might receive training on administering rectal diazepam or intranasal midazolam, which are commonly prescribed rescue medications. Additionally, staff members in direct contact with the student, such as teachers and bus drivers, are trained on how to follow the action plan.[7,9,11] Administering rescue medications is not uniform globally. Availability varies from country to country, based on resources.

Having a seizure action plan in place reduces anxiety for both students and parents, knowing that the school is prepared to handle seizures appropriately. It also reassures teachers and staff, providing them with clear guidelines and minimizing hesitation in emergencies. Schools must invest time in training staff and ensuring that all stakeholders understand the seizure action plan. Furthermore, regular updates are necessary as the student's medical needs or medications change over time. Some of these facilities may not be available in under-resourced countries.

Additional considerations for academic accommodations

Beyond the specific examples outlined above, schools should foster an environment of inclusivity and support through broader initiatives, such as:

Peer education: Educating classmates about epilepsy can reduce stigma and promote empathy. For example, students can learn that epilepsy is a neurological condition and that witnessing a seizure requires staying calm and seeking help.

Counseling services: Access to school counselors trained to support students with epilepsy can help address emotional and social challenges, such as bullying or isolation.

Technological support: Providing access to assistive technology, such as note-taking devices or audio-recorded lectures, can compensate for memory or attention difficulties associated with seizures or medication.[10]

Academic accommodations, when implemented effectively, not only support students in managing their condition but also empower them to achieve their full potential. These strategies demonstrate the importance of collaboration among students, families, educators, and healthcare providers in creating a safe and equitable learning environment.

Workplace accommodations

Some young PWE often face challenges in gaining and keeping jobs, especially when the condition begins during their working years, potentially leading to long-term unemployment.
Hanneke M. De Boer[12]

Workplace accommodations are essential for enabling individuals with epilepsy to thrive professionally, contributing their skills and talents while minimizing barriers related to their condition. These accommodations are mandated by laws such as the ADA in the USA, which requires employers to provide reasonable adjustments to ensure individuals with disabilities have equal opportunities.[5] The specific type of accommodations an individual will ask for are specific to them. Just as in education accommodations, these workplace accommodations should be tailored to work for the impacted individual. Below, several types of accommodations, including flexible work schedules, job restructuring, accessible workspaces, and education for coworkers, are detailed to illustrate their implementation and importance.

Flexible work schedules

Epilepsy often affects energy levels, cognitive function, and the ability to adhere to rigid schedules, particularly if seizures or medication side effects occur during specific times of the day. Flexible work schedules allow employees to tailor their hours to align with their health needs. Employers might permit employees to work earlier or later than standard hours to accommodate recovery periods after seizures or manage drowsiness caused by medications. Telecommuting options can also be offered, enabling employees to work from home on days when traveling or being in the office poses risks. For example, an employee prone to seizures triggered by fatigue might benefit from a reduced or staggered work schedule.[13,14]

This flexibility reduces stress and enables employees to maintain productivity without compromising their health. It also allows individuals to manage appointments with healthcare providers without penalization.[5] Employers might need to adapt team workflows to accommodate flexible schedules, but open communication and planning can often address these concerns effectively.

Job restructuring

Some job tasks may be unsafe or impractical for employees with epilepsy, especially those involving heavy machinery, high-risk environments, or long hours of intense concentration. Job restructuring ensures employees can focus on tasks that align with their abilities while avoiding unnecessary risks. Employers might reassign non-essential duties or adjust workloads to remove tasks that could pose safety risks. For example, an employee with frequent seizures might be excused from operating machinery or driving, while other team members take over these responsibilities. Instead, the employee could focus on administrative or planning roles that do not require physical exertion or high-risk activities.[13,15]

By modifying job roles, employers retain valuable talent and ensure workplace safety. Employees with epilepsy can work without fear of injury or seizure-related incidents, fostering a sense of security and inclusion.[16] Successful job restructuring requires collaboration between the employee and employer to identify essential and non-essential tasks. In small teams, reassigning responsibilities may require additional planning or hiring.

Accessible workspaces

An accessible workspace is critical for ensuring the safety and comfort of employees with epilepsy, particularly in the event of a seizure. This involves creating an environment where seizures can be managed without endangering the individual or others. Modifications may include:
- Removing sharp objects, heavy furniture, or other hazards from work areas to prevent injury during a seizure
- Providing cushioned flooring or anti-fatigue mats for employees prone to falls
- Equipping offices with emergency response tools, such as seizure-alert devices, and ensuring quick access to first aid supplies
- Establishing quiet, private spaces where employees can recover after a seizure.[14,17]

For example, an open-plan office might include a designated rest area where employees can lie down or seek privacy if they feel a seizure coming on. Employers may also provide specialized desks with adjustable heights to accommodate post-seizure fatigue.[15]

Accessible workspaces reduce the risk of injury and create a supportive environment that prioritizes employee well-being. Such modifications also benefit overall workplace safety, as they are often aligned with universal design principles.[14] Employers may face upfront costs for workspace modifications, but these investments typically yield long-term benefits by improving employee retention and satisfaction.

Education and training for coworkers

Misunderstandings and stigma surrounding epilepsy can create barriers for employees in the workplace. Education and training programs for coworkers promote awareness, empathy, and preparedness, fostering an inclusive work culture. Employers can organize training sessions or workshops on epilepsy, covering topics such as seizure first aid, common triggers, and the importance of supporting colleagues with the condition. For example, co-workers might learn how to recognize the signs of a seizure, how to assist without interfering, and when to seek medical help.

Educating co-workers reduces stigma and fear, helping them view epilepsy as a manageable condition rather than a liability. This improves teamwork, morale, and support for employees with epilepsy.[9,16] Effective education programs require time and resources. Employers must ensure that training is accurate and delivered by qualified professionals, such as healthcare providers or epilepsy advocacy groups.[5]

Seizure action plans in the workplace

Like their use in schools, seizure action plans outline clear steps for responding to a seizure, ensuring that both the affected employee and their co-workers feel prepared and supported. Employers, in collaboration with the employee and healthcare professionals, can develop a plan tailored to the individual's needs. The plan might include:

- Information on the employee's seizure type and typical symptoms
- A protocol for providing first aid during a seizure, such as ensuring the individual's safety, timing the episode, and calling emergency services if necessary
- Guidance on post-seizure recovery, including allowing the employee time to rest before resuming work.[14,17]

Having a seizure action plan increases confidence among all staff members, ensuring a swift and appropriate response. Employees with epilepsy benefit from reduced anxiety, knowing that their colleagues understand how to help in an emergency.[14]

Additional accommodations

Other accommodations include allowing service animals trained to assist with epilepsy, offering breaks for medication or rest, and implementing assistive technology such as seizure-alert devices. Employers should also establish clear anti-discrimination policies and grievance procedures to address any issues related to stigma or unfair treatment. Workplace accommodations are not one size fits all: they must be tailored to the individual's specific needs and job requirements. By investing in these accommodations, employers can unlock the potential of employees with epilepsy, creating a more diverse and inclusive workforce while complying with legal standards.

Accommodations in social and family settings

Accommodations in social and family settings are crucial for supporting individuals with epilepsy, fostering an environment that promotes safety, emotional well-being, and independence. Families and social networks often serve as the primary support systems for PWE, yet they may face challenges in understanding and addressing the needs of their loved ones. By implementing thoughtful accommodations, family members and friends can help individuals with epilepsy navigate daily life while reducing the risk of isolation or stigma. This section explores key areas where accommodations can be provided, including fostering open communication, creating safe environments, planning for social activities, and addressing emotional and psychological needs.

Fostering open communication

Open communication between individuals with epilepsy and their family members or friends is foundational for effective support. It helps clarify expectations, reduce misunderstandings, and promote mutual understanding. Encourage discussions about the individual's condition, seizure triggers, and specific needs. For example, family members can learn about the type of seizures their loved one experiences and how to respond appropriately.

- Establish regular check-ins to discuss any changes in seizure patterns, treatment plans, or daily challenges
- Educate family members and friends about epilepsy to reduce misconceptions and enhance their confidence in providing support.[18,19]

Open communication fosters a sense of trust and reassurance, allowing individuals with epilepsy to feel more comfortable sharing their needs and concerns. It also equips family members with the knowledge necessary to provide informed care.[19] Families may initially struggle with discussing epilepsy openly, particularly if stigma or cultural barriers are present. Overcoming these challenges requires patience, education, and a commitment to destigmatizing the condition.

Creating safe home environments

Ensuring that the home environment is safe and seizure-friendly is essential for minimizing risks associated with seizures. This requires

proactive measures to prevent injuries and facilitate quick responses during seizures.
- Remove or cushion sharp edges on furniture to reduce the risk of injury during a seizure
- Install safety equipment, such as grab bars in bathrooms, to prevent falls
- Use non-slip mats in areas prone to moisture, such as kitchens and bathrooms
- Place soft surfaces, such as rugs or padded mats, in areas where the individual spends significant time
- Incorporate assistive devices, such as seizure-monitoring systems, to alert family members or caregivers if a seizure occurs during sleep or when the individual is alone.[12,20]

A safe home environment allows PWE to move about freely without constant supervision, promoting independence while reducing the risk of injury. Implementing safety measures can involve costs and may require modifications to the home. However, many changes are low-cost or covered by community resources or advocacy organizations.

Planning social activities with inclusion in mind

Social activities are vital for maintaining emotional well-being and a sense of normalcy, but they often require accommodations to ensure inclusivity for individuals with epilepsy. Choose venues that are safe and accessible, avoiding environments with potential seizure triggers. Allow flexibility in schedules to accommodate recovery time after seizures or medication side effects.[4,19] Inclusive social planning helps PWE feel valued and included, reducing feelings of isolation and promoting stronger relationships with family and friends. Social activities may need to be adapted on short notice if the individual experiences a seizure or fatigue. Family members and friends must remain flexible and understanding to ensure a supportive atmosphere.

Addressing emotional and psychological needs

Living with epilepsy often takes an emotional and psychological toll, not only on the individual but also on their family members. Providing emotional accommodations is essential for fostering resilience and maintaining mental health. Encourage the individual to express their feelings and seek professional counseling if needed. Family members might also consider therapy to learn coping strategies and improve communication. Support the individual in joining peer support groups or epilepsy communities where they can share experiences and connect with others facing similar challenges. Address stigma within the family by openly discussing epilepsy and promoting acceptance. For example, family members can counter misconceptions by sharing accurate information about the condition.[7,16] Help manage stress by encouraging relaxation techniques, such as mindfulness or yoga.[7] Emotional accommodations help individuals with epilepsy build self-confidence and reduce feelings of anxiety or depression. They also strengthen familial bonds and improve the overall well-being of the household.[7] Families may initially find it difficult to discuss epilepsy-related emotions due to cultural or generational differences. Overcoming these challenges requires a commitment to empathy and open-mindedness.

Financial and practical support

Families often bear financial and logistical responsibilities related to managing epilepsy, such as covering medical costs or coordinating appointments. Designate a family member to assist with managing medical appointments, insurance paperwork, and medication schedules. Explore financial assistance programs offered by epilepsy foundations or government agencies to offset the costs of treatment and accommodations. Share caregiving responsibilities among family members to prevent burnout and ensure consistent support for the PWE.[12,20] Practical support relieves stress for both the individual with epilepsy and their caregivers, enabling them to focus on their relationships and personal growth. Balancing practical responsibilities with personal obligations can strain family dynamics. Families may benefit from external resources, such as respite care or community support programs.

Accommodations in social and family settings go beyond physical adjustments, encompassing emotional, social, and practical aspects of support. By fostering open communication, creating safe environments, planning inclusive activities, addressing emotional needs, and providing practical assistance, families and friends can empower individuals with epilepsy to lead fulfilling lives. These accommodations also strengthen relationships and promote a deeper understanding of epilepsy, ultimately reducing the stigma and isolation often associated with the condition.

Barriers to effective accommodations

Despite the necessity of accommodations for individuals with epilepsy, several barriers hinder their effective implementation. These barriers can stem from societal attitudes, knowledge gaps, systemic challenges, and personal factors. Understanding these obstacles is essential to overcoming them and ensuring that PWE receive the support they need in academic, workplace, social, and family contexts. Some of the barriers are as follows:

Societal stigma and discrimination

One of the most significant barriers to effective accommodations is societal stigma surrounding epilepsy. Misconceptions about the condition, often rooted in outdated or inaccurate beliefs, continue to influence how individuals with epilepsy are perceived and treated. Many people associate epilepsy with diminished capabilities, leading to biased attitudes in educational settings, workplaces, and social environments.[1,17] Discrimination based on these misconceptions can discourage PWE from seeking accommodations, fearing judgment or exclusion.[8] Stigma fosters an environment where individuals with epilepsy may feel compelled to hide their condition, thus missing out on necessary support.[8,11] Public education campaigns about epilepsy can help dispel myths and promote greater acceptance. Advocacy efforts by epilepsy organizations can highlight success stories of individuals thriving with proper accommodations, reducing stigma at a broader level.[17]

Lack of awareness and education

A widespread lack of knowledge about epilepsy among educators, employers, family members, and peers can impede effective accommodations. Without a clear understanding of the condition, those in supportive roles may struggle to implement appropriate measures. Educators may not know how to adapt classroom settings for students with epilepsy, such as accommodating for absences due to seizures or allowing for flexible deadlines.[7] Employers may misunderstand the types of workplace adjustments required or mistakenly believe accommodations would impose excessive costs.[12] Family members might lack the information necessary to create safe environments or recognize seizure triggers.[19] Insufficient education can lead to inadequate or inappropriate accommodations, leaving individuals with epilepsy unsupported in critical areas. It can also perpetuate stigma, as those who lack knowledge may harbor unfounded fears or biases.[4] Training programs for educators, employers, and caregivers can provide essential knowledge about epilepsy and its management. Schools and workplaces can partner with epilepsy advocacy organizations to offer informational workshops and resources.[4,17]

Systemic and policy-level challenges

Even when laws and policies mandate accommodations, systemic issues can hinder their implementation. These challenges often arise from bureaucratic inefficiencies, resource constraints, or gaps in legal enforcement. Bureaucratic processes for requesting and approving accommodations can be lengthy and complicated, discouraging individuals from pursuing them.[6,14] Limited funding for disability services in schools and workplaces can result in inadequate resources for implementing accommodations.[13] Inconsistent enforcement of disability rights laws, such as the ADA, leaves many individuals without the support they are entitled to.[5] Systemic barriers create disparities in access to accommodations, particularly for individuals from marginalized or low-income backgrounds. They also contribute to frustration and a sense of injustice among PWE and their families.[14] Streamlining accommodation request processes and providing clear guidance on eligibility criteria can make support more accessible. Increasing funding for disability programs and enforcement mechanisms can ensure that accommodations are consistently provided.[4,5]

Individual-level factors

In some cases, individuals with epilepsy themselves may face barriers to accessing accommodations due to personal circumstances or internalized stigma. Individuals may hesitate to disclose their condition due to concerns about privacy, discrimination, or being treated differently.[3,21] Some individuals, particularly students or those newly diagnosed, may not know how to request accommodations or advocate for their rights.[19] Costs associated with transportation, medical care, or assistive devices may limit an individual's ability to utilize available accommodations.[16] These barriers can prevent individuals from seeking the support they need, leading to avoidable challenges in academic, workplace, or social settings. Internalized stigma can exacerbate feelings of isolation and reduce confidence in pursuing opportunities that require accommodations.[21] Counseling and peer support groups can help PWE build self-confidence and develop self-advocacy skills. Providing clear information about legal rights and available resources can empower individuals to navigate accommodation processes effectively.[16,19]

Barriers to effective accommodations for individuals with epilepsy are multifaceted, encompassing societal, systemic, and personal factors. Overcoming these obstacles requires a coordinated effort involving education, advocacy, policy reform, and community support. By addressing these barriers, we can create environments where PWE are empowered to achieve their full potential and live without undue limitations.

Perspectives on accommodation needs

Understanding the perspectives of individuals with epilepsy, as well as the views of educators, employers, healthcare professionals, and families, is essential for identifying gaps in current accommodations and improving support systems. These perspectives highlight the diverse and nuanced needs of PWE, as well as the challenges faced by those responsible for implementing accommodations. This section explores the insights gained from these key stakeholders.

Perspectives of individuals with epilepsy

PWE often express the need for accommodations that address both their medical and social challenges. Their perspectives emphasize the importance of autonomy, safety, and equality in various aspects of life. Individuals with epilepsy prioritize accommodations that enhance safety during seizures, such as the presence of trained personnel or access to medical alerts.[21] They also value adjustments that mitigate seizure triggers, including modifications to lighting, noise levels, and schedules in both academic and workplace settings.[19]

Many PWE stress the importance of accommodations that enable independence, such as flexible work arrangements or access to assistive technology that allows them to perform tasks without constant supervision.[12] They also value opportunities to participate fully in social and family activities without being treated as fragile or incapable.[4] Some individuals with epilepsy report hesitance in requesting accommodations due to fear of stigma, discrimination, or being perceived as a burden.[3] They emphasize the need for confidentiality and sensitivity in accommodation processes to ensure they feel secure in disclosing their condition.[17]

Perspectives of educators and employers

Educators and employers often recognize the need to support individuals with epilepsy but may face challenges due to limited resources or knowledge. Their perspectives shed light on areas where training and guidance can improve accommodation practices. Educators note difficulties in managing the academic needs of students with epilepsy, particularly when seizures lead to frequent absences or cognitive impairments.[7] Many people report feeling unprepared to handle medical emergencies or to adapt instructional materials effectively. Employers highlight concerns about productivity and safety, particularly in industries involving heavy machinery or high-risk environments.[5] Some employers may overestimate the costs or logistical complexities of implementing accommodations.[8] Both groups emphasize the importance of clear guidelines and training programs to help them understand epilepsy and their responsibilities under disability laws like the ADA.[6] They also value case studies or examples of successful accommodations to provide practical insights into what works in real-world scenarios.[13]

Perspectives of families

Families of individuals with epilepsy play a vital role in providing support but often express their own needs for education and resources to fulfill this role effectively. Family members, particularly parents of children with epilepsy, report feelings of anxiety and uncertainty about how to best support their loved ones.[11] They may worry about seizure management, educational progress, or career prospects. Some families also express frustration with societal stigma, which can limit their ability to advocate for accommodations without facing prejudice.[19] Families often emphasize the need for accommodations that promote inclusion and reduce isolation, such as social activities designed to be accessible for PWE.[4] They also highlight the importance of coordinated efforts among schools, workplaces, and healthcare providers to ensure consistent support.[14]

Perspectives of healthcare professionals

Healthcare providers, including neurologists and epilepsy specialists, offer unique insights into the medical and psychosocial aspects of accommodation needs. Providers advocate for accommodations that go beyond medical management, addressing mental health, cognitive challenges, and social integration.[21] They also stress the importance of individualized approaches, as the needs of individuals with epilepsy vary widely depending on seizure type, frequency, and personal circumstances.[7] Healthcare professionals often emphasize the importance of collaboration between medical teams, educators, employers, and families to create comprehensive accommodation plans.[13] They also encourage the use of seizure action plans in schools and workplaces, which outline specific steps to take during and after a seizure.[7]

Insights from advocacy organizations

Organizations like the Epilepsy Foundation in the US provide critical perspectives on accommodation needs, informed by years of experience advocating for individuals with epilepsy. Advocacy groups stress the importance of empowering PWE to advocate for their own needs through education and access to resources.[4] They also highlight the role of public awareness campaigns in reducing stigma and fostering supportive environments in schools, workplaces, and communities.[17] These organizations advocate for stronger enforcement of disability rights laws and increased funding for accommodation programs.[14] They also push for mandatory training on epilepsy for educators, employers, and first responders to improve understanding and preparedness.[6]

Summary of perspectives

The perspectives on accommodation requirements underscore the complexity and individuality of support requirements for PWE. By integrating the insights of individuals with epilepsy, their families, educators, employers, healthcare providers, and advocacy organizations, we can develop more effective and inclusive accommodations.

Addressing these diverse perspectives requires a combination of education, collaboration, and systemic reform to ensure that the rights and needs of PWE are fully met.

Recommendations for improvement

While many accommodations for individuals with epilepsy are effective, there is significant room for improvement in their implementation, accessibility, and sustainability. These recommendations aim to address existing gaps and enhance the quality of life for PWE across all domains of life.

Enhancing awareness and education: Improving accommodations requires greater epilepsy awareness among the public, employers, educators, and peers. Targeted education on seizure first aid and triggers, combined with large-scale awareness campaigns, can reduce stigma. Periodic training for healthcare professionals and educators ensures up-to-date practices for managing epilepsy.[1,2,7,13]

Improving accessibility to resources and support: Accessing resources for epilepsy accommodations can be challenging. Local or online hubs could centralize information on issues such as seizure plans and legal rights. Financial aid from governments, non-profits, or employers can help cover costs. Support networks can also connect families to shared resources and strategies.[6,10,14]

Enhancing collaboration across stakeholders: Collaboration among families, schools, employers, and healthcare providers is crucial for effective epilepsy support. Healthcare providers can help create tailored action plans, such as seizure protocols in schools. Employers should involve employees in workplace adjustments, while multidisciplinary teams in schools can ensure appropriate accommodations.[6,7,10,12,17]

Strengthening legal protections and enforcement: Legal protections like the ADA exist but lack consistent enforcement and awareness. Governments should improve compliance monitoring and provide clearer guidelines. Advocacy groups can raise awareness through workshops and legal aid, while global standards could address regional inconsistencies.[4,6,7,17,21]

Promoting technological innovation: Technology can improve epilepsy accommodations through seizure-monitoring wearables, seizure-safe educational tools, and workplace innovations like adjustable lighting and ergonomic systems.[2,10,14]

Encouraging inclusive practices in social and community settings: Inclusivity should extend to community settings. Events can be made epilepsy-friendly with practices like avoiding strobe lights and providing quiet zones. Adaptive activities at sports centers promote health and engagement, while platforms for sharing experiences foster empathy and understanding.[4,10,12,21]

Encouraging research and policy development: Research and policy initiatives are vital for improving epilepsy accommodations. Studies on effective practices like flexible work schedules can guide policies. Advocacy groups should collaborate with policymakers to prioritize equity and inclusion. Metrics to evaluate accommodations can help refine and replicate successful models.[6,7,13,15]

Promoting self-advocacy and empowerment: Empowering individuals with epilepsy through communication workshops, advocacy leadership roles, and resilience programs is key to long-term success. These initiatives build confidence, promote rights awareness, and equip PWE to navigate challenges and request accommodations effectively.[1,10,21]

Conclusion

Improving accommodations for individuals with epilepsy requires education, accessibility, collaboration, legal protections, and inclusive practices. These efforts promote inclusion, independence, and quality of life. Ongoing advocacy and collaboration are essential to ensure PWE can thrive.[2,4,8] Through a combination of tailored strategies and systemic improvements, we can create an inclusive world where epilepsy is no longer a barrier to success. By addressing barriers, enhancing public awareness, and fostering collaboration, society can ensure that individuals with epilepsy are empowered to reach their full potential.[2,5,20]

References:

1. Jacoby, A., Gorry, J., & Baker, G. A. (2005). Employers' attitudes to employment of people with epilepsy: still the same old story? *Epilepsia*, *46*(12), 1978-1987. https://doi.org/10.1111/j.1528-1167.2005.00345.x
2. Ballasiotes, M. (2020). Academic and Workplace Accommodations for People with Epilepsy. https://doi.org/10.17615/6dj2-0g15
3. Troxell, J. (1997). Epilepsy and employment: The Americans with Disabilities Act and its protection against employment discrimination, *Med Law, 16*(2):375-84. PMID: 9212629. https://pubmed.ncbi.nlm.nih.gov/9212629/
4. Smeets, V. M., van Lierop, B. A., Vanhoutvin, J. P., Aldenkamp, A. P., & Nijhuis, F. J. (2007). Epilepsy and employment: Literature review. *Epilepsy & Behavior*, *10*(3), 354-362. https://doi.org/10.1016/j.yebeh.2007.02.006
5. Epilepsy Foundation. (2024). Employer accommodations for epilepsy. https://www.epilepsy.com/lifestyle/employment/accomodation
6. U.S. Equal Employment Opportunity Commission. (2013). Epilepsy in the workplace and the ADA. https://www.eeoc.gov/laws/guidance/epilepsy-workplace-and-ada
7. Johnson, P. A. (2022). School nurses' participation in accommodations for children with epilepsy: a quality improvement project. https://ir.library.louisville.edu/dnp/41
8. Majkowska-Zwolińska, B., Jędrzejczak, J., & Owczarek, K. (2012). Employment in people with epilepsy from the perspectives of patients, neurologists, and the general population. *Epilepsy & Behavior*, *25*(4), 489-494. https://doi.org/10.1016/j.yebeh.2012.10.001
9. Barnett, J. E. H., & Gay, C. (2015). Accommodating students with epilepsy or seizure disorders: effective strategies for teachers. *Research, Advocacy, and Practice for Complex and Chronic Conditions*, *34*(1), 1-13. https://doi.org/10.14434/pders.v34i1.13258
10. Chimedza, M. (2021). *Exploring the lived experiences of students with disclosed epilepsy in accessing support services at a teachers' college in Zimbabwe* (Doctoral dissertation, Stellenbosch: Stellenbosch University). http://hdl.handle.net/10019.1/123729
11. Johnson, E., Atkinson, P., Muggeridge, A., Cross, J. H., & Reilly, C. (2022). Impact of epilepsy on learning and behaviour and needed supports: Views of children, parents and school staff. *European Journal of Paediatric Neurology*, *40*, 61-68. https://doi.org/10.1016/j.ejpn.2022.08.001
12. De Boer, H. M. (2005). Overview and perspectives of employment in people with epilepsy. *Epilepsia*, *46*, 52-54. https://doi.org/10.1111/j.0013-9580.2005.461016.x
13. Johnson, E. K. (2016). Perspectives on work for people with epilepsy. In *Handbook of Return to Work: From Research to Practice* (pp. 617-632). Boston, MA: Springer US. https://doi.org/10.1007/978-1-4899-7627-7_33
14. Wo, M. C. M., Lim, K. S., Choo, W. Y., & Tan, C. T. (2016). Factors affecting the employability in people with epilepsy. *Epilepsy Research*, *128*, 6-11. https://doi.org/10.1016/j.eplepsyres.2016.10.003
15. Bishop, M. (2002). Barriers to employment among people with epilepsy: report of a focus group. *Journal of Vocational Rehabilitation*, *17*(4), 281-286. https://content.iospress.com/articles/journal-of-vocational-rehabilitation/jvr00167
16. Brown, I. (2024). Epilepsy, employment, and work. *Comorbidities and Social Complications of Epilepsy and Seizures: The cognitive, psychological and psychosocial impact of epilepsy*, 242. https://books.google.com/books?hl=en&lr=&id=l8sVEQAAQBAJ&oi=fnd&pg=PA242&dq=people+with+epilepsy+perspectives+of+employment&ots=MahsXxZwom&sig=jnT42dTIy3Vv-

mIUihqxF4jv0CE#v=onepage&q=people%20with%20epilepsy%20perspectives%20of%20employment&f=false
17. Epilepsy Association of the Big Bend. (2021). Epilepsy and employment. https://eabb.org/epilepsy-and-employment/
18. Scambler, G., & Hopkins, A. (1988). Accommodating epilepsy in families. In *Living with chronic illness* (pp. 156-176). Routledge. ISBN: 9781003508175, https://www.taylorfrancis.com/chapters/edit/10.4324/9781003508175-8/accommodating-epilepsy-families-graham-scambler-anthony-hopkins
19. Pembroke, S., Higgins, A., Pender, N., & Elliott, N. (2017). Becoming comfortable with "my" epilepsy: Strategies that patients use in the journey from diagnosis to acceptance and disclosure. *Epilepsy & Behavior*, 70, 217-223. https://doi.org/10.1016/j.yebeh.2017.02.001
20. Cramer, J. A. (1994). Quality of life for people with epilepsy. *Neurologic clinics*, 12(1), 1-13. https://www.neurologic.theclinics.com/article/S0733-8619(18)30107-5/abstract
21. Fisher, R. S., Vickrey, B. G., Gibson, P., Hermann, B., Penovich, P., Scherer, A., & Walker, S. (2000). The impact of epilepsy from the patient's perspective I. Descriptions and subjective perceptions. *Epilepsy research*, 41(1), 39-51. https://doi.org/10.1016/S0920-1211(00)00126-1

PERSONAL ACKNOWLEDGEMENTS

While many people supported me throughout the years, I wish to extend my deepest gratitude to those who stood steadfastly by my side during the most challenging moments of my epilepsy journey. Your unwavering support, love, and sacrifice gave me the strength to endure and the courage to share my story.

- To my husband, **Vitalis** - you are the partner I always hoped for. Through every seizure and every setback, you remained by my side, honoring our vows with grace and devotion. I am forever grateful.
- To my beloved children, **Kudzaishe, Kudakwashe, Kundai-Munashe, and Kuzivakwashe** - thank you for walking this journey with me. Your unwavering love and support through the years have been a constant source of strength.
- To **Betina Zimhunga-Mutunami**, my dear daughter - you were my anchor during the most confusing and vulnerable period of my life. Thank you for caring for me and ensuring that Kuzivakwashe and the other children were looked after so well. I truly appreciate you.
- To my mother, **Scolastica Ruzvidzo-Kwesvu** - your ceaseless prayers, love, and hope have carried me through many dark days. Thank you, Mom, for being a pillar of faith and comfort.
- To my late aunt, **Viola Kwenda** - your love and dedication were unmatched. You traveled over 200 kilometers just to be there for me after every seizure. Your presence alone brought immense comfort.
- To my dear late aunts, **Auxilia Nyanhemwa** and **Kiriana Sandra Chiroodza** - your love uplifted me in ways words cannot express. You are remembered with deep affection and gratitude.
- To my sisters, **Maselyn, Roselyn, and Vivian** - thank you for your love and support. A special thank you to Roselyn, who never hesitated to leave her own family behind to care for me whenever the situation demanded it.
- To my late brother, **Fidelis Ruzvidzo** - your quiet presence was always reassuring. You were there in your own way, and I hold those memories close.
- To my pastors, **Dr. Isaiah Musafare Magaya and Amai** - thank you for the times when I did not understand what was happening to me.

Your spiritual guidance and encouragement provided clarity, comfort, and strength when I needed it most.
- To the special group of women and staff at the **Epilepsy Support Foundation in Zimbabwe** - thank you for the many years of collaboration, friendship, and shared purpose. Your dedication to the epilepsy community continues to inspire me.
- To my amazing team of doctors - I extend my sincere gratitude for your professionalism, clinical expertise, and thoughtful care over the years. You have consistently treated me as a person, not just a case, and involved me in every step of my treatment journey. I am deeply grateful.

Each of you played a vital role in helping me live with hope, dignity, and purpose. This book is as much yours as it is mine.

With deepest gratitude,

Dr. Clotilda Mujeyi Chinyanya (DBA)

ABOUT THE AUTHOR

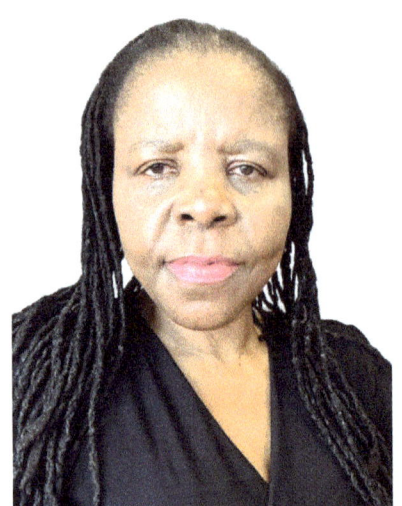

Dr. Clotilda Mujeyi Chinyanya is an epilepsy advocate and author. She is committed to changing the narrative around epilepsy through education, awareness, and empowerment. She is an Epilepsy Awareness Ambassador with the Epilepsy Foundation, a committee member of the Zimbabwe chapter of the International League Against Epilepsy (ILAE), and an active voice in global efforts to end epilepsy stigma.

Driven by both personal experience and professional insight, Clotilda approaches epilepsy from a multidimensional perspective that recognizes not only the medical aspects of the condition but also the emotional, cultural, and societal impacts. Her work is grounded in the belief that accurate information and open dialogue are powerful tools in breaking down misconceptions and improving quality of life for people with epilepsy.

In *Demystifying Epilepsy*, she brings together the latest research, expert perspectives, and real-life experiences to provide a clear, and accessible guide to understanding epilepsy. The book reflects her commitment to making complex information understandable and relatable, especially for those often left out of medical conversations — patients, caregivers, and communities.

Clotilda's advocacy is rooted in her work across disciplines and borders, where she continues to promote policies and practices that support epilepsy inclusion, care, and dignity. She believes that when people are informed, they are empowered, not only to manage the condition more effectively but also to challenge the stigma that still surrounds it.

Demystifying Epilepsy is a call to awareness and action, and Clotilda is leading that charge with empathy, expertise, and unshakable purpose.

www.ingramcontent.com/pod-product-compliance
Lightning Source LLC
Chambersburg PA
CBHW070613030426
42337CB00020B/3780